Download Your Included Ebook Today!

W9-DCV-398

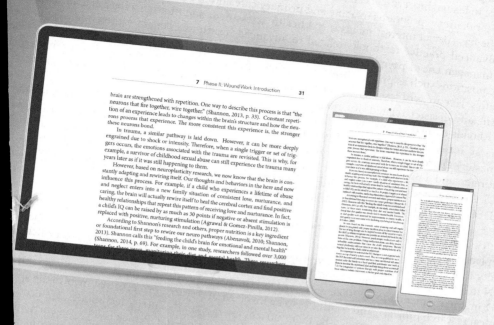

our print purchase of *Formulating a Differential Diagnosis for the Advanced Practice Provider, Second Edition*, **includes an ebook download** the device of your choice—increasing cessibility, portability, and searchability!

wnload your ebook today at:
p://connect.springerpub.com/content/
k/978-0-8261-5223-7 or scan the QR code
e right with your smartphone
enter the access code below:

CX7DJ6

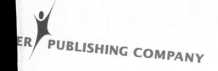

ER PUBLISHING COMPANY

springerpub.com

Jacqueline Rhoads, PhD, APRN-BC, CNL-BC, PMHNP-BE, FAANP, holds three board certification as an acute care nurse practitioner, adult gerontology nurse practitioner, and clinical nurse leader. Sh is board eligible as a psychiatric mental health nurse practitioner. She has more than 30 years of clinic experience in leadership, critical care, acute care, and primary care nursing. Dr. Rhoads teaches in grad ate and baccalaureate programs in acute and primary care and in the family and adult nurse practition tracks. She has special interest in advanced health assessment and pharmacology. She has authored major advanced practice textbooks related to advanced health assessment, differential diagnoses, clinical management of psych/mental health, as well as numerous peer-reviewed articles. She has research positions such as project director, principal investigator, and project coordinator in three m universities. Her areas of research include investigating posttraumatic stress disorder post-Vietnam, ert Storm, and disaster-related situations.

Dr. Rhoads earned her bachelor's from University of the Incarnate Word, her master's in Burn Trauma at Texas Woman's University, her PhD in Nursing at University of Texas in Austin, an post-master's degrees: as an acute care nurse practitioner, an adult nurse practitioner, a gerontology practitioner, and a psychiatric mental health nurse practitioner. She is especially proud of her ser the U.S. Army Nurse Corps where she held strategic leadership positions as chief nurse, deployabl ical (DEPMED) training officer, nuclear biological chemical officer, and head nurse.

Julie C. Penick, DNP, PhD, MSN, FNP-BC, maintains both an active family practice, specia complementary and alternative medicine modalities, and an education practice where she is faculty in a competency-based MSN program at Western Governors University. Dr. Penick ea MSN in adult health nursing in 1992, her post-master's family nurse practitioner certificate in PhD in energy medicine in 2003, and her DNP in 2011. Dr. Penick has been involved with clinical research projects, and continues to be involved in research projects that involve the app "energy" as healing approaches—be that nutrient energy, subtle energy techniques, applicatio netic field energy, and application of direct or indirect current—Dr. Penick is active in curricul and conducting continuing professional education for nurses. Dr. Penick has been a certified titioner through the American Nurse Credentialing Center (ANCC) for more than 20 years.

FORMULATING A DIFFERENTIAL DIAGNOSIS FOR THE ADVANCED PRACTICE PROVIDER

Second Edition

Jacqueline Rhoads, PhD, APRN-BC, CNL-BC, PMHNP-BE, FAANP
Julie C. Penick, DNP, PhD, MSN, FNP-BC

Editors

SPRINGER PUBLISHING COMPANY

Copyright © 2018 Springer Publishing Company, LLC

All rights reserved.

No part of this publication may be reproduced, stored in a retrieval system, or transmitted in any form or by any means, electronic, mechanical, photocopying, recording, or otherwise, without the prior permission of Springer Publishing Company, LLC, or authorization through payment of the appropriate fees to the Copyright Clearance Center, Inc., 222 Rosewood Drive, Danvers, MA 01923, 978-750-8400, fax 978-646-8600, info@copyright.com or on the Web at www.copyright.com.

Springer Publishing Company, LLC
11 West 42nd Street
New York, NY 10036
www.springerpub.com

Acquisitions Editor: Margaret Zuccarini
Compositor: Exeter Premedia Services Private Ltd.

ISBN: 978-0-8261-5222-0
ebook ISBN: 978-0-8261-5223-7

18 19 20 21 22 / 7 6 5 4 3

The author and the publisher of this Work have made every effort to use sources believed to be reliable to provide information that is accurate and compatible with the standards generally accepted at the time of publication. Because medical science is continually advancing, our knowledge base continues to expand. Therefore, as new information becomes available, changes in procedures become necessary. We recommend that the reader always consult current research and specific institutional policies before performing any clinical procedure. The author and publisher shall not be liable for any special, consequential, or exemplary damages resulting, in whole or in part, from the readers' use of, or reliance on, the information contained in this book. The publisher has no responsibility for the persistence or accuracy of URLs for external or third-party Internet websites referred to in this publication and does not guarantee that any content on such websites is, or will remain, accurate or appropriate.

Library of Congress Cataloging-in-Publication Data

Names: Rhoads, Jacqueline, 1948- editor. | Penick, Julie C., editor.
Title: Formulating a differential diagnosis for the advanced practice
    provider / Jacqueline Rhoads, Julie C. Penick [editors].
Other titles: Differential diagnosis for the advanced practice nurse
Description: Second edition. | New York, NY : Springer Publishing Company,
    LLC, [2018] | Preceded by Differential diagnosis for the advanced practice
    nurse / Jacqueline Rhoads, Marilee Murphy Jensen, editors. 2015. |
    Includes index.
Identifiers: LCCN 2017029620| ISBN 9780826152220 (paperback) | ISBN
    9780826152237 (ebook)
Subjects: | MESH: Nursing Diagnosis—methods | Diagnosis, Differential |
    Physical Examination—nursing | Case Reports
Classification: LCC RT48 | NLM WY 100.4 | DDC 616.07/5—dc23
LC record available at https://lccn.loc.gov/2017029620

Contact us to receive discount rates on bulk purchases.
We can also customize our books to meet your needs.
For more information please contact: sales@springerpub.com

Printed in the United States of America by McNaughton & Gunn.

CONTENTS

CONTRIBUTORS

Patricia Abbott, PhD, MSN, FNP-C, Assistant Professor, Regis University College of Nursing, Lakewood, Colorado

Barbara Bjeletich, ARNP, Emergency Room Provider, University of Washington, Seattle, Washington

Dorothy Cooper, MN, ARNP, ANP-BC, WHNP-BC, Nurse Practitioner, The Everett Clinic, Everett, Washington

Patricia Cox, DNP, MPH, FNP-BC, Assistant Professor, DNP Clinical Coordinator, University of Portland, School of Nursing, Portland, Oregon

John Cranmer, DNP, MPH, MSN, ANP-BC, Senior Research Fellow, Department of Global Health, University of Washington, Internal Medicine Nurse Practitioner, SeaMar Community Health Centers, Seattle, Washington

Lynda Hillman, DNP, FNP-BC, Nurse Practitioner, Multiple Sclerosis Center/ Rehabilitation Medicine, University of Washington Medical Center, Seattle, Washington

Marilee Murphy Jensen, ARNP, MSN, Family Nurse Practitioner, Northwest Hospital, University of Washington, Seattle, Washington

Sarah Kooienga, PhD, ARNP, FNP, Assistant Professor, Washington State University College of Nursing, Vancouver, Washington

Patricia Mathis, MSN, FNP-BC, Overlake Hospital Medical Center and Swedish Medical Center, Issaquah, Washington

Melody Rasmor, EdD(c), APRN-BC, COHN-S, Assistant Professor, Washington State University College of Nursing, Vancouver, Washington

Jacqueline Rhoads, PhD, APRN-BC, CNL-BC, PMHNP- BE, FAANP, Professor, Graduate Nursing Department, University of Texas Medical Branch School of Nursing, Galveston, Texas

Christie Rivelli, MSN, FNP, Family Nurse Practitioner, Coastal Family Health Center, Battle Ground, Washington

Kumhee Ro, DNP, ARNP, FNP, Clinical Assistant Professor, Biobehavioral Nursing and Health Systems, School of Nursing, University of Washington, Seattle, Washington

Melody Stringer, MSN, ARNP-BC, Nurse Practitioner, The Vancouver Clinic (Urgent Care), Vancouver, Washington

Diane Switzer, DNP, ARNP, FNP-BC, ENP-BC, CCRN, CEN, Emergency Department, Harborview Medical Center, University of Washington, Bellevue, Washington

Charles Wiley, MSN, ARNP, FNP-BC, Adjunct Faculty, Puget Sound Physicians Group, Emergency Department, Harborview Medical Center, University of Washington, Bellevue, Washington, Adjunct Faculty, Seattle Pacific University ARNP Program, Issaquah, Washington

FOREWORD

Formulating a Differential Diagnosis for the Advanced Practice Provider is a well-thought-out, clinically relevant text that is ideal for both novice and seasoned physician assistants and nurse practitioners. The ability to extract historical information, perform a focused physical examination, and critically analyze the collected data are vital skills that must be mastered and maintained in order to be an effective health care provider.

This updated second edition features a directed approach to many new symptoms commonly encountered in every day practice. The authors present a chief complaint, which is skillfully woven into a case study in order to replicate a real-life approach. The focus is placed on pertinent subjective and objective information that must be gleaned from each patient. Red flags and inclusive charts help to guide the selection of diagnostic studies and the formulation of a differential diagnosis. The authors' collective knowledge and clinical experience is evidenced by the clinical decision-making explanation that accompanies each case, culminating in a final diagnosis and treatment plan.

The straightforward, well-organized presentation of this text provides quick access to the critical thinking process that is necessary in the evaluation of the most commonly encountered symptoms in medicine today, and is sure to be relied on as a trusted resource in clinical practice by advanced practice providers.

Maureen A. Knechtel, MPAS, PA-C
Assistant Professor of Physician Assistant Studies
Milligan College
Johnson City, Tennessee
Physician Assistant
The Wellmont Cardiovascular Associates Heart Institute
Kingsport, Tennessee

PREFACE

Establishing *differential diagnosis* can be challenging even for the expert advanced practice provider (APP). For the APP student, establishing the diagnosis is even more of a challenge. It is the goal of the authors to present a clinically useful guide for both the student and the clinical provider to use in discerning a reliable diagnosis. Much of the diagnosis is based on patient input, so standard methods of communicating with the patient are important in eliciting a useful history and background that can accurately point the APP to a likely diagnosis. Using this as a platform from which to conduct and order appropriate diagnostic tests is the next logical step for the clinician. How does one learn to formulate such a platform? Currently, there are very few textbooks available that would provide such a guide to the development of a differential diagnosis for common patient/client complaints. This book is designed to bridge the gap between common chief complaints and the formulation of a correct diagnosis by providing a step-by-step approach to eliciting useful patient responses through an unfolding case study approach. We have attempted to include the more commonly occurring symptoms that present in the clinical setting.

The second edition of this handy clinical reference presents a standard method of formulating a differential diagnosis that the APP can use throughout clinical practice. Seventy-five common symptoms are organized and presented in alphabetical order, starting with abdominal pain and moving through to cough, ear discharge, fatigue, hand and joint swelling, headache, low back pain, shortness of breath, and skin rashes, to vomiting and wrist pain (last symptom). These symptoms, or chief complaints, represent the symptoms most frequently presented by patients to the primary care practitioner.

PATIENT-BASED CASE SCENARIOS

The patient-based case scenario is used to present each symptom. The case unfolds systematically and is followed consistently as each symptom is explored, as it would in a clinical setting. This systematic approach helps the student to structure her or his approach to a patient, supporting the idea of establishing a method of clinical decision making. Each symptom exploration follows the same format, which includes a "Case Presentation" followed by:

1. Introduction to Complaint (includes background, usual cause, additional causes)
2. History of Complaint (includes symptomatology, directed questions to ask, assessment: cardinal signs and symptoms, medical history: general, medical history: specific to complaint)
3. Physical Examination (includes vital signs, general appearance, visual examination of area concerning chief complaint, additional related inspection and examination, areas to palpate and areas to auscultate)

4. Case Study: History and Physical Examination Findings (includes responses to directed questions, findings of physical examination)
5. Differential Diagnosis (a table that compares typical symptoms associated with conditions that might present similarly and need to be compared with the results of the patient's history and physical examination findings)
6. Diagnostic Examination (a table that presents diagnostic tests that the APP can consider performing or ordering to facilitate arriving at the correct diagnosis)
7. Clinical Decision Making (a summary of the case study and statement of the likely diagnosis)

UNIQUE FEATURES

Case Study: History—This two-column table presents the directed question posed to the patient in the first column and the patient's response to the question in the second column.

Case Study: Physical Examination Findings—This section presents the actual findings of the physical examination. Together, the case study history table and the case study physical examination findings lead the examiner to the differential diagnosis table, which clearly compares the relative differences among the more usual and customary diagnoses.

Differential Diagnosis Table—This table presents the more usual diagnostic choices that can be made based on the client's chief complaint and provides the clinician significant clues as to which diagnoses might be most accurate.

Diagnostic Examination Table—This table presents the diagnostic tools available to further clarify or confirm a diagnosis related to the presenting symptom. It includes the estimated cost and codes to be considered when determining which tests to order. Some of the tests are common tests that are included in the office visit, such as the otoscopy, which provides visualization of the ear canal and tympanic membrane to assess for the presence of foreign body, signs of trauma, erythema, effusion, or rupture. Other tests provide more insight into a possible diagnosis and often are more costly.

Clinical Decision Making—This section describes the APP's analysis of the patient's health history (including responses to directed and nondirected questions), the physical exam, results of the diagnostic tests, and the scrutiny of the differential diagnosis table (comparing common symptoms for possible diagnoses). Decision making is laid out for the reader, indicating the salient points that surfaced during the analysis process, and offers the most likely diagnosis.

Clinical information presented in this book is considered generally accepted practice. Although every effort has been made to present correct and up-to-date information, the health care field is rapidly changing and the idea of "common knowledge" today might be different tomorrow, based on new developments and research findings. For this reason, readers are encouraged to keep up with all available resources to help ensure accurate decision making.

Establishing differential diagnoses for client complaints is a critical step in the delivery of optimum health care. It is our hope that this book will serve as a useful guide for nurse practitioners in practice. We feel it will be a wonderful adjunct to APP curricula in nursing programs across the globe.

Jacqueline Rhoads
Julie C. Penick

ACKNOWLEDGMENTS

I would like to express my gratitude to the many people who saw me through this book; to all those who provided support, talked things over, read, wrote, offered comments, allowed me to quote their remarks, and assisted in the editing, proofreading, and design.

I would like to thank Amanda Devine for helping me in the process of topic selection and editing. Thanks to Margaret Zuccarini, my editor, who encouraged me. Without them this book would have never found its way to the advanced practice faculty and providers.

Above all, I want to thank my mother, who supported and encouraged me in spite of all the time it took me away from her.

Jacqueline Rhoads

I would like to express my gratitude to my friend and professional colleague, Dr. Jacqueline Rhoads, for seeing something in me that allowed her to invite me to come alongside her on this project. I am in hopes that the professionals who engage with this resource find it to be a valuable tool for their practice—educational, leadership, or clinical.

I also want to thank my mother, who passed away at 93 years of age while I was working on my contributions for the book.

Julie C. Penick

ACKNOWLEDGMENTS

INTRODUCTION TO DIFFERENTIAL DIAGNOSIS AND DIAGNOSIS OF COMMON PROBLEMS

Diseases are defined by a pattern of symptoms the patient reports, signs observed during physical examination, and diagnostic testing. Determining the differential diagnosis is the process of distinguishing one disease from another that presents with similar symptoms. With the chief complaint established, information is gathered through the history and physical examination. When the patient presents with a chief complaint, such as cough, the provider considers the most common diseases that present with cough, forming a working differential diagnosis list. The provider analyzes the data obtained, eliminates some diseases, and narrows down the differential diagnosis. At times, further diagnostic testing is needed to make the final diagnosis. The construction of a differential diagnosis is essential in making an accurate diagnosis.

PATIENT HISTORY
Identification/Chief Complaint

The first piece of information obtained is the chief complaint or the patient's reason for seeking medical attention. This statement gives the provider a general idea of possible diagnoses. For example, "a healthy 16-year-old boy presents with a nonproductive cough he's had for 3 days."

Subjective

The most common etiology of the disease is in the ears, nose, throat, and respiratory system. With this in mind, the provider asks the patients a series of *open-ended questions* to gather data related to the presenting problem. These questions form the basis of the symptom analysis:

- Onset
- Location/radiation
- Duration/timing
- Character
- Associated symptoms
- Aggravating or triggering factors
- Alleviating factors
- Effects on daily life

Once a general history is obtained, the provider moves on to obtain more details through a *directed history*. Patients may not offer pertinent symptoms unless prompted. These questions are focused on the diagnostic possibilities related to the presenting problem. For example, a patient who presents with chest pain may not recall that the pain is much better when he or she leans forward, indicating possible pericarditis.

Once questions regarding the symptom are completed, the provider moves on to obtain data regarding the patient's general health status, and relevant past medical, family, and social history. The patient's past medical history and family history outline risk factors for diseases. The social history may reveal occupational exposures or habits that influence the presence of diseases, such as heart and lung disease from smoking, or liver disease from alcohol or drug use.

PHYSICAL EXAMINATION

The physical examination starts when you walk into the room and observe the patient's general appearance. Visual clues include facial expression, mood, stress level, hygiene, skin color, and breathing pattern. Although they may seem trivial, the assessment of vital signs is critical, and their accuracy is imperative. The presence of fever, tachycardia, or low blood pressure is cause for concern and alerts the provider that the patient may have a serious disease.

Unlike the patient who comes in for a comprehensive physical examination, the patient who presents with a symptom requires a *focused* physical examination. The examination is directed by the chief complaint and history. For example, a 16-year-old with a recent cough requires examination of the ears, eyes, nose, throat, neck (for lymphadenopathy), heart, lungs, and abdomen (for an enlarged liver or spleen). Attention is given to the skin to look for cyanosis, the nails for clubbing, and the vascular system for edema. Neurologic examination is limited to mental status, and other parts of the examination are not relevant.

The physical examination provides positive and negative findings, and may provide the diagnosis without the need for further testing. For example, if the examination of a patient who reports a painful skin rash yields findings of a cluster of vesicles on an erythematous base following a dermatome, this is a positive physical finding confirming a clinical diagnosis of herpes zoster. On the other hand, the lack of a rash would be a negative physical finding and further exploration would be needed. The physical examination may also reveal unsuspected findings, or may be completely normal despite the presence of disease.

DIFFERENTIAL DIAGNOSIS

Once the chief complaint, history, and physical examination are established, a list of possible diseases is formed ranking the most common diagnoses and the most serious or "not to miss" diagnoses. The axiom that common diseases present commonly and uncommon diseases are uncommon cannot be overstressed. Keeping an open mind, and exploring all possibilities, is important. Premature closure or discarding a diagnosis too early may result in diagnostic error. The depth of one's differential diagnosis is determined by the breadth of knowledge of the provider. A disease cannot be diagnosed and treated unless it is known to the provider. This can be a challenge for the novice who is faced with a mountain of information to learn about thousands of diseases. It results in a chronic sense of dissatisfaction with one's knowledge base, and can be a source of great fear and frustration. However, it serves to stimulate exploration and learning, and with experience and guidance, knowledge grows. The novice will find that a solid reference enables him or her to master the task of differential diagnosis as his or her clinical experience matures.

DIAGNOSTIC TESTING

When the diagnosis cannot be made on history and physical data alone, diagnostic testing is the next step in determining the correct diagnosis. Diagnostic testing should be done only if necessary to yield an impact on the diagnosis, and ultimate treatment of the problem. Ordering unnecessary tests is enormously expensive. When possible, order basic tests to screen for disease, and if the diagnosis remains unclear, move on to more elaborate testing.

Consider the sensitivity and specificity of a test as well. "Sensitivity" is the proportion of patients with the diagnosis who will test positive. "Specificity" is the proportion of patients without the diagnosis who will test negative.

If the diagnosis is not defined by the history, physical examination, and diagnostic testing, the provider then needs to reevaluate the patient over time, reformulating new diagnostic possibilities as new signs or symptoms arise.

STEPS TO WRITING A DIFFERENTIAL DIAGNOSIS

Knowledge of how to write a medical diagnosis comprises several critical steps.

1. Obtain the patient's chief complaint, such as "cough for 2 weeks" and list three common problems that present with that symptom. For example, acute cough is most likely viral bronchitis, pneumonia, or viral rhinosinusitis with postnasal drip.
2. Obtain a detailed history as outlined previously. Make a list of the patient's symptoms and pertinent risk factors. Note the pertinent positive and negative associated symptoms. For example, a patient with a cough who has a high fever and shortness of breath (positives) likely has pneumonia. A patient who has a cough without a high fever or shortness of breath (negatives) may have viral bronchitis. Based on the information from your history, direct your physical examination to look for significant signs of illness. For example, is there sinus tenderness? Is there a postnasal drip in the posterior pharynx? Are there wheezes or crackles present?
3. Review your differential diagnosis list of possible diagnoses based on the history and physical examination. Determine whether you need additional diagnostic testing based on your findings. For example, a patient with a fever of 102°F, heart rate of 120, and respiratory rate of 30 with diminished breath sounds in the right lower lobe and crackles will benefit from a chest x-ray to confirm the presence or absence of pneumonia. A complete blood count will identify whether there is a significant leukocytosis or elevated white blood cell count. A basic metabolic panel will ascertain whether there is an electrolyte imbalance or dehydration.
4. Establish a clear determination that shows why this particular diagnosis is accurate for the patient. Review your rationale for why you chose this diagnosis as opposed to others on your list of possibilities. Keep an open mind as you review your facts for any other diagnostic possibilities you may have missed, including a life-threatening illness.
5. Develop a treatment plan, including diagnostic testing, pharmacologic agents, patient education, and follow-up. If your diagnosis remains unclear, consider appropriate referral for further evaluation.

SUMMARY

This book is written to help the reader learn the process of formulating a differential diagnosis using the skills of gathering appropriate data from the history, physical examination, and relevant diagnostic testing. Each chapter is interspersed with cases describing an initial chief complaint, history, and physical examination. Tables outlining the common diagnosis with cardinal signs and symptoms as well as diagnostic testing are provided for the reader's review. Clinical diagnostic reasoning for the final diagnosis is outlined. The approach is to give pertinent information as well as demonstrate the process of clinical reasoning. It is well known that the process of differential diagnosis takes years to master. It is especially challenging for new students learning the complexities of diagnosis. It is our hope that this book will help you start your journey with the tools to make this learning process interesting and relevant.

ABDOMINAL PAIN

Case Presentation: A 25-year-old female presents to the emergency department (ED) with complaints of severe abdominal pain.

INTRODUCTION TO COMPLAINT

- Abdominal pain is a subjective feeling of discomfort in the abdomen caused by nausea, vomiting, or constipation.
- It is caused by a variety of problems including diverticulitis, gastrointestinal (GI) ulcers, and constipation.
- The goal of the initial assessment is to distinguish acute life-threatening conditions from chronic/recurrent or mild, self-limiting conditions.
- It can be caused by tension in the GI tract:
  - Muscle contraction or distention
  - Ischemia
  - Inflammation of the peritoneum

Colic Pain

- Tension-type pain
- Associated with forceful peristaltic contractions
- Most characteristic type of pain arising from the viscera
- Produced by an irritant substance, from infection or bacteria, or the body's attempt to force its luminal contents through an obstruction

Stretching Pain

- Tension-type pain
- Caused by acute stretching of an organ, such as the liver, spleen, or kidney, due to enlargement
- Patient is restless, moves about, and has difficulty getting comfortable

Ischemic Pain

- Intense, continuous pain
- Strangulation of bowel from obstruction is a common cause

Inflammatory Pain

- Visceral peritonitis
- Aching
- Patient lies still and does not want to move
- Pain may be referred from abdomen to other parts of the body via common neural pathways

HISTORY OF COMPLAINT
Symptomatology

Ask about the following characteristics of each symptom using open-ended questions:

- Onset (sudden or gradual)
- Chronology
- Current situation (improving or deteriorating)
- Location
- Radiation
- Quality
- Timing (frequency, duration)
- Severity
- Precipitating and aggravating factors
- Relieving factors
- Associated symptoms
- Effects on daily activities
- Previous diagnosis of similar episodes
- Previous treatments
- Efficacy of previous treatments

Directed Questions to Ask

- How long ago did your pain start?
- Was the onset gradual or sudden?
- What word would describe your pain; is it dull, sharp, crampy, or grabbing?
- Does your pain come and go or is it constant?
- How long does it last?
- Is the pain getting worse?
- Does your pain radiate into your back, groin, or legs?
- Do you have a change in your appetite?
- Do you have any nausea, or vomiting?
- Do you have any burning sensation in the abdomen or chest?
- Do you have any constipation or diarrhea?
- Do you have any pain or difficulty with urination?
- Have you had any blood in your urine?
- Have you been sexually active?
- Have you had any pain with sexual activity?
- When was your last menstrual period (LMP)?
- Have you missed any periods?
- Have you had any abnormal spotting?
- Have you had any vaginal discharge that is different than usual?
- Is there any unusual vaginal odor?
- Have you had any new stressors or life changes prior to your new onset of pain?

Assessment: Cardinal Signs and Symptoms

In addition to the general characteristics outlined previously, the location of the pain provides an important clue to the possible etiology of the pain.

Pain Location
- EPIGASTRIC: esophagus, stomach, duodenum, liver, gallbladder, pancreas, spleen
- UPPER ABDOMINAL: esophagus, stomach, duodenum, liver, gallbladder, pancreas, thorax

- RIGHT UPPER QUADRANT (RUQ): usually esophagus, stomach, duodenum, liver, gallbladder, pancreas, thorax; often indicates cholecystitis
- LEFT UPPER QUADRANT (LUQ): spleen

Medical History: General

- Medical conditions and surgeries
- Allergies
- Current medications
- Bowel pattern
- LMP

Medical History: Specific to Complaint

- Previous abdominal surgeries
- Pregnancies
- Miscarriages
- Abortions
- Recent use of new prescribed medications
- Recent use of over-the-counter medications, such as ibuprofen or Naprosyn
- Family history of cancer of the stomach, bowel, uterus, or ovaries

PHYSICAL EXAMINATION

Vital Signs

- Temperature
- Pulse
- Respiration
- Oxygen saturation (SpO_2)
- Blood pressure (BP)

General Appearance

- Apparent state of health
- Appearance of comfort or distress
- Color
- Nutritional status
- Hygiene
- Match between appearance and stated age
- Difficulty with gait or balance

Abdominal Inspection

- SKIN: color, lesions, masses, or hernias
- SIZE/SHAPE: distention, shape, symmetry, surgical scars, hernias, pulsations

Abdominal Examination

- AUSCULTATION: for frequency, intensity, pitch of bowel sounds (BS), determine presence of bruits, friction rub
- RECTAL: if rectal bleeding or change in bowel habits; testing of stool as positive or negative

Pelvic Examination

- EXTERNAL: observe for redness or lesions
- INTROITUS: observe for discharge or lesions

- VAGINA: observe for presence or absence of rugae, discharge, bleeding, or odor
- CERVIX: inspect for lesions, discharge from os; note whether there is pain with motion of the cervix from side to side
- UTERUS: note size, shape, and position and whether there is any tenderness with movement
- OVARIES: note if palpable; if palpable, note whether they are enlarged, tender, or masses are present
- PERCUSSION: look for patterns of dullness and tympany
- PALPATION: locate masses or organomegaly, pulsations
  - Light palpation: tenderness, pain, presence of guarding, rigidity, and rebound tenderness
  - Deep palpation: locate masses or organomegaly, pulsations

CASE STUDY

History

Directed Question	Response
When did the pain start?	*2 weeks ago.*
On a scale of 0 to 10 what number would you give the intensity of the pain?	*8 to 10.*
Is the pain sharp, dull, or crampy?	*The pain is sharp and crampy.*
Is it constant or does it come and go?	*It comes and goes.*
What triggers the pain?	*It hurts if I run, sit down hard, or if I have sex.*
Do you have any nausea or vomiting?	*No.*
How is your appetite?	*It is good.*
Do you have constipation or diarrhea?	*No.*
Do you have fever or chills?	*No.*
When was your last period?	*5 days ago.*
Was it at the normal time?	*Yes.*
Are you using birth control?	*Yes, I take the shot each month.*
Was your period associated with more pain or cramping?	*Yes, it was the worst period pain I ever had.*
Have you ever had an infection in your ovary or uterus before?	*No, never.*
Have you ever been pregnant?	*No, never.*
Have you had a new partner?	*Yes, we started up about 2 months ago.*
Do you feel safe with your new partner?	*Yes, he's really good to me.*
Do you use condoms?	*No, he hates them.*
Do you have anything else to tell me?	*No, I just want to get rid of this pain.*

Physical Examination Findings

- VITAL SIGNS: temperature 99°F; respiratory rate (RR) 20; heart rate (HR) 110, regular; BP 138/90; oxygen saturation (SpO$_2$) 96%; pain 5/10
- GENERAL APPEARANCE: female in acute distress and severe pain
- HEAD, EYES, EARS, NOSE, THROAT (HEENT): within normal limits; eyes: anicteric; pupils equal, round, and reactive to light and accommodation (PERRLA); nose: no discharge; mouth/throat: moist membranes, no lesions
- CHEST: lung clear in all fields; S1S2, no murmurs, gallops, or rubs
- ABDOMEN: soft, diffuse tenderness
- SKIN: no rashes
- EXTREMITIES: range of motion (ROM) × 4, no joint pain or swelling

Abdominal Examination

- INSPECTION: no masses or thrills noted; no discoloration and skin is warm to the touch; no tattoos or piercings; abdomen is nondistended and round
- AUSCULTATION: BS are normal in all four quadrants, no bruits noted
- PALPATION: on palpation, abdomen is tender to touch in four quadrants; tenderness noted on light palpation, deep palpation reveals no masses, spleen and liver unremarkable
- PERCUSSION: tympany heard in all quadrants, no dullness noted in abdominal area

Pelvic Examination

- EXTERNAL: mature hair distribution; no external lesions on labia
- INTROITUS: slight green-gray discharge, no lesions
- VAGINAL: normal rugae; moderate amount of green discharge on vaginal walls
- CERVIX: nulliparous os with small amount of purulent discharge from os with positive cervical motion tenderness (CMT)
- UTERUS: ante-flexed, normal size, shape, and position
- ADNEXA: bilateral tenderness with fullness; both ovaries without masses
- RECTAL: deferred
- VAGINAL DISCHARGE: green in color

DIFFERENTIAL DIAGNOSIS

Clinical Observations	Pelvic Inflammatory Disease	Sexually Transmitted Disease	Septic Abortion	Ectopic Pregnancy	Appendicitis
Onset	Gradual	Gradual	Sudden	Sudden	Sudden
Pain	Yes	Yes	Yes	Yes	Yes
Location	Pelvic area/ right and left lower quadrant	Pelvic area/ right and left lower quadrant	Localized	Pelvic area/ right and left lower quadrant	Epigastric or per umbilical/right lower quadrant
Fever	High	High or low	High	If ruptured	Possible
Discharge	Common	Common	Common with infection	Possible	No

(continued)

Clinical Observations	Pelvic Inflammatory Disease	Sexually Transmitted Disease	Septic Abortion	Ectopic Pregnancy	Appendicitis
Inguinal nodes	Yes	Yes	Yes	Yes	Yes
Vaginal bleeding	Possible	Rare	Common	Common	No
CMT	Very common	Common	Common	Common	No

CMT, cervical motion tenderness.

DIAGNOSTIC EXAMINATION

Exam	Code	Cost	Results
CBC with differential	85025	$75	High white blood cells (WBCs)
Quantitative pregnancy test	81025		Done to rule out the possibility of a tubal/ectopic pregnancy
Wet mount (saline)	87070	$23.26	If pH <4.5, wet mount reveals up to 3 to 5 WBCs/high-power field and presence of epithelial cells and lactobacilli (may be physiological discharge) WBCs high in the presence of a foreign body
Chlamydia and gonococcus (STI test)	V73.88, V74.5	$28 each	Common link to PID
Urinalysis and urine culture if UA shows leukocytes	81000	$55	Screens for infection
Pelvic and vaginal ultrasound	76830	$390	Examines margins of pelvic structures to determine size
Culdocentesis	57020	$125	Determines hemoperitoneum (ruptured ectopic pregnancy from pelvic sepsis)
Laparoscopy	58541–58544	$1,700	Definitive test to diagnose PID but due to invasiveness it is not done often Usually indicated when the diagnosis is in doubt or the results of the procedure are questionable

CBC, complete blood count; PID, pelvic inflammatory disease; STI, sexually transmitted infection, UA, urinalysis; WBC, white blood cell.

CLINICAL DECISION MAKING
Case Study Analysis

Pertinent positives are:

- Fever, lower abdominal pain above pubic bone that is band-like
- Dyspareunia
- Greenish vaginal discharge with dysuria
- Burning on urination

Pertinent negatives are:

- Normal, regular menses
- Negative pregnancy test
- No fever or chills

Diagnosis: *Pelvic inflammatory disease*

The advanced practice provider notes that the client's abdomen is nonpalpable for masses and bowel sounds are normal. The pain has been slowly becoming worse over the past two weeks, which is consistent with pelvic inflammatory disease. Additional information that suggests this client is experiencing pelvic inflammatory disease includes pain with intercourse (dyspareunia) and a green discharge. Burning with urination commonly occurs as well. Although a fever can be associated with other health problems, the combination of a fever with diffuse abdominal pain, pain with intercourse, and a green vaginal discharge all support the diagnosis of pelvic inflammatory disease.

Treatment will be provided with antibiotics and if the symptoms continue, a urinalysis and additional diagnostic testing might be required to determine the source of the patient's symptoms.

ABDOMINAL SWELLING

Case Presentation: *A 42-year-old female reports to the clinic with a complaint of significant abdominal swelling.*

INTRODUCTION TO COMPLAINT

Abdominal "swelling" is also known as a "distended abdomen." The defining characteristic of abdominal swelling is the "stomach area/belly" being larger than usual. Abdominal swelling can result from a wide variety of causes. Most commonly, it is caused by overeating and/or the formation of "gas" secondary to inadequate digestive processes. Besides overeating, some of the more common causes of abdominal swelling include:

- Lactose intolerance
- Irritable bowel syndrome (IBS)
- Intestinal blockage(s)
- Intestinal dysbiosis
- Uterine fibroids
- Ovarian cyst(s)
- Ascites (can be a sign of a serious medical condition)
- Pregnancy

HISTORY OF COMPLAINT

Symptomatology

Ask about the following characteristics of each symptom using open-ended questions:

- Onset (sudden or gradual)
- Chronology
- Current situation (improving or deteriorating)
- Location
- Radiation
- Quality
- Timing (frequency, duration)
- Severity
- Precipitating and aggravating factors
- Relieving factors
- Associated symptoms
- Effects on daily activities
- Previous diagnosis of similar episodes
- Previous treatments
- Efficacy of previous treatments

Directed Questions to Ask

- When did the abdominal "swelling" start?
- Do you have any abdominal pain along with the swelling?
- Have you experienced this type of abdominal swelling before?
- Is it possible that you are pregnant?
- Are you lactose intolerant?
- How often do you have a bowel movement (BM)? When was your last BM?
- Do you have IBS?
- Have you had any menstrual cycle problems?
- Have you ever had any ovarian cysts?
- Do you have uterine fibroids?
- Do you have any medical problem or other medical diagnoses?
- Are you taking any medications or over-the-counter (OTC) supplements?

Assessment: Cardinal Signs and Symptoms

- Distended abdomen
- Abdominal pain/cramping

Medical History: General

- Medical conditions and surgeries
- Allergies (seasonal as well as others)
- Medication currently used (prescription, birth control pill [BCP] and OTC)
- Herbal preparations and traditional therapies

Medical History: Specific to Complaint

- Onset of abdominal swelling
- Lactose intolerance
- IBS
- Uterine fibroids or ovarian cysts
- Medical problem known to cause ascites or swelling

PHYSICAL EXAMINATION
Vital Signs

- Temperature
- Pulse
- Respiration
- Oxygen saturation (SpO_2)
- Blood pressure (BP)

General Appearance

- Apparent state of health
- Appearance of comfort or distress
- Color
- State of hydration

Neck
- Inspect for symmetry, swelling, masses
- Palpate for tenderness, size of thyroid, and presence of any nodules/cysts

Cardiovascular
- Auscultate for heart sounds; check for murmurs, gallops, rubs
- Palpate peripheral pulses

Respiratory
- Auscultate lungs for crackles and wheezing

Abdomen
- Inspect for contour, symmetry, scars
- Auscultate for bowel sounds, bruits
- Palpate for pain, masses, organomegaly

Pelvis
- Inspect external genitalia, condition of vaginal tissues, appearance of cervix
- Palpate for cervical motion tenderness, adnexal tenderness/masses, size/shape/position of uterus

CASE STUDY
History

Directed Question	Response
When did the abdominal "swelling" start?	*About 3 weeks ago. My belly is just getting bigger and bigger and nothing I am doing seems to be helping.*
Do you have any abdominal pain along with the swelling?	*Just feel "sore" all across my abdomen.*
Have you experienced this type of abdominal swelling before?	*No.*
Is it possible that you are pregnant?	*No, I had a hysterectomy 3 years ago.*
Are you lactose intolerant?	*No.*
How often do you have a BM? When was your last BM?	*I had a BM this morning. I have been having a decent BM every day or every other day since this started.*
Do you have IBS?	*No.*
Have you had any menstrual cycle problems?	*Not anymore . . . was having irregular periods and heaving bleeding/cramping before my hysterectomy.*
Have you ever had any ovarian cysts?	*No.*
Do you have uterine fibroids?	*I did—that's why they did the hysterectomy.*
Do you have any medical problem or other medical diagnoses?	*No.*
Are you taking any medications or OTC supplements?	*No. I just finished a couple rounds of antibiotics for severe bronchitis. Thought I would never get over it.*

Physical Examination Findings

- VITAL SIGNS: temperature 99.0°F; respiratory rate (RR) 20; heart rate (HR) 65, regular; BP 128/74; SpO$_2$ 97%
- GENERAL APPEARANCE: well developed, healthy appearing female who presents with obvious non-verbal cues of discomfort
- NECK: no thyroid enlargement or nodules/masses
- CARDIOVASCULAR: heart regular/rhythm, no murmur or gallop
- RESPIRATORY: lungs clear
- ABDOMEN: distended; non-localized, diffuse pain with palpation; no organomegaly; hyperactive bowel sounds in all four quadrants
- PELVIS: external genitalia normal, vaginal tissue supple, no cervical motion tenderness, uterus not enlarged, no uterine or adnexal tenderness or masses appreciated

DIFFERENTIAL DIAGNOSIS

Clinical Observations	Decreased BP	Distension	Pain	Nausea/ Vomiting	Diarrhea	Elevated Temp
Lactose intolerance	No	Yes	Yes	No	No	No
IBS	No	No	Yes	Yes/No	Yes	Yes
Intestinal blockage	Yes	Yes	Yes	Yes	Yes	Yes
Intestinal dysbiosis	Yes	Yes	Yes	Yes	No	No
Uterine fibroid	No	No	No	No	No	No
Ovarian cyst	No	Yes	No	No	No	No
Pregnancy	No	Yes	No	No	No	No
Ascites	No	Yes	Yes	Yes	No	No

IBS, irritable bowel syndrome.

DIAGNOSTIC EXAMINATION

Exam	Code	Cost	Results
Lactose tolerance test	82951, 82952	$175	To evaluate if serum glucose level increases at several time intervals after the ingestion of the lactose product
Hydrogen breath test	91065	$175	To evaluate for rise in hydrogen of at least 20 ppm above baseline measurement

(*continued*)

Exam	Code	Cost	Results
Stool acidity test	83986	Varies, $40 to $100	Most often used in infants and children, to check the pH of the stool (which normally is alkaline)
Stool for parasites/bacteria	87506 multi-panel test	Varies by market and lab	To check for the presence of parasitic or pathologic organisms
Comprehensive digestive stool analysis	Multiple CPT codes are used for the individual elements of the test	Varies by market and lab	Testing done to evaluate if there is an intestinal dysbiosis. This stool analysis evaluates: • Digestion/absorption markers • Gut metabolic markers • Gut microbiology markers
Pregnancy test	81025 urine 84703 serum	OTC urine strips, $0.50 to $10 Serum, $49	Testing to determine if pregnant
Abdominal x-ray	74000	$280 (national average)	To evaluate possible etiologies of the abdominal swelling
Ultrasound	76700 abdominal 76856 pelvic 76817 transvaginal	$390 (national average, abdominal) $525 (national average, pelvic or transvaginal)	To evaluate possible etiologies of the abdominal swelling
Lower GI series/BE/barium–air contrast enema	74270 lower GI/BE 74280 combination	$618 (national average)	To evaluate possible etiologies of the abdominal swelling
CT scan	74150 abdomen, without contrast	Varies by market and type of scanner, $270 to $4,800	To evaluate possible etiologies of the abdominal swelling
Flexible sigmoidoscopy	45330	Varies by market and provider, $2,393 (national average)	To evaluate possible etiologies of the abdominal swelling
Colonoscopy	45378	Varies by market and provider, $3,081 (national average)	To evaluate possible etiologies of the abdominal swelling

BE, barium enema; CPT, Current Procedural Terminology; GI, gastrointestinal.

CLINICAL DECISION MAKING

Case Study Analysis

The advanced practice provider (APP) performs the assessment and physical exam on the patient and finds the following data: 42-year-old, surgically menopausal female, who has an abdominal appearance that would parallel a full gestational pregnancy. Physical exam findings positive for hyperactive bowel sounds and diffuse abdominal tenderness.

The APP provides the patient with an anti-yeast dietary model to follow and recommends aggressive supplementation with pre and probiotics.

Diagnosis: *Intestinal dysbiosis, suspected etiology recent heavy antibiotic use*

ANKLE PAIN

Case Presentation: A 48-year-old female avid runner presents to your clinic with a complaint of ankle pain on the left ankle present for 3 days.

INTRODUCTION TO COMPLAINT

- The ankle is a base, a lever, and a shock absorber
- Ankle pain can be acute or chronic
- Acute pain is usually caused by an injury due to ankle ligament injuries
- Assessment of acute ankle pain should be focused on the mechanism of injury
- The necessity for radiography is determined by clinical presentation
- When pain and swelling have diminished 3 to 5 days later, reexamination could be completed for differentiating diagnosis of a partial tear from frank ligament rupture. Assessment before that time could be inconclusive

Acute Pain

- Fracture
- Trauma to the ligament or tendon
- Inflammation due to arthritis or bursitis

Chronic Pain

- Most often caused by degenerative joint disease, usually osteoarthritis
- Is a slow progression, not a result of recent injury or trauma
- Overuse of the joint can cause inflammation and edema, and some inflammation to the bursa can be involved
- Could be infectious (osteonecrosis)
- Could be related to loss of bone due to metabolic disorders as with parathyroid disease, osteoporosis, and Paget's disease

HISTORY OF COMPLAINT

Symptomatology

Ask about the following characteristics of each symptom using open-ended questions:

- Determine the onset and mechanism of the injury
- The mechanism of injury is helpful in guiding decision making
- The ankle is a complex joint; the two directions of injury include:
  - Inversion/supination and eversion/pronation
    - Stretched areas usually fracture or tear prior to those areas being compressed
    - With an inversion injury the lateral ankle is stretched
    - In an eversion injury the medial aspect is stretched

- Internal and external rotation of the talus: rotational forces stress supporting structures and can guide injury examination
- The position of the ankle at the time of the injury
- The force applied to the ankle that causes the injury
- The amount of force

Directed Questions to Ask

- How did you injure your ankle?
- Where is the site of the most significant pain?
- Do you have other injured areas on the body (hip, knee)?
- How long has it been since the injury?
- Can you put weight on it? Range of motion (ROM); none to full?
- Any numbness or tingling or other symptoms characteristic of compartment syndrome?
- Any history of injury or intervention to lower extremities?
- Do you smoke?
- High body mass?
- Do you have diabetes?
- Are you on chronic steroids?
- What medications have you taken for systemic disease or previous ankle injury or disability?

Assessment: Cardinal Signs and Symptoms

- Does the patient need surgery to repair area?
- Is there an open fracture?
- Neurovascular compromise
- Fracture dislocation

Medical History: General

- Past medical or surgical history
- Medications
- Allergies to food or medications
- Family history
- Social history

Medical History: Specific to Complaint

- Family history of musculoskeletal disease

PHYSICAL EXAMINATION

Vital Signs

- Blood pressure (BP)
- Temperature
- Pulse
- Respiration
- Oxygen saturation (SpO$_2$)

General Appearance

- Amount of distress

- Pain, 0 to 10 and location
- Difficulty with gait or balance

Inspection

- Swelling
- Ecchymosis
- Deformity
- Skin (blisters, abrasions): any open or penetrating wound increases the risk for cellulitis

Palpation

- Area of maximal tenderness
- Tibia
- Fibula
- Fibular neck
- Test for ligament laxity *after acute fracture is ruled out*
- ROM
- Joint stability

Associated Systems for Assessment

- Dorsalis pedis and posterior tibialis pulses
- Distal capillary refill
- Any indication of vascular compromise: cold, dusky, loss of sensation
- Motor function

CASE STUDY

History

Directed Question	Response
Can you describe what happened when you were injured?	I was stepping off of the curb and I twisted my ankle.
Can you remember if you stepped on the inside of the ankle or the outside?	I stepped on the outside of my foot.
Was there pain right away?	Yes, there was; it hurt.
On a scale of 0 to 10 what number would you give the pain?	Oh, about a 5.
How long did the pain last?	Well it is still hurting but now it is about a 2 or 3.
Was there immediate swelling?	Yes, there was, but it has gone down from what it was initially.
Were you able to walk on your foot?	Yes, I was able to walk to my car okay.
Do you have pain now when you walk on it?	Yes, I do.
Is there any weakness?	No, not really weak, just pain.

Directed Question	Response
Is there any numbness?	No, there is not.
Have you ever injured your ankle before?	No.
Do you have any other joint pains?	No.
Is there any family history of arthritis?	My mother had it when she was in her 80s.
Do you smoke?	No.
Do you have any medical illnesses such as diabetes or gout?	No.
Have you ever taken prednisone or steroids?	No.

Physical Examination Findings

- VITAL SIGNS: temperature 98.2°F; RR 18, regular; heart rate (HR) 62; BP 120/80
- GENERAL APPEARANCE: 48-year-old female, body mass index (BMI) 25, no apparent distress, ambulating to the examination room with a limp, inversion injury
- MUSCULOSKELETAL: lateral ankle anterior talofibular tenderness to palpation, but no pain to posterior edge of medial or lateral malleolus and no midfoot pain; positive swelling present; negative anterior drawer test; talar tilt negative
- SKIN: ecchymosis; skin warm, dry, intact
- EXTREMITIES: distal perfusion intact

Assessing Ankle Injury Severity

Any ankle sprain needs to be assessed as to severity of injury. By using a grade scale the provider can determine the degree of injury and subsequent treatment.

MILD SPRAIN
- Occurs with slight stretching and minimal damage to the fibers (fibrils) of the ankle ligaments
- Patient can place pressure on foot and walk
- Minimal joint instability
- Mild pain
- Mild swelling
- Some joint stiffness

MODERATE SPRAIN
- Partial tearing of the ligament
- Abnormal looseness (laxity) of the ankle joint
- Moderate tearing of the ligament fibers
- Some instability of the joint
- Moderate to severe pain and difficulty walking
- Swelling and stiffness
- Minor bruising

SEVERE SPRAIN
- Complete tear of the ligament occurs
- Total rupture of a ligament
- Gross instability of the joint
- Severe pain initially followed later by no pain
- Severe edema
- Extensive bruising

DIFFERENTIAL DIAGNOSIS

Clinical Observations	Fracture or Dislocation: Stable or Unstable	Sprain or Contusion	Achilles Tendonitis
Onset	Abrupt	Abrupt	Abrupt
Bilateral	No	No	No
Deformity	Yes	No	No
Warmth	Yes	Yes	No
Edema	Yes	Yes	No
Skin	Compound fracture	Ecchymosis	Clear intact
Stiffness	No	Yes	Yes
Neurovascular	Yes	Yes	No
Pain	Yes	Yes	Yes

DIAGNOSTIC EXAMINATION

Exam	Code	Cost	Results	Notes
Ankle series	73610	$90	Fractures or ligament tears	Imaging is indicated if the patient has pain in the malleolar zone and bone tenderness at specific sites or experiences the inability to bear weight
Foot series	74022	$100	Fractures	Imaging is indicated if the patient has midfoot pain and bone tenderness at specific sites or experiences the inability to bear weight immediately
MRI	73630	$400–$3,500	Highly effective for early detection and should be ordered early if there is a high level of suspicion for cellulitis, soft tissue abscess, osteomyelitis	Identifies redundant and inflamed soft tissue Recommendation is to limit MRI in the ankle ligament for athletes at the advanced competitive level, patients with history of chronic ankle instability, and if suspected deltoid ligament injury
CT	73700	$400–$3,500	Fractures	If suspected fracture of the talus

(*continued*)

Exam	Code	Cost	Results	Notes
Bone scan	77080	Between $200 and $600 depending on location	Highly effective for early detection and should be ordered early if there is a high level of suspicion for cellulitis, soft tissue abscess, osteomyelitis	Indicated if stress fracture is present; useful for unexplained bone pain, bone infection, injuries undetectable on standard x-ray
MR arthrogram	23350	Between $1,090 and $2,339 depending on location	Talofibular and calcaneal ligament tears, talus defects	Used to diagnose and for minor intervention to shave away redundant soft tissue and bone Appropriate for chronic anterior talofibular and calcaneal ligament tears Osteochondral defect of talus Anterior ankle impingement due to repetitive stress, usually identified by bone spurs on standard x-ray Posterior ankle impingement due to overuse Synovitis, the procedure is used to remove the synovium

MR, magnetic resonance.

CLINICAL DECISION MAKING

Case Study Analysis

The advanced practice provider performs the assessment and physical examination on the patient and finds the following: minor trauma, single site of injury, and no neurovascular impairment. Although rating the injury as a 3 on a pain rating scale of 0 to 10, the patient is able to bear weight, which indicates the absence of a fracture. The area is ecchymotic, which supports the diagnosis of a sprain. Overall assessment results suggest no indication for imaging at this time. Even though the patient sustained the injury when walking, this type of injury is associated with sports. The anterior talofibular ligament is the weakest part of the ankle and the most likely area affected by trauma. Treatment should be symptomatic to include rest, support with walking, mild over-the-counter analgesics as required, and progressive ambulation. Should symptoms persist or worsen, the patient is advised to return for further investigation to include x-rays and possible immobilization.

Diagnosis: *Lateral ankle sprain: mild sprain*

ANXIOUS MOOD

Case Presentation: A 23-year-old African American male presents with a complaint of being in an anxious mood.

INTRODUCTION TO COMPLAINT

- Many physical problems that manifest or present with anxiety such as arrhythmias, drug reactions, metabolic disorders, cancers, asthma, subdural hematoma, vitamin B12 deficiency, among others.
- Anxiety affects approximately 15% of the adult population, and is more common in those who have experienced trauma and/or abuse, drugs, and alcohol.
- Many individuals can experience symptoms of depression.
- Thyroid disorders can cause anxiety. Hyperthyroidism results from the oversecretion of the thyroid hormones. It occurs in about 1.2% of the U.S. population and peaks between ages 20 and 40. It is more common in women than men and its symptoms are often mistaken for a psychiatric illness. Patients generally experience heart palpitations, diaphoresis, heat intolerance, anxiety, and tachycardia.

HISTORY OF COMPLAINT

Symptomatology

Ask about the following characteristics of each symptom using open-ended questions:

- Onset
- Current situation
- Timing
- Severity
- Precipitating factors
- Relieving factors
- Associated symptoms
- Effects on daily activities
- Previous diagnosis of similar episodes

Directed Questions to Ask

- When did this feeling begin?
- Is there anything that makes it better? Worse?
- Have you had any big changes recently? (such as a move, new job, breakup, birth of a child, etc.)
- Do you have a support network? Family or friends?
- Any childhood or recent trauma?
- What other symptoms accompany the anxious mood?

- Any unexpected weight loss?
- Do you do any excessive exercise?
- Do you eat a balanced diet?
- Do you drink a lot of caffeine, alcohol, or energy drinks? Use tobacco products?
- Do you have any shortness of breath during these episodes? Pain?
- Does anyone in your family suffer from anxiety or depression?
- Any difficulty falling or staying asleep at night?

Assessment: Cardinal Signs and Symptoms

HEENT
- Lymphadenopathy
- Thyroid swelling
- Headache
- Pupillary response

Respiratory
- Lung sounds
- Wheezing
- Dyspnea

Cardiovascular
- Rate and rhythm
- Murmurs

Gastrointestinal (GI)
- Nausea

Neurologic
- Steady gait

Psychology
- Eye contact
- Fidgeting

Medical History

- Medical conditions and surgeries
- Allergies
- Medication use, including illicit drugs
- Family history of anxiety
- History of abuse (physical, sexual, psychological)
- History of trauma (natural disaster, war, insecure housing or food)
- Exercise and diet

PHYSICAL EXAMINATION

Vital Signs

- Temperature
- Pulse
- Blood pressure (BP)
- Oxygen saturation (SpO_2)
- Respiration

General Appearance

- Appearance
- Coloring
- Nutritional status
- Sleep pattern
- Gait
- Orientation

HEENT
- No lymphadenopathy
- Thyroid not enlarged
- Symmetrical
- Nontender

Respiratory
- Lung sounds
- Dyspnea

Cardiovascular
- Rate and rhythm
- No murmurs
- Gallops, or rubs
- Capillary refill
- Distal pulses

Musculoskeletal
- Range of motion (ROM)
- Pain
- Masses, or deformities of extremities

CASE STUDY

History

Directed Question	Response
When did this feeling begin?	*3 months ago.*
Is there anything that makes it better? Worse?	*It's worse before I get ready for work and in the mornings. It's somewhat better on the weekend.*
Have you had any big changes recently? (such as a move, new job, breakup, birth of a child, etc.)	*I moved to a new apartment and started a new job about 5 months ago.*
Do you have a support network? Family or friends?	*I talk to my mom regularly and see my brother on some weekends. I was playing basketball with friends, but now I feel too worn out.*
Any childhood or recent trauma?	*No.*
What other symptoms accompany the anxiety?	*Sometimes I feel a little lightheaded or dizzy, maybe have some nausea.*

Directed Question	Response
Any unexpected weight loss?	*No.*
Do you do any excessive exercise? Eat a balanced diet?	*I try to eat well, but sometime I have fast food or Chinese. I don't like to eat in the mornings. I don't exercise enough!*
Do you drink a lot of caffeine, alcohol, or energy drinks? Use tobacco products?	*I probably drink too much coffee. And I'll have an energy drink when I get to work. I don't smoke or drink alcohol.*
Do you have any shortness of breath during these episodes? Pain?	*No, just anxiety.*
Does anyone in your family suffer from anxiety or depression?	*Not that I know of.*
Any difficulty falling or staying asleep at night?	*Sometimes. I worry about the anxiety I'm going to feel in the morning and it stresses me out.*

Physical Examination Findings

- VITAL SIGNS: temperature 98.9°F; respiration 18; pulse 62/irregularly irregular; BP 110/74; SpO_2 100% on room air
- GENERAL APPEARANCE: well-appearing male in no acute distress, A + O × 4 (alert and oriented times four)
- HEENT: PERRLA, extraocular movements intact, lymph nodes nonpalpable, thyroid not enlarged
- RESPIRATORY: lungs clear bilaterally to auscultation
- CARDIOVASCULAR: heart rhythm irregularly irregular, rate 62, cap refill <2 seconds, peripheral pulses 2+ bilaterally
- GASTROINTESTINAL: bowel sounds present in all four quadrants, nontender, soft abdomen
- MUSCULOSKELETAL: full ROM of extremities, neck, back, no crepitus or deformities noted
- SKIN: intact, dry, no ecchymosis, lesions, rashes, or discoloration noted

DIFFERENTIAL DIAGNOSIS

Clinical Observations	Generalized Anxiety	Arrhythmia	Hypoglycemia	Thyroid Disease
Onset	Gradual, more days than not	Sudden	Sudden or gradual	Gradual
Timing	Constant, interferes with daily life, worse	Intermittent or constant	After eating carbs, after exercise, if not eating	Constant
Eye symptoms	No	No	Diplopia, blurred vision	Lid lag, ophthalmopathy

(*continued*)

Clinical Observations	Generalized Anxiety	Arrhythmia	Hypoglycemia	Thyroid Disease
Weight changes	Possible gain or loss	No	No	Weight loss with increased appetite
Heart rate and rhythm	Tachycardia, palpitations	Irregular, may have palpitations, angina, may be tachycardic, bradycardic	Tachycardia w/ or w/o PVCs, palpitations	Tachycardia, palpitations
Weakness, fatigue	Yes	Yes/No	Yes	Yes
Dizziness	No	Yes/No	Yes	No
Tremors	Yes/No	No	Yes	Yes
Other possible symptoms	Nausea, diaphoresis	Syncope, hypotension	Seizures, diaphoresis	Goiter

PVC, premature ventricular contraction.

DIAGNOSTIC EXAMINATION

Exam	Code	Cost	Result
EKG	R94.31	$41	Normal sinus rhythm—regular PR interval <0.2 seconds, QRS interval <0.12 seconds, regular PP and RR intervals, Hr between 60 and 100 Arrhythmia—Atrial—may demonstrate absence of P wave with irregular QRS intervals, multiple P waves to QRS complexes, or dyssynchronous P wave complex to QRS complex
			Ventricular—may show absence of P wave with regular QRS interval, wide QRS intervals (either frequent or infrequent), notched QRS waves indicative of a block, multifocal QRS complexes, or irregular, nonuniform QRS complexes (which may be life-threatening)
PRIME-MD screening tool	NK	$0	Helps with the recognition and diagnosis of mental disorders Patients fill out the form before the visit and clinician reviews answers and clarifies during the appointment Differentiates between major depressive disorder, other depressive disorder, anxiety disorder, and somatic disorders and offers treatment suggestions based on scoring

(*continued*)

Exam	Code	Cost	Result
Blood glucose	R73.09	$11	Should be performed after patient fasts for 8 hours Determines if the blood glucose level falls below the normal range of 70–100 mg/dL However, a normal blood glucose level at a single time point does not exclude the possibility of hypoglycemia at other times
Thyroid panel	R94.6	$44	Measures the amount of TSH and thyroid hormones (T3 and T4) present in the bloodstream. A low level of TSH (<0.4 uIU/mL) is indicative of hyperthyroidism

PRIME-MD, Primary Care Evaluation of Mental Disorders; TSH, thyroid-stimulating hormone; T3, serum triiodothyronine; T4, free thyroxine.

CLINICAL DECISION MAKING

Case Study Analysis

After assessing the patient and obtaining a detailed history, the advanced practice provider (APP) found the patient to be experiencing mild anxiety as per the Patient Health Questionnaire-9* assessment tool. EKG showed a sinus rhythm with frequent premature ventricular contractions (PVCs), which the patient described as the feeling he normally had when he felt dizzy and nauseated. Thyroid-stimulating hormone (TSH) levels were 1.8 uIU/mL and fasting glucose was 80 mg/dL. These test results are considered normal.

> *Diagnosis:* Anxiety related to arrhythmia due to excessive caffeine ingestion

From this assessment, the APP and patient discussed cutting back on caffeine intake from coffee and energy drinks and incorporating stress-reduction techniques. Patient felt these were reasonable changes and follow-up was set for 1 month later.

Follow-up: At the 1-month follow-up the patient reported improvement of symptoms and only occasional anxiety related to work. EKG at this time demonstrated a normal sinus rhythm. Patient was counseled to return if symptoms recurred or if he began to feel overwhelmed or depressed.

BLOOD IN URINE

Case Presentation: A 46-year-old male reports to the clinic with a complaint of blood in his urine.

INTRODUCTION TO COMPLAINT

- Hematuria can be visible (gross) or nonvisible (microscopic). Forty-five percent of all cases are attributable to infection (25%) and kidney stones (20%)
- Urinary tract infections: invasion of bacteria via the urethra into the bladder
- Urge to urinate, pain with urination, burning with urination
- Foul smelling urine
- Kidney infections: bacteria reach the kidneys via the ureters or via the bloodstream. Symptoms similar to urinary tract infection, often accompanied by fever and flank pain
- Kidney stones: precipitation of minerals in the urine in the kidney forming stones; movement of stones often causes excruciating pain; can cause microscopic or gross hematuria
- Kidney trauma: from a contact sport or other injury
- Kidney disease: glomerulonephritis, primary or secondary to viral or strep infections
- Ingested substances: ingestion of toxic substances can cause inflammation and damage to the filtration system of the kidney; cytoxan and penicillin can cause hematuria; ingestion of anticoagulants leads to hematuria, particularly if there is an underlying condition that causes the bladder to bleed
- Inherited conditions: sickle cell anemia and Alport syndrome
- Strenuous exercise: intense workouts can result in hematuria thought to be secondary to dehydration or breakdown of red blood cells (RBCs), which occurs with sustained aerobic activity
- Cancer: kidney, bladder, or prostate

HISTORY OF COMPLAINT

Symptomatology

Ask about the following characteristics of each symptom using open-ended questions:

- Onset (sudden or gradual)
- Chronology
- Current situation (improving or deteriorating)
- Location

- Radiation
- Quality
- Timing (frequency, duration)
- Severity
- Precipitating and aggravating factors
- Relieving factors
- Associated symptoms
- Effects on daily activities
- Previous diagnosis of similar episodes
- Previous treatments
- Efficacy of previous treatments

Directed Questions to Ask

- When did you first see blood in your urine?
- How much blood would you say was in your urine?
- Do you have any urinary frequency?
- Do you have any pain?
- Have you had a problem with diarrhea or loose stools recently?
- Have you had a sore throat?
- Have you been exposed to anyone with a sore throat or strep throat?
- Have you seen any "sand-like," granular material in the commode after you urinated?
- Are you exposed to any chemicals or known toxic substances at work or home?
- Have you had an accident or an injury recently that impacted your kidney area?
- Any known family history of kidney disease?
- What is your exercise routine?

Assessment: Cardinal Signs and Symptoms

- Urinary frequency
- Urinary urgency
- Pain with urination
- Burning with urination
- Fever
- Flank pain
- Visible blood in urine

Medical History: General

- Medical conditions and surgeries
- Allergies (seasonal as well as others)
- Medication currently used (prescription, birth control pill [BCP] and over the counter (OTC)
- Herbal preparations and traditional therapies

Medical History: Specific to Complaint

- Frequent sore throats
- Known strep throat
- Blood in urine
- Kidney stones

PHYSICAL EXAMINATION
Vital Signs
- Temperature
- Pulse
- Respiration
- Oxygen saturation (SpO_2)
- Blood pressure (BP)

General Appearance
- Apparent state of health
- Appearance of comfort or distress
- Color
- State of hydration

Mouth and Throat
- Inspect oral cavity for breath odor, color, lesions; throat and pharynx for color, exudates, tonsillar enlargement

Neck
- Inspect for symmetry, swelling, masses
- Palpate for tenderness, enlargement, lymph node chain

Abdomen
- Inspect for contour, heaves, scars, bruising, contusions
- Auscultate for bowel sounds, bruits
- Palpate for pain, masses, costovertebral (CVA) angle tenderness

CASE STUDY
History

Directed Question	Response
When did you first see blood in your urine?	*Yesterday.*
How much blood would you say was in your urine?	*Lots of red water in the commode every time I pee.*
Do you have any urinary frequency?	*No.*
Do you have any pain?	*No.*
Have you had a problem with diarrhea or loose stools recently?	*No.*
Have you had a sore throat?	*No.*
Have you been exposed to anyone who has a sore throat or strep throat?	*No.*
Have you seen any "sand-like," granular material in the commode after you urinated?	*No.*

Directed Question	*Response*
Are you exposed to any chemicals or known toxic substances at work or home?	*No.*
Have you had an accident or an injury recently that impacted your kidney area?	*No.*
Any known family history of kidney disease?	*No.*
What is your exercise routine?	*I walk a couple miles about three times a week.*

Physical Examination Findings

- VITAL SIGNS: temperature 98.4°F; respiratory rate (RR) 16; heart rate (HR) 74, regular; BP 116/67; SpO$_2$ 98%
- GENERAL APPEARANCE: well-developed; healthy-appearing male in no acute distress
- MOUTH: no oral lesions; teeth and gums in good repair
- PHARYNX: no erythema; no tonsillar enlargement; no exudate
- NECK: no palpable lymph node
- ABDOMEN: soft, nontender without mass or organomegaly; no CVA tenderness

DIFFERENTIAL DIAGNOSIS

Clinical Observations	Urinary Tract Infection	Kidney Infection	Kidney Stone	Kidney Trauma	Other Etiologies
Gross hematuria	Possible, not typical	Possible	Possible	Possible	Possible
Microscopic hematuria	Possible, not typical	Not uncommon	Not uncommon	Not uncommon	Possible
Urinary frequency	Typical	Typical	Not typical	Not typical	Possible
Pain with urination	Typical	Typical	Common	Possible	Possible

DIAGNOSTIC EXAMINATION

Exam	Code	Cost	Results
Urine dip stick	81000	$10	For microscopic blood—will be negative

(*continued*)

Exam	Code	Cost	Results
Complete urinalysis, includes microscopy	81015	$49	For microscopic blood—presence of >4 RBCs per field high power field For gross blood—too numerous to count RBCs per high power field Presence of RBC casts indicative of kidney infection For kidney stone etiology—may see calcium oxalate crystals (about 80% of stones are of this nature)
Comprehensive metabolic panel	80053	$49	For evaluation of kidney function—creatinine, BUN, and electrolytes
CT Scan	74150	Varies by market, $270–$4,800	Can be used to diagnose both kidney stones and traumatic injury to the kidney

BUN, blood urea nitrogen; RBC, red blood cell.

CLINICAL DECISION MAKING

Case Study Analysis

The advanced practice provider performs the assessment and physical exam on the patient and finds the following data: history of seeing blood in urine, urine dipstick evaluation negative, urine microscopy reveals too numerous to count RBCs per high power field, urine for culture and sensitivity are negative, CT scan and cystoscopy are negative.

Given that this is the patient's first episode of gross hematuria, and advanced testing (CT and cystoscopy) did not reveal any pertinent findings, referral will be made to a urologist for further evaluation and management.

Additional testing may be recommended to include urine for cytology to rule out an infectious cause, intravenous pyelogram to rule out kidney stones after an abdominal flat plate, and additional laboratory tests to evaluate for an acute kidney injury. Further assessment may be required to examine the patient's exercise routine as a possible contributing factor to hematuria. Provided with contact information to schedule an appointment with a urologist. The urologist will proceed to determine which diagnostic testing is most appropriate.

Diagnosis: Gross hematuria, etiology unknown

BREAST LUMPS

Case Presentation: A 55-year-old African American female social worker presents to your clinic with a finding of a lump in her left breast while in the shower this past week.

INTRODUCTION TO COMPLAINT

- Family history and other factors can affect a women's perception of this finding
- Several other conditions can cause breast lumps
- All breast lumps need a thorough and systematic approach to history and physical examination

Fibroadenoma

- A fibroadenoma is the most common cause of a breast lump
- It is always benign and is made up of a combination of glandular breast tissue and fibroconnective tissue
- Often it can be influenced by hormones and becomes large enough that it is easily felt and sometimes easily visible
- Age as well as definite characteristics will help differentiate the diagnosis of a fibroadenoma as a cause of a breast lump

Cyst

- Cysts are generally fluid filled
- They can be singular or appear in clusters
- Generally, breast cysts decline with menopause and may be present, more frequently, during the luteal phase of a women's menstrual cycle
- Because cysts are influenced by hormones, they may continue to be present in postmenopausal women who are on hormone replacement therapy

Cancer

- Cancer can be another cause of a breast lump
- Often cannot be diagnosed based on physical examination findings alone
- A breast lump that is a cancer may have characteristics that are a cause for concern but it cannot be diagnosed without a diagnostic evaluation, which will include a biopsy of the mass

HISTORY OF COMPLAINT

Symptomatology

Ask about the following characteristics of each symptom using open-ended questions:

- Onset (sudden or gradual)
- Chronology
- Current situation (improving or deteriorating)
- Location
- Radiation
- Quality
- Timing (frequency, duration)
- Severity
- Precipitating and aggravating factors
- Relieving factors
- Associated symptoms
- Effects on daily activities
- Previous diagnosis of similar episodes
- Previous treatment
- Efficacy of previous treatment

Directed Questions to Ask

- What was your age of menarche?
- What was your age of menopause (if applicable)?
- Do you have a family history of breast cancer (first-degree relative [mother, sister, or daughter] on either mother's or father's side, age of diagnosis, family history of breast cancer in any male relative)?
- Have you had screening for breast cancer mutations (*BR/CA1/2*)?
- Do you have a personal history of breast cancer?
- How old were you with your first pregnancy?
- Do you use alcohol?
- Do you have a history of chest or neck radiation?
- Do you have a history of breast biopsies and diagnoses?
- Do you use hormones (oral contraceptives or hormone replacement therapy)?
- Are you on a high-fat diet?
- Do you do any physical activities?
- Have there been any changes since initially finding the lump either in its size, or in pain, skin changes, nipple discharge, change with menstrual cycle?
- Have you had any weight changes, palpable lumps in armpit or under clavicle?

Assessment: Cardinal Signs and Symptoms

In addition to the general characteristics outlined previously, additional characteristics of specific symptoms should be elicited.

General
- Weight changes
- Recent fever
- Chills
- General malaise

Neck and Axilla
- Recent palpable lumps/tenderness

Breasts
- Noticeable skin changes, pain, tenderness, nipple discharge
- A complete assessment should include the chest wall, heart, and lungs

Medical History: General
- Relevant past medical conditions and surgeries
- Allergies
- Current medications: prescription, oral contraceptives, hormone replacement, over-the-counter herbal products (dosage and length of treatment)

Medical History: Specific to Complaint
- Previous breast lump
- Breast biopsy or surgery
- Ovarian or colon cancer

PHYSICAL EXAMINATION
Vital Signs
- Temperature
- Blood pressure (BP)
- Pulse
- Respiration

General Appearance
- Apparent state of health
- Appearance of comfort or distress
- Color, temperature of skin
- General nutritional status
- Hygiene

Neck
- Chest wall
- Axillae
- Supraclavicular, infraclavicular, and axillary adenopathy (sitting and supine)

Breasts
- VISUAL: sitting and supine
- Observe outline and contour of breasts: look for any bulging or asymmetrical areas
- Movement of breasts with arms above head and at side, flexion of pectoral muscles with hands on hips, and pressing in to contract muscles
- SKIN CHANGES: check for dimpling or retraction of the breast tissue, edema, ulceration, erythema or scaling, irritated skin changes, peau d'orange (orange-peel appearance)
- NIPPLES: look for asymmetry, inversion, or retraction; evidence of discharge or crusted exudates

Palpation
- REGIONAL LYMPH NODES: With patient in sitting position, palpate the axillae and infraclavicular and supraclavicular nodes. This is best done with the patient in a relaxed position. Document any findings, observing for position, mobility, tenderness.

- BREAST EXAMINATION: This should be done initially in the sitting position, supporting the breast with one hand and examining with the other. The breasts should then be examined with the patient in the supine position, with the arm on the side you are examining above her head. For a woman with large breasts, it may be helpful for her to roll onto the contralateral hip so that you can better palpate the upper and lower lateral quadrants of the breast you are examining and then complete the examination with her on her back.

The entire breast should be examined using a systematic approach: either using small concentric circles with varying degrees of pressure (light, medium, and deep) or the up and down approach also known as the "lawnmower" method. The finger pads should be used for palpation rather than the fingertips. It is important to cover all breast tissue, imagining a rectangle rather than a circle. Assess for consistency of tissue, presence of tenderness, nodularity, dominant masses, and borders of the mass. Compare asymmetry between breasts.

Documentation
- Document size, shape, and borders of lump. Size should be measured in centimeters, the clock position of the mass should be recorded, and the number of centimeters from the areola should be measured (e.g., 4 × 4 cm circular mass with smooth borders, 10 o'clock position, 5 cm from the nipple)
- Document as much details as possible, including negative findings

CASE STUDY
History

Directed Question	Response
Was the onset sudden or gradual?	Sudden, I found it while showering.
Where is the lump located?	Left breast, upper outer quadrant.
How big is it?	It feels like a small pea.
Can you move it around?	No, it doesn't feel like it will move.
Are the borders palpable?	No, I can't seem to feel the borders easily.
Is there tenderness or pain?	No, there is no tenderness or pain.
Have you noticed any skin changes or nipple discharge from the left breast?	No, I have not.
Have you felt any lumps or tenderness in your left armpit?	No.
When was the last time you had a mammogram?	I got a negative-screening mammogram 2 years ago.
How old were you when your periods started?	I was 13 years old.
At what age did you go into menopause?	I was 52.
Have you ever been pregnant? How old were you when you had your first child?	I was 26 with my first child.
Did you breastfeed? How long?	Yes, for 4 months.

Directed Question	Response
Did you ever take hormones, either birth control pills or postmenopausal hormone replacement?	*I took birth control pills for 10 years, starting when I was 20. I am not on hormone replacement.*
Have you ever had breast surgeries or a breast biopsy?	*No.*
Do you have a family history of breast disease or breast cancer?	*My grandmother had breast cancer when she was 76 years old.*
Do you do self-breast exams?	*On occasion.*
How has your recent health been?	*I've been very healthy.*
Do you drink alcohol?	*I drink an occasional glass of wine two times a week.*
Do you exercise?	*Yes, three to four times a week for 30 minutes.*
Do you have a high-fat diet?	*No.*

Physical Examination Findings

- VITAL SIGNS: temperature 98.6°F; respiratory rate (RR) 16; heart rate (HR) 80, regular; BP 120/80; height: 5'8"; weight 160 lb; body mass index (BMI) 24
- GENERAL APPEARANCE: well-developed, nourished, healthy-appearing female
- NECK: supple, no cervical adenopathy
- BREASTS: Examined in sitting and supine positions; in sitting position, no evidence of skin changes, right breast is slightly larger than the left, symmetrical movement with the arms above the head and at the side and with flexion of the pectoral muscles; 5-mm nonmobile, nontender, firm mass felt at 10 o'clock position, 5 cm from the areola; right breast without dominant masses or tenderness; nipples without inversion or evidence of nipple discharge; breast lump is palpated in the supine position in the same manner as in the sitting position
- LYMPH: negative axillary, infraclavicular, and supraclavicular lymphadenopathy
- RESPIRATORY: lungs clear to auscultation
- CARDIOVASCULAR: regular rate and rhythm (RRR)
- CHEST WALL: symmetrical, no tenderness over intercostal spaces

DIFFERENTIAL DIAGNOSIS

Clinical Observations	Cyst	Fibroadenoma	Cancer
Onset	Sudden	Gradual	Gradual/sudden
Age	15–55	15–25 (puberty/young adult)	30–90: more common >50, postmenopause
Cyclic	Can be cyclic	Usually not	Not related

(*continued*)

Clinical Observations	Cyst	Fibroadenoma	Cancer
Hormone influenced	Can be	Can be	Can be/but not caused by
Shape	Round or elongated	Round or elongated	Irregular
Borders	Well defined	Smooth, well defined	Difficult to define
Tenderness	Usually tender	Nontender	Nontender
Skin changes	Not present	Not present	May be present; peau d'orange
Nipple discharge	Not present	Not present	Usually not present
Mobility	Mobile	Very mobile	Nonmobile, may be fixed to chest wall

DIAGNOSTIC EXAMINATION

Exam	Code	Cost*	Results
Mammogram	77055	$385	Noninvasive medical imaging involves exposing breasts to a small dose of ionizing radiation to produce pictures of the breast.
			Three recent advances in mammography include digital mammography, computer-aided detection, and breast tomosynthesis.
			Digital mammography • Also called full-field digital mammography (FFDM) • The x-ray film is replaced by electronics that convert x-rays into mammographic pictures of the breast
			Computer-aided detection (CAD) • Search digitized mammographic images for abnormal areas of density, mass, or calcification that may indicate the presence of cancer
Ultrasound	76645	$279	• Ultrasound imaging of the breast uses sound waves to produce pictures of the internal structures of the breast • Primarily used to help diagnose breast lumps or other abnormalities your doctor may have found during a physical exam, mammogram or breast MRI; ultrasound is safe, noninvasive

*These are approximate fees that may vary by facility and region.

CLINICAL DECISION MAKING
Case Study Analysis

The advanced practice provider performs the assessment and physical examination on a patient with a sudden onset of a lump in the upper outer quadrant of the left breast found while in the shower. It is nontender and nonmobile. There are no skin changes or evidence of nipple discharge. She has no other symptoms. She cannot feel any lumps under her arm or under her collarbone. She has never had a positive-screening mammogram, nor does she have a history of breast biopsies or surgeries. She is menopausal and not currently taking hormone replacement. She has a family history of a maternal grandmother with breast cancer diagnosed in her 70s. She is worried and concerned as a coworker was recently diagnosed with breast cancer. Her physical examination reveals a 5-mm-size firm, nonmobile lump at the 10 o'clock position in the left breast, 5 cm from the nipple. A nontender fixed nodule is associated with breast cancer. There is negative lymphadenopathy.

> **Diagnosis:** *Pending mammogram results*

Depending upon the results of the mammogram the patient may need a diagnostic mammogram and ultrasound followed by a biopsy. Further treatment will depend upon the results of all diagnostic testing.

In women under 30 years of age, further diagnostic testing includes a unilateral breast ultrasound and in women over 30 years of age, it includes a diagnostic mammogram and ultrasound.

It should never be assumed by the clinician that a diagnosis can be made based on the history and physical examination alone. In young women, it may be advisable to observe the breast lump over a menstrual cycle to see if there are changes, especially if tenderness is a symptom and the lump is found during the luteal phase of the menstrual cycle.

A negative clinical examination is not conclusive of a negative diagnosis of cancer even in light of a negative mammogram and ultrasound. All palpable lumps with negative imaging should be referred to a breast surgeon for final diagnosis and management.

CHEST PAIN

Case Presentation: *A 70-year-old female reports experiencing pain in her chest while walking up steps today.*

INTRODUCTION TO COMPLAINT

Chest pain can be caused by several serious, life-threatening disorders, such as cardiac ischemia, pulmonary embolism, or pneumonia. However, chest pain is a common complaint and may also be caused by non-life-threatening problems, such as arthritis, acid reflux, or panic disorder.

Cardiac Chest Pain

- Chest pain triggered by exertion, eating a meal, emotional distress; is relieved with rest
- Usual risk factors for coronary disease are present, such as hypertension, diabetes, or hyperlipidemia
- Pericarditis, or inflammation of the sac around the heart, causes chest pain, which becomes worse when lying down and is relieved when leaning forward

Pulmonary

- Chest pain that increases with a deep breath is termed pleuritic chest pain
- It is usually sharp, stabbing, and associated with inflammation of the pleural lining
- It is associated with pneumonia, pulmonary embolus, autoimmune disease, and viral infections

Musculoskeletal

- Pain in the joints of the costochondral junction is common with increased movement
- It is always reproducible by movement or pressure

Gastrointestinal

- Acid reflux can cause a burning pain or spasm in the midchest and mimics cardiac pain
- It may be precipitated by eating a fatty meal and then lying down, especially if obese
- It is relieved with antacids or acid blockers

HISTORY OF COMPLAINT

Symptomatology

Ask about the following characteristics of each symptom using open-ended questions:

- Onset: sudden or gradual
- Location/radiation

- Duration, timing
- Characteristics of the pain
- Associated symptoms
- Aggravating factors
- Alleviating factors
- Effect on daily activities

Directed Questions to Ask

- Is the pain worse with exertion?
- Is it relieved with rest?
- Does the pain radiate to the neck, jaw, or arm?
- Is the pain worse with a deep breath?
- Are you having difficulty breathing because of the pain?
- Does movement make the pain worse?
- Have you had heartburn?
- Is the pain worse after eating a meal?
- Is the pain worse when lying down? If so, is it better when sitting up or leaning forward?
- Have you had this pain in the past?
- If so, how did you treat it?

Assessment: Cardinal Signs and Symptoms

The following signs and symptoms are highly associated with some types of chest pain.

Symptom and Signs	Disorder
Constitutional	
Fever, chills, and sweats	Pneumonia, pericarditis
Respiratory	
Chest pain with deep breath	Pleurisy, pulmonary embolus, pneumonia
Shortness of breath	Pneumonia, pulmonary embolus, cardiac disease, CHF
Cardiovascular	
Hypertension, high cholesterol, diabetes	Ischemic heart disease
Exertional chest pain relieved with rest	Ischemic heart disease, valvular heart disease
Palpitation	Cardiac arrhythmia
Gastrointestinal	
Heartburn or acid reflux	GERD, esophageal spasm, atypical ischemia
Nausea, vomiting	Ischemic heart disease, GERD, or peptic ulcer

(*continued*)

Symptom and Signs	Disorder
Vascular	
Swelling of both lower extremities	CHF
Swelling of one lower extremity	DVT and subsequent pulmonary embolus
Skin	
Cyanosis	Pneumonia, ischemic heart disease, COPD
Clubbing of nails	COPD, lung cancer

CHF, congestive heart failure; COPD, chronic obstructive pulmonary disease; DVT, deep vein thrombosis; GERD, gastroesophageal reflux disease.

Medical History: General

- Past medical conditions: ask about history of high cholesterol, smoking, hypertension, type 2 diabetes, other chronic illness
- Medications: ask if the patient is taking aspirin, nitroglycerin, a nonsteroidal anti-inflammatory drug (NSAID), or any new drug
- Family history: ask about family history of early heart disease, stroke, transient ischemic attack (TIA), diabetes, high cholesterol, or sudden death
- Social history: ask about occupation, stressors, habits such as smoking, alcohol, exercise, diet habits

Medical History: Specific to Complaint

- Pain
- Redness
- Swelling

PHYSICAL EXAMINATION

Vital Signs

- Temperature/pulse/respiration
- Blood pressure (BP)
- Pulse oximetry

General Appearance

- Does the patient appear to be in acute distress, fearful, or diaphoretic? Is there obvious shortness of breath?
- Does the patient appear to be healthy and relaxed?

Neck

- Palpate carotid arteries for symmetry of stroke and listen for bruit
- Evaluate the jugular venous pressure at a 45-degree angle

Cardiopulmonary

HEART

- Listen for S1 and S2 and identify any abnormal sounds, such as a murmur, gallop, or friction rub
- Palpate the point of maximum impulse (PMI)
- Determine whether rhythm is regular or irregular
- Count the heart rate (HR) and note if it is excessively slow or rapid

LUNGS

- Observe character of respiration and confirm whether it is labored, rapid, or shallow
- Listen for quality of breath sounds: Are they clear, diminished, or absent?
- Listen for adventitious sounds, such as crackles (rales), rhonchi, or friction rubs
- Percuss the chest to identify dullness indicating pleural effusion or pneumonia
- Perform E to A testing. If there is a consolidation, when the patient says "E" it will sound like an "A." Tactile fremitus is increased if there is a lobar pneumonia. If there is dullness to percussion, this indicates fluid rather than air in the lungs

Abdomen

- Observe the abdominal aorta for abnormally wide or prominent pulsations
- Listen to the abdomen for bowel tones and bruits
- Percuss the abdomen to identify areas of tympany, dullness, or tenderness
- Palpate the abdomen to identify areas of tenderness, organomegaly, or masses

Vascular/Extremities

- Observe lower extremities for edema; check capillary refill and distal pulses

Skin

- Observe for pallor or cyanosis
- Check nails for clubbing or cyanosis of nail bed

Neurologic

- Describe mental status
- Is the patient alert and oriented or confused and somnolent?

CASE STUDY

History

A 70-year-old female presents to the urgent care walk-in clinic stating that she woke up at about 3 a.m. with pain in the center of her chest. It went away after a few hours, but was there when she woke up in the morning. She reports no shortness of breath, diaphoresis, or fatigue. She has not had fever or chills.

Directed Question	Response
Are you having the discomfort right now?	*Yes, but very little now.*
Can you describe it?	*It is like an ache or a burning sensation.*
Where is it? Can you put a finger on it?	*Yes, right here [center of sternum].*
Does it go anywhere else in the chest?	*Up into my throat.*

Directed Question	*Response*
Does it go into the arms at all?	*No, my arms feel fine.*
On a scale of 0 to 10, what was it?	*Oh, I'd say an 8 or so.*
What is it now?	*Oh, a 2 or so.*
Does anything make it worse?	*Yes, I couldn't sleep last night.*
Was the pain worse when you were lying down?	*Oh yes, much worse.*
Did anything make it better?	*Yes, sitting up helped.*
Did anything else help?	*Yes, drinking a glass of water.*
Was it worse when you walked around today?	*No, can't say it was.*
Was it worse going up steps?	*No, it wasn't.*
Did you feel weak or sweaty with the pain?	*Yes, a little bit.*
Did you feel nauseated?	*Yes, a little bit.*
Did you vomit?	*No, I didn't.*
Do you have a history of a stomach ulcer?	*No, I never have.*
Do you have a history of acid reflux?	*No, I never have that I know of.*
Do you have high blood pressure?	*Yes, I take medication for it.*
What is the name of the medication?	*Procardia, I just started this new one.*
Do you have high cholesterol?	*No, my doctor said that is fine.*
Do you have heart disease, like angina?	*No, I don't think so.*
Do you ever have to stop what you are doing due to chest pain, pressure, nausea, or heartburn?	*No, I never have had to do that.*
Does your heart ever race fast, or beat irregularly?	*Not that I have ever noticed.*
Do your legs ever swell up?	*No, they don't do that.*
Do you feel short of breath?	*No, I breathe just fine.*
Does the pain feel worse when you take in a deep breath?	*[Takes deep breath] No, it doesn't.*
Does it hurt when you press on the chest?	*[Presses] No, it doesn't.*
What did you eat last night before bed?	*Mexican food, chips, and salsa.*

Physical Examination Findings

- VITAL SIGNS: temperature 98.8°F; respiratory rate (RR) 16 unlabored; HR 72 and regular; BP 129/70; oral pulse oximetry is 99%
- GENERAL APPEARANCE: pleasant obese female, alert, in no acute distress
- SKIN: warm, dry, color is normal
- NECK: carotids are 2+ without bruits; thyroid is not palpable; no lymphadenopathy
- HEART: S1 and S2 normal without murmur, gallop, or rub
- LUNGS: clear and resonant
- CHEST WALL: nontender along the sternal border and rib areas
- ABDOMEN: bowel tones are normal, no abdominal bruit; abdomen is soft, slightly tender in the epigastric area, no masses or organomegaly
- RECTAL: rectal vault nontender; stool is negative for blood
- EXTREMITIES: radial and pedal pulses 2+ and equal; no edema, cyanosis, or clubbing of the nails

DIFFERENTIAL DIAGNOSIS

Clinical Observations	History	Physical Examination	Diagnostic Tests
Angina	Triggered by exertion and relieved by rest in <30 minutes	Often normal; listen for S3, S4, or murmurs; or abnormal BP	EKG, stress test, lipid panel, cardiac enzymes
Acute coronary syndrome	Substernal, radiates to neck, jaw, lasts >30 minutes, diaphoretic, nausea, vomiting	Pale, sweaty; may have S3, S4, rales, murmur; or normal examination	EKG, troponin, CK-MB, coronary angiogram
Pericarditis	Chest pain that is stabbing, worse lying down, better leaning forward	Hallmark is pericardial friction rub; increased JVP or edema LE	EKG, CXR, echo, MRI, pericardial tap, high ESR, plus blood cultures or plus ANA
Pleuritic	Pain worse with deep respirations	Pleural friction rub	CXR or EKG, CBC, ESR, ANA, D-dimer
Pneumonia	Fever, cough	Crackles over lobe	CXR, CBC/white blood cell count
Pulmonary embolism	Dyspnea, pleuritic pain, leg swelling, calf pain, risk factors	Rapid RR, and HR, pleural friction rub, unilateral edema LE	CT angiography or V/Q scan, ABGs, D-dimer, venous Doppler
Pneumothorax	Sudden dyspnea running or trauma	Decreased or absent breath sounds	CXR shows loss of lung markings
Musculoskeletal	Worst with motion or pressure to local area	Pain reproducible	Physical examination

(*continued*)

Clinical Observations	History	Physical Examination	Diagnostic Tests
GERD/esophageal	Pain lying down, after eating fatty meal	Better sitting up or with antacid/lidocaine	Endoscopy or upper gastrointestinal scan
Aortic dissection	Male:female 3:1; age 60 to 80; sudden onset of severe, sharp chest pain radiating into back, syncope	Severe hypertension; >20 mmHg in BP between arms; absent distal pulses; early manifestations: Horner's syndrome, sudden hoarseness	EKG to rule out MI; CXR, TEE, MRI, and helical CT are options

ABGs, arterial blood gases; ANA, antinuclear antibodies; BP, blood pressure; CBC, complete blood count; CK-MB, creatinine kinase isoenzyme MB; CXR, chest x-ray; ESR, erythrocyte sedimentation rate; GERD, gastroesophageal reflux disease; HR, heart rate; JVP, jugular venous pressure; LE, lower extremities; MI, myocardial infarction; RR, respiratory rate; TEE, transesophageal echo; V/Q, ventilation/perfusion.

DIAGNOSTIC EXAMINATION

Exam	Code	Cost	Results
Electrocardiogram	93000	$150	If cardiac risk factors are present, exertional chest pain may reveal classic changes of ischemia; a normal EKG does not rule out ischemia
Cardiac troponins	84484	$300	Elevated in ischemic as well as other cardiac disease
CK-MB isoenzymes	82553	$300	Evidence of ischemic heart disease
BNP	83880	$250	Secreted by ventricles in response to volume overload in CHF, high in renal failure
CBC	85025	$75	Identifies anemia or elevated white blood cell count
Comprehensive metabolic panel	83516	$120	Evaluates electrolytes, renal and liver status
Chest x-ray	71020	$250	Shortness of breath, fever, ischemic or pleuritic chest pain; may reveal pulmonary congestion from CHF, pneumonia, pleural thickening, or effusion
Cardiac echo-cardiogram	93351	$1,500	Evaluate patients with ischemic heart disease for structural abnormalities, abnormal wall motion, abnormal valves, and ejection fraction
Stress testing	93015	$800	If cardiac chest pain is present, conduct exercise treadmill, stress echocardiogram, or radionuclide testing
Coronary angiography	75574	$2,500	Invasive but gold standard for ruling in or ruling out the presence of CAD

(*continued*)

Exam	Code	Cost	Results
CT spiral	74000	$1,200	If a pulmonary embolus is suspected due to sudden shortness of breath
Chest CT	71275	$1,800	If aortic dissection, pneumonia, effusion are suspected

BNP, beta natriuretic peptide; CAD, coronary artery disease; CBC, complete blood count; CHF, congestive heart failure; CK-MB, creatinine kinase isoenzyme MB.

Basic Interpretation of Electrocardiogram (EKG)

T wave inversion, ST segment elevation, or Q waves are diagnostic of an ST elevation MI (STEMI), indicating damage through the entire wall of the ventricle. The leads that are abnormal indicate the area of cardiac injury. "Q waves" develop over 12 to 16 hours and indicate an older cardiac injury.

EKG Leads	Ischemic Area of Heart
V1 through V6	Anterior or anterolateral
Leads I and aVL	Lateral
Leads II, III, and AVF	Inferior
No cardiac changes	No ischemia or non-STEMI

AVF, augmented voltage foot.

Diagnostic testing reveals the following:

- EKG, troponins, creatinine kinase isoenzyme MB (CK-MB), complete blood count (CBC), renal and liver studies are normal.
- Echocardiogram reveals no abnormalities.

CLINICAL DECISION MAKING

Case Study Analysis

A 70-year-old female, after eating a fatty, spicy meal, wakes up at 3 a.m. with substernal chest pain associated with burning in the chest that was relieved on sitting up and also on taking antacids. Her pertinent negatives are the absence of exertional chest pain, dyspnea, and lower extremity edema. She started taking a new medication, Procardia, which can cause relaxation of the lower esophageal sphincter, leading to acid reflux and esophageal spasm. Her differential diagnosis includes atypical chest pain, cardiac ischemia, or gastric acid reflux. Her cardiac enzymes, EKG, and echocardiogram are normal.

The combination of high-fat content meal, and pain relieved when sitting up and after taking an antacid all indicate acute onset or exacerbation of GERD. In addition, the adverse effect of Procardia may have precipitated the episode.

The advanced practice provider provides teaching about the need to avoid foods with a high-fat content and that are spicy. The patient should also sit upright for at least 60 minutes after eating, avoid eating for several hours before going to sleep, and limit the intake of alcohol and caffeine. Should the symptoms continue, the cardiologist should be notified of the patient's adverse effect to determine if a medication change would be indicated.

Diagnosis: *Likely side effect of new medication Procardia, which can cause relaxation of the lower esophageal sphincter, leading to acid reflux and esophageal spasm*

CONFUSION

Case Presentation: *An 85-year-old woman presents to the acute care office with new onset of confusion. She lives by herself; her husband died 2 years ago. Her two children check on her weekly. She was found five blocks from her house wandering around not knowing where she was. She has been brought in by her daughter.*

INTRODUCTION TO COMPLAINT

- Disturbed orientation in regard to time, place, or person, sometimes accompanied by disordered consciousness
- Confusion may result from drug side effects or from a relatively sudden brain dysfunction
- Acute confusion is often called delirium (or "acute confusional state"), although delirium often includes a much broader array of disorders than simple confusion
- These disorders include the inability to focus attention; various impairments in awareness; and temporal or spatial disorientation.
- Mental confusion can also result from chronic organic brain pathologies, such as dementia, as well

HISTORY OF COMPLAINT

Symptomatology

Ask about the following characteristics of each symptom using open-ended questions:

- Onset (sudden or gradual)
- Chronology
- Current situation (improving or deteriorating)
- Location
- Radiation
- Quality
- Timing (frequency, duration)
- Severity
- Precipitating and aggravating factors
- Relieving factors
- Associated symptoms
- Effects on daily activities
- Previous diagnosis of similar episodes
- Previous treatments
- Efficacy of previous treatments

Directed Questions to Ask

- When did the confusion start?
- Have you had any fevers?
- Have you had any shortness of breath (SOB)?
- Have you had any nausea and vomiting (N/V)?
- Have you noticed any fatigue?
- Have you noticed a change in appetite?
- What medications have changed?
- Any stressful events?
- Any change in environment?
- Have you had any trauma to your head?
- Have you been in a recent accident?
- Have you noticed any headaches?
- Are you diabetic?

Assessment: Cardinal Signs and Symptoms

- Mental
  - Disoriented
  - Confused
- Possible signs of infection if that is the source, such as fever, cough, SOB, painful urination or malaise

Medical History: General

- CABG X 2 in 2001
- Hypertension (HTN)
- No known allergies
- Current medications:
  - Metoprolol 50 mg PO BID for HTN
  - Soma 250 mg PO TID for back pain

Medical History: Specific to Complaint

- Confusion

PHYSICAL EXAMINATION

Vital Signs

- Temperature
- Heart rate (HR)
- Respiration
- Oxygen saturation (SpO_2)
- Blood pressure (BP)

General Appearance

- State of health, color, appearance of comfort or distress

Neurologic Exam

- Alert and oriented, National Institutes of Health (NIH) stroke exam, ability to follow commands and characteristics of speech

Heart

- Measure pulses, HR, rhythm, heart sounds, swelling

Lungs
- Appearance of SOB, lung sounds in all fields, percussion of lung fields

CASE STUDY
History

Directed Question	Response
When did the confusion start?	*In the past 2 days (per daughter).*
Have you had any fevers?	*No, I don't know of any fevers.*
Have you had any shortness of breath?	*No.*
Have you had any nausea or vomiting?	*No.*
Have you noticed any fatigue?	*I have some tiredness from the new medication.*
Have you noticed a change in appetite?	*No.*
What medications have changed?	*I take Soma for back pain.*
Any stressful events?	*No.*
Any change in environment?	*No.*
Have you had any trauma to your head?	*No.*
Have you been in a recent accident?	*No.*
Have you noticed any headaches?	*No.*
Are you diabetic?	*Not that I'm aware of.*

Physical Examination Findings
- VITAL SIGNS: temperature 98.2°F; respiratory rate (RR) 15; heart rate (HR) 65; BP 134/74; SpO$_2$ 96% on room air
- GENERAL APPEARANCE: slightly disheveled (hair not recently combed and clothes not matching but clean), tired looking
- NEUROLOGIC EXAM: oriented to self but not time, place, or situation; NIH stroke scale of 0; able to follow commands and speech is clear
- HEAD: no head trauma noted, skin intact, no bumps, lacerations or bruising noted
- NECK: supple, nontender, no carotid bruit, no jugular venous distention
- RESPIRATORY: clear throughout all lung fields
- CARDIOVASCULAR: normal rate, regular rhythm, no murmur, rubs, or gallops +1 pitting edema lower ext
- GASTROINTESTINAL: soft, nontender, nondistended, normal bowel sounds
- GENITOURINARY: no costovertebral angle tenderness
- MUSCULOSKELETAL: normal range of motion, normal strength
- INTEGUMENTARY: warm, dry
- COGNITION AND SPEECH: speech clear, but she is slow to respond
- PSYCHIATRIC: cooperative, appropriate mood and affect

DIFFERENTIAL DIAGNOSIS

Clinincal Observations	Low Glucose	Delirium (Medication Induced)	Delirium (Infection Induced)	Thyroid
Onset	Abrupt	Abrupt	Abrupt	Gradual
Fever	No	No	Yes	No
SOB	No	No	Yes	No
Cough	No	No	Yes	No
Fatigue	No	Possible	Yes	Yes
Memory loss	Gradual	Abrupt	Abrupt	Gradual
Leveled WBC	No	No	Yes	No
Positive urine culture	No	No	Yes, possible	No
Low GBS	Yes	No	No	No
TSH level	Normal	Normal	Normal	Abnormal

GBS, Guillain–Barré syndrome; SOB, shortness of breath; TSH, thyroid-stimulating hormone; WBC, white blood cell.

DIAGNOSTIC EXAMINATION

Exam	Code	Cost	Results
Glucose fasting	R73.01	$1	The normal range for a fasting glucose is 60–99 mg/dl. According the 2003 ADA criteria, diabetes is diagnosed with a *fasting* plasma glucose of 126 mg/dL or more. A precursor, IFG, is defined as reading of fasting glucose levels of 100–125 mg/dL. Sometimes a glucose tolerance test, which involves giving you a sugary drink followed by several blood glucose tests, is necessary to properly sort out normal from IFG from diabetes. In addition, the glycohemoglobin (see the following) may now be used to diagnose diabetes. Be aware that variations in lab normals exist. Also, Europeans tend to use a 2-hour after eating definition of diabetes rather than a fasting glucose. Using the European standards tends to increase the number of people who are classified as having diabetes.
Thyroid hormones; thyroid-related tests	R94.6	$39	There are two types of thyroid hormones easily measurable in the blood, thyroxine (T4) and triiodothyronine (T3). For technical reasons, it is easier and less expensive to measure the T4 level, so T3 is usually not measured on screening tests. Additionally, most diseases impact both T4 and T3 similarly, so T4 is typically measured first.

(*continued*)

Exam	Code	Cost	Results
			Please be clear on which test you are looking at. We continue to see a tremendous amount of confusion among doctors, nurses, laboratory technicians, and patients on which test is which. In particular, the "total T3", "free T3," and "T3 uptake tests" are very confusing, and are not the same test.
	R94.6	$45	**Thyroxine (TT4).** This shows the total amount of T4. The total T4 consists of two Portions: T4, which is bound to carrier proteins and is inactive, and "free" or unbound T4 that is available to cells and therefore active. High levels may be due to hyperthyroidism; however, technical artifact occurs when the bound/inactive T4 is increased. This can occur when estrogen levels are higher from pregnancy, birth control pills, or estrogen replacement therapy. An FT4 (see the following) can avoid this interference.
	R94.6		**FT4.** This test directly measures the free T4 in the blood rather than estimating it like the FTI. Because it is a more reliable test than the TT4, many labs such as ours do the FT4 routinely rather than the TT4. High levels suggest hyperthyroidism, and low levels are found in hypothyroidism and chronic illness.
	R94.6		**TT3.** This is usually not ordered as a screening test, but rather when thyroid disease is being evaluated. T3 is the more potent and shorter lived version of thyroid hormone. Some people with high thyroid levels secrete more T3 than T4. In these (overactive) hyperthyroid cases the T4 can be normal, the T3 high, and the TSH low. The TT3 reports the total amount of T3 in the bloodstream, including T3 bound to carrier proteins plus freely circulating T3.
	S23.122		**FT3.** This test measures only the portion of thyroid hormone T3 that is "free," that is, not bound to carrier proteins.
	S84479		**Thyroid uptake (T3RU).** This is a test that confuses doctors, nurses, and patients. First, this is not a specific thyroid test, but a test on the proteins that carry thyroid hormone around in your bloodstream. Not only that, a high test number may indicate a low level of the protein! The method of reporting varies from lab to lab. The proper use of the test is to compute the FTI.
	S22.069A		**FTI or T7.** A mathematical computation allows the estimation of the FTI from the T4 and T3 uptake tests. The results reveal how much thyroid hormone is free in the bloodstream. In contrast to the TT4 alone, it is less affected by estrogen levels. While this test is less commonly ordered, it is still of use in special situations, such as pregnancy.
	R94.6		**TSH.** This protein hormone is secreted by the pituitary gland and regulates the thyroid gland. A high level suggests your thyroid is underactive, and a low level suggests your thyroid is overactive. This test can vary by time of day, so a single abnormal measurement does not always mean there is a problem. Also, levels tend to be higher in older people, so it is not uncommon to see mild elevations in people in their 70s or 80s, which do not necessarily indicate a medical problem.

(*continued*)

Exam	Code	Cost	Results
CBC	R68.89	$33	**WBC** count is the number of white cells. High WBC count can be a sign of infection. WBC is also increased in certain types of leukemia. Low white counts can be a sign of bone marrow diseases or an enlarged spleen. Low WBC is also found in HIV infection in some cases. **Hgb and Hct.** The hemoglobin is the amount of oxygen carrying protein contained within the RBCs. The hematocrit is the percentage of the blood volume occupied by RBCs. In most labs the Hgb is actually measured, while the Hct is computed using the RBC measurement and the MCV measurement. Thus purists prefer to use the Hgb measurement as more reliable. Low Hgb or Hct suggests an anemia. Anemia can be due to nutritional deficiencies, blood loss, destruction of blood cells internally, or failure to produce blood in the bone marrow. High Hgb can occur due to lung disease, living at high altitude, or excessive bone marrow production of blood cells. **MCV.** This helps diagnose a cause of an anemia. Low values suggest iron deficiency, high values suggest either deficiencies of B_{12} or folate, ineffective production in the bone marrow, or recent blood loss with replacement by newer (and larger) cells from the bone marrow. **PLT.** This is the number of cells that plug up holes in your blood vessels and prevent bleeding. High values can occur with bleeding, cigarette smoking or excess production by the bone marrow. Low values can occur from premature destruction states such as ITP, acute blood loss, drug effects (such as heparin), infections with sepsis, entrapment of platelets in an enlarged spleen, or bone marrow failure from diseases such as myelofibrosis or leukemia. Low platelets also can occur from clumping of the platelets in a lavender colored tube. You may need to repeat the test with a green top tube in that case.
Sputum culture	R09.3	$47.52	A normal Gram stain of sputum contains polymorphonuclear leukocytes, alveolar macrophages, and a few squamous epithelial cells. The presence of normal flora does not rule out infection. Examination of a Gram-stained smear of the specimen frequently reveals whether the specimen is satisfactory or not. The quality of sputum samples is determined by the minimum number of squamous epithelial cells and polymorphonuclear leukocytes per low power field. An acceptable specimen has more than 25 leukocytes and fewer than 10 epithelial cells per low power field. An unacceptable sample can be misleading and should be rejected by the laboratory. Culture of the sputum on blood agar frequently reveals characteristic colonies, and identification is made by various serologic or biochemical tests. Cultures of *Mycoplasma* are infrequently done; diagnosis is usually confirmed by a rise in antibody titer. If Legionella pneumonia is suspected, the organism can be cultured on charcoal-yeast agar, which contains the high concentrations of iron and sulfur required for growth.

(continued)

Exam	Code	Cost	Results
			If tuberculosis is suspected, an acid-fast stain should be performed immediately, and the sputum cultured on special media, which are incubated for at least 6 weeks.
			In diagnosing aspiration pneumonia and lung abscesses, anaerobic cultures are important.
Urine culture	R82.7	$29	Urine tests are typically evaluated with a reagent strip that is briefly dipped into your urine sample. The technician reads the colors of each test and compares them with a reference chart. These tests are semiquantitative; there can be some variation from one sample to another on how the tests are scored.
			pH. This is a measure of acidity for urine.
			SG. This measures how diluted urine is. Water would have a SG of 1.000. Most urine is around 1.010, but it can vary greatly depending on fluids last taken.
			Glucose. Normally there is no glucose in urine. A positive glucose occurs in diabetes.
			Protein. Normally there is no protein detectable on a urinalysis strip. Protein can indicate kidney damage, blood in the urine, or an infection. Up to 10% of children can have protein in their urine.
			Blood. Normally there is no blood in the urine. Blood can indicate an infection, kidney stones, trauma, or bleeding from a bladder or kidney tumor.
			Bilirubin. Normally there is no bilirubin or urobilinogen in the urine. These are pigments that are cleared by the liver. In liver or gallbladder disease they may appear in the urine as well.
			Nitrate. Normally negative, this usually indicates a urinary tract infection.
			Leukocyte esterase. Normally negative. Leukocytes are a type of WBCs (or pus cells). This looks for WBCs by reacting with an enzyme in the white cells. WBCs in the urine suggest a urinary tract infection.
			Sediment. Items such as mucous and squamous cells are commonly seen. Abnormal findings would include more than 0–2 RBCs, more than 0–2 WBCs, crystals, casts, renal tubular cells, yeast, or bacteria. (Bacteria can be present if there was contamination at the time of collection.) Squamous cells may indicate contamination by skin cells if the specimen was not collected carefully.

ADA, American Diabetes Association; CBC, complete blood count; FTI, free thyroxine index; FT3, free T3; FT4, free T4; GBS, Guillain–Barré syndrome; Hct, hematocrit; Hgb, hemoglobin; IFG, impaired fasting glucose; ITP, immune thrombocytopenia; MCV, mean corpuscular volume; PLT, platelet count; RBC, red blood cell; SG, specific gravity; T3RU, T3 resin uptake; TT3, total T3; TT4, total T4; WBC, white blood cell.

CLINICAL DECISION MAKING

Case Study Analysis

The exam of the patient showed fatigue, memory loss, and confusion, but was negative for SOB, fever, and cough. Onset of symptoms was abrupt. Urine was negative for leukocytes. Complete blood count and sputum culture were normal. There is no history of diabetes thus testing for this health problem was deferred. It is unlikely that the acute onset of delirium is due to an undiagnosed infection or other disease process.

> **Diagnosis:** *Delirium due to medication*

The advanced practice provider will notify the primary care provider of the patient's onset of symptoms as being related to the medication prescribed for back pain. Will recommend discontinuing the prescribed medication and suggest conservative treatment to include physical therapy and the application of heat to the area.

The patient should not be left alone and this will be discussed with the daughter. Depending upon the half-life and clearance of the medication, the patient's mentation should improve in a few days. The patient should make an appointment to see the primary care physician to discuss the findings from this examination and the recommended approach for further treatment of the back pain.

COUGH

Case Presentation: A 75-year-old female with chronic obstructive pulmonary disease (COPD) presents to the clinic with a cough she has had for the past 2 weeks.

INTRODUCTION TO COMPLAINT

A cough is the body's natural response to stimuli that irritate the larynx, trachea, and large bronchi. It can be caused by a problem in the upper and lower airways, disruptions in the cardiovascular system, and side effects from certain medications. It is the fifth most common symptom prompting physician visits.

Acute Cough

Cough that lasts less than 3 weeks.

- Viral rhinosinusitis
- Viral bronchitis
- Postnasal drip due to allergy or sinus disease
- COPD or asthma exacerbation
- Pneumonia

Chronic Cough

Cough that lasts longer than 8 weeks.

- Chronic bronchitis
- Postnasal drip
- Airway hyperresponsiveness after resolution of a viral or bacterial respiratory infection (i.e., postinfection cough)
- Asthma
- Medications, especially angiotensin converting enzyme (ACE) inhibitors
- Gastroesophageal reflux disease

Red Flags
The following findings are of particular concern:

- Dyspnea
- Hemoptysis
- Weight loss
- Risk factors for tuberculosis (TB) or HIV infection
- Wheezing
- Fever, night sweats, and weight loss

Allergies

- Dust
- Smoke
- Pollen or mold
- Pets
- Plants
- Cleaning agents and room deodorizers
- Chemical fumes

Medicines

- ACE chronic cough

Other Causes

- Compression in air passage from a tumor
- Enlarged peribronchial lymph nodes
- Impacted cerumen or a foreign body in the external auditory canal triggers reflex cough through stimulation of the auricular branch of the vagus nerve
- Pulmonary embolism

HISTORY OF COMPLAINT

Symptomatology

Ask about the following characteristics of each symptom using open-ended questions:

- Current situation (improving or deteriorating)
- Onset (acute or gradual)
- Characteristics of the cough (i.e., whether dry or producing sputum or blood)
- Associated symptoms
- Aggravating factors or triggers
- Alleviating factors
- Effect on daily activities

Directed Questions to Ask

- What time does the cough occur (i.e., primarily at night)?
- Do you have any shortness of breath?
- Do you have difficulty swallowing?
- Do you have pain with swallowing?
- Do you have a sore throat?
- Do you have heartburn?
- Do you have the need to clear your throat frequently? Postnasal drainage?
- Is it worse at night when lying down?
- Are there any precipitating factors (i.e., cold air, strong odors)?
- Do you experience any pain with your cough? When and where is the pain?
- Are you coughing up phlegm?
- Is the cough dry, brassy, or high pitched and unproductive?
- Are you wheezing (making a whistling sound when you breathe)?
- Are you feeling feverish? Have you taken your temperature?
- Are you losing weight without trying?

- Are you having drenching sweats in bed at night? (the sheets and your pajamas get soaking wet)
- Does anything relieve your cough?
- Does anything trigger your cough, such as running, talking, or laughing?
- Are there any other associated symptoms?
- How does the cough affect your daily activities?
- Have you had a previous diagnosis of similar episodes?
- Have you had previous treatments for your cough?
- What medications do you take?
- Do you have a history of allergies?
- Do you smoke? If so, how many packs per year?
- Do you drink alcohol?
- Do you have family members who have a cough now or in the past?

Assessment: Cardinal Signs and Symptoms

In addition to the general characteristics outlined previously, additional characteristics of specific symptoms should be elicited.

General
- Fever
- Chills
- Sweats
- Malaise
- Weight loss

Eyes
- Itching, watery

Ears
- Pain
- Drainage
- Hearing loss

Nose/Oropharynx
- Cobblestone appearance (postnasal drainage)
- Runny nose

Sinuses
- Palpate
- Percuss
- Transilluminate

Mouth/Throat/Pharynx
- Pale
- Boggy
- Swollen
- Difficulty swallowing
- Choking episodes while eating or drinking (aspiration)
- Sore throat (upper respiratory infection [URI], postnasal drip)

Neck
- Pain
- Swelling
- Enlarged lymph nodes

Trachea/Larynx
- Inspiratory strider

Lungs
- Hyperresonant on percussion
- Distant breath sounds, scattered rhonchi, or wheezing on auscultation
- Prolonged expiration
- Bilateral expiratory wheezes
- Unilateral wheezing
- Basilar rales
- Crackles
- Rales
- Pleuritic chest pain

Cardiovascular
- Edema or weight loss (tumor, TB)
- Tachycardia
- Gallop

Gastrointestinal
- Heartburn (gastroesophageal reflux disease)

Skin
- Color
- Temperature
- Turgor
- Capillary refill response

Other Associated Symptoms
- Night sweats
- Fever
- Chills

Medical History: General

- History of allergies
- Smoking history
- Drug history (should specifically include use of ACE inhibitors)
- Past surgical history
- Past medical history

Medical History: Specific to Complaint

- Recent respiratory infections (i.e., within previous 1–2 months)
- Asthma
- COPD
- Gastroesophageal reflux disease
- Exposure to TB
- HIV infection
- Exposure to potential respiratory irritants
- Exposure to known allergens
- Travel to regions with endemic fungal illnesses

PHYSICAL EXAMINATION

Note: If the patient is coughing during the examination, document character and frequency.

Vital Signs

- Respiration
- Temperature
- Pulse
- Oxygen saturation (SpO_2)
- Blood pressure (BP)

General Appearance

- Apparent state of health
- Appearance of comfort or distress
- Skin color
- Nutritional status
- State of hydration
- Hygiene
- Match between appearance and stated age
- Difficulty with gait or balance
- Signs of respiratory distress
- Chronic illness (i.e., wasting, lethargy)

Inspection

Nose and Throat

- Focus on appearance of the nasal mucosa (i.e., color, congestion)
- Presence of discharge (external or in posterior pharynx)
- Drainage, redness, and edema
- Illuminate sinuses
- Swollen tonsils
- Exudate on tonsils

Ears

- Exam for triggers of reflex cough

Neck

- Symmetry
- Swelling
- Masses
- Active range of motion
- Thyroid enlargement
- Swallowing
- Tracheal deviation
- Cervical and supraclavicular areas inspected and palpated for lymphadenopathy

Respiratory

- Adequacy of air entry and exit
- Symmetry of breath sounds
- Presence of crackles, wheezes, or both
- Signs of consolidation (e.g., egophony, dullness to percussion)

Cardiovascular
- Pulse strength
- Murmurs
- S1 S2
- S3 S4, gallop, pericardial effusion, muffled heart tones

CASE STUDY
History

Directed Question	Response
When did the symptoms start?	*They started about 2 weeks ago.*
Did the cough start suddenly or was it gradual over time?	*I did not pay much attention to it. My husband noticed.*
What time does the cough occur (i.e., primarily at night)?	*Worse at night.*
Do you have any shortness of breath?	*Yes, I feel short of breath.*
Do you have difficulty swallowing?	*No.*
Do you have pain with swallowing?	*No.*
Do you have a sore throat?	*No.*
Do you have heartburn?	*No.*
Do you have the need to clear your throat frequently?	*No.*
Is it worse at night when lying down?	*No.*
Are there any precipitating factors (i.e., cold air, strong odors)?	*No.*
Are you coughing up anything?	*Yes, yellow-green stuff.*
Do you experience any pain with your cough?	*No.*
Are you wheezing (making a whistling sound when you breathe)?	*No.*
Are you running a temperature?	*Yes, I didn't take it, I just feel hot.*
Are you having drenching sweats in bed at night? (the sheets and your pajamas get soaking wet)	*Yes, for the past 3 days.*
Does anything relieve your cough?	*Cough drops, but they don't help.*
Are there any other associated symptoms?	*I feel very weak and tired.*
How does the cough affect your daily activities?	*Yes, I just can't do much.*

Directed Question	Response
Have you had a previous diagnosis of similar episodes?	*No.*
Have you had previous treatments for your cough?	*Just the cough drops.*
What medications do you take?	*A water pill for blood pressure.*
Do you have a history of allergies?	*No, I never had allergies.*
Do you smoke? If so, how many packs per year?	*No I do not. My husband smokes outside of the house.*
Do you drink alcohol?	*Socially, a glass of wine occasionally.*
Do you have family members who have a cough now or in the past?	*No.*

Physical Examination Findings

- VITAL SIGNS: temperature 102°F; respiratory rate (RR) 30; heart rate (HR) 120; BP 120/88; O_2Sat 92
- GENERAL APPEARANCE: patient appears tired; skin color pale, patient diaphoretic and sweaty, short stature, and overweight; height 5'4"; weight 170 lb
- EARS: no drainage, no tenderness
- EYES: no drainage; pupils equal, round, and reactive to light and accommodation (PERRLA)
- NOSE: clear nasal discharge, turbinates clear, nares clear, nasal sinuses clear, no septum deviation, mucus pink not boggy, and no tenderness
- MOUTH: no oral lesions; membranes dry; teeth and gums in good repair
- PHARYNX: posterior pharynx without redness or postnasal drip; tonsils absent
- NECK: no lymphadenopathy in any nodes; no other cervical nodes palpable; neck is supple; thyroid is not enlarged
- CHEST: lung crackles left lower base without wheezes or rhonchi; do not clear with coughing; dullness to percussion over the left lower lobe (LLL); RR is 30, shallow, no use of accessory muscles
- ABDOMEN: soft, round, nontender; no organomegaly or masses
- SKIN: skin color pale, warm, and moist; no rashes
- EXTREMITIES: no clubbing, cyanosis, or edema

DIFFERENTIAL DIAGNOSIS

Clinical Observations	Sore Throat	Fever	Productive Cough	Dyspnea	Headache	Chest Pain	Weight Loss	Hemoptysis	Dry Cough	Night Sweat
URI (including acute bronchitis)	Yes	Low	Yes/No	Mild	Yes/No	No	No	No	Yes	No
Pneumonia (viral, bacterial, aspiration, rarely fungal)	Rare	Yes, high	Yes/No	Yes	Yes/No	Yes/No	No	Yes/No	Yes/No	Yes
Postnasal drip (allergic, bacterial origin)	Yes, scratchy	No	No	No	Yes/No	No	No	No	Yes	No
COPD exacerbation	No	No	Yes/No	Yes	No	No	No	No	Yes/No	No
PE	No	No	Yes/No	Yes, severe	No	Yes, with deep breath	No	Occasional	Yes	No
Asthma	No	No	No	Yes	No	No	No	No	Yes	No
ACE inhibitors	No	No	No	No	No	No	No	No	Yes	No
Tumor	No	Yes/No	Yes/No	No	No	Yes/No	No	Yes/No	Yes	Yes/No
TB or fungal infections	No	Yes	No	No	No	No	Yes	Yes	No	Yes/No

ACE, angiotensin converting enzyme; COPD, chronic obstructive pulmonary disease; PE, pulmonary embolism; TB, tuberculosis; URI, upper respiratory infection.

DIAGNOSTIC EXAMINATION

Exam	Code	Cost	Results
Chest radiography (x-ray)	71020	$300	<ul><li>Shows heart, lungs, airway, blood vessels, and lymph nodes</li><li>Bones of spine and chest, including breastbone, ribs, collarbone, and the upper part of spine</li><li>The most common imaging test or x-ray used to find pathology</li></ul>
CT scan thorax with contrast (testing to be performed only if positive chest x-ray and high suspicion for PE or lung cancer)	71260	$1,400	Cross-sectional images of a part of the body are formed through computerized axial tomography and shown on a computer screen
CBC	85025	$75	The CBC test typically has several parameters. These are the most relevant: WBC<ul><li>High WBC count can be a sign of infection</li><li>WBC can be increased in certain types of leukemia</li><li>Decreased WBCs can be a sign of bone marrow diseases or an enlarged spleen or HIV</li></ul>Hgb and Hct<ul><li>Hgb is the amount of oxygen-carrying protein contained within the RBCs</li><li>Hct is the percentage of the blood volume occupied by RBCs</li><li>Low Hgb or Hct suggests an anemia</li><li>High Hgb can occur due to lung disease, living at high altitudes, or excessive bone marrow production of blood cells</li></ul>MCV<ul><li>This helps diagnose a cause of anemia; low values suggest iron deficiency; high values suggest deficiencies of either vitamin B_{12} or folate, ineffective production in the bone marrow, or recent blood loss with replacement by newer (and larger) cells from the bone marrow</li></ul>Platelet count<ul><li>High values can occur with bleeding, cigarette smoking; low values can occur from premature destruction or excess production by the bone marrow</li><li>States such as immune thrombocytopenia, acute blood loss, drug effects (such as heparin), infections with sepsis, entrapment of platelets in an enlarged spleen, or bone marrow failure from diseases such as myelofibrosis or leukemia</li></ul>

(*continued*)

Exam	Code	Cost	Results
TB skin test (testing to be performed only if high suspicion for TB)	86580	$20	The TB skin test is used to determine whether someone has developed an immune response to the bacterium that causes TB; this response can occur if someone currently has TB, if he or she was exposed to it in the past, or if he or she received the BCG vaccine against TB Negative: Induration of <2 mm Positive: Induration >15 mm normal immune system, >10 mm induration health care worker or personal contact of someone with active TB, >5 mm induration immunocompromised
D-dimer (testing to be performed only if there is high suspicion for PE)	85379	$80	A normal or negative D-dimer result means that it is most likely that the person tested does not have an acute condition or disease that is causing abnormal clot formation and breakdown A positive D-dimer result may indicate the presence of an abnormally high level of fibrin degradation products. It tells the doctor that there may be significant blood clot (thrombus) formation and breakdown in the body
EKG (testing to be performed only if high suspicion of cough related to cardiac causes, such as CHF)	93000	$800	An EKG is used to measure: • Any damage to the heart • How fast your heart is beating and whether it is beating normally • The effects of drugs or devices used to control the heart (such as a pacemaker) • The size and position of your heart chambers • Normal heart rate: 60 to 100 beats per minute • Heart rhythm: consistent and even Abnormal EKG results may be a sign of: • Abnormal heart rhythms (arrhythmias) • Damage or changes to the heart muscle • Changes in the amount of sodium or potassium in the blood • Congenital heart defect • Enlargement of the heart • Fluid or swelling in the sac around the heart • Inflammation of the heart (myocarditis) • Past or current heart attack
Pulse oximetry	94760	$15	Oximetry measures the concentration of oxygen in the blood; the test is used for the evaluation of various medical conditions that affect the function of the heart and lungs Normal results: between 95% and 100% at room temperature Low normal: 90%–95% at room temperature Abnormal results: below 90% at room temperature

(*continued*)

Exam	Code	Cost	Results
Bronchoscopy (testing to be performed only if high suspicion for lung cancer)	31622	$800	Bronchoscopy is a procedure that allows the doctor to look at the patient's airway through a thin viewing instrument called a bronchoscope
			Bronchoscopy may be done either to diagnose problems with the airway, the lungs, or the lymph nodes in the chest or to treat problems such as an object or growth in the airway

BCG, bacillus Calmette-Guerin; CBC, complete blood count; CHF, congestive heart failure; Hct, hematocrit; Hgb, hemoglobin; HR, heart rate; MCV, mean corpuscular volume; PE, pulmonary embolism; RBC, red blood cell; TB, tuberculosis; WBC, white blood cell.

CLINICAL DECISION MAKING

Case Study Analysis

The patient's symptoms of a rapid heart and respiratory rate in addition to a fever indicated a chest x-ray. Radiologic examination confirmed that the patient has left lower lobe pneumonia. The patient also has a white blood cell count of 20,000/mm^3, which supports the diagnosis of bacterial pneumonia. Additional assessment findings included no hemoptysis, no change in weight, and no evidence of sinus pain, nasal discharge, or wheezing or rhonchi upon chest auscultation.

Treatment should include antibiotics and a mucolytic agent. The patient should schedule an appointment with the primary care provider or return for a follow-up examination in 2 weeks. Depending upon the antibiotic prescribed, the patient should be instructed to complete the entire course of the medication, ensure an adequate intake of oral fluids, obtain adequate rest, and engage in respiratory hygiene when coughing and expectorating. The patient should also be encouraged to seek medical attention if the symptoms worsen or continue beyond the course of prescribed antibiotics. Should this occur, further testing may include sputum culture, sputum culture and sensitivity (C&S), Mantoux test, and possible bronchoscopy.

Diagnosis: Left lower lobe pneumonia

COUGHING UP BLOOD

> *Case Presentation:* *A 38-year-old African American woman presents with hemoptysis.*

INTRODUCTION TO COMPLAINT

- Hemoptysis is the expectoration of blood
  - It can be blood-streaked sputum or gross blood, bright red or rust-colored, from the bronchial arteries or pulmonary arteries
  - Called pseudohemoptysis if blood comes from the upper respiratory tract or gastro-intestinal (GI) tract
- Considered massive hemoptysis if there is >500 mL of blood expectorated in 24 hours or more than 100 mL in 1 hour
  - Requires a prompt response if they also have respiratory distress to protect the airway and manage the blood loss
- Most often blood comes from the bronchial arteries, which have a high systemic pressure but only carry a small portion of the blood volume; the rest of lower respiratory bleeding comes from the pulmonary arteries, which supplies most of the body's blood with oxygen but is a low pressure system
- Many potential causes of hemoptysis exist including infections (pneumonia, tuberculosis, lung abscess), airway diseases (bronchitis, bronchiectasis, neoplasms, airway trauma, fistulas, cystic fibrosis), immune disorders (Goodpasture's syndrome, lupus, granulomatosis), coagulopathic, cocaine-induced, pulmonary vascular disorders (pulmonary embolism, elevated pulmonary capillary pressure, pulmonary aneurysm), and idiopathic
- Bronchitis, lung cancer, and bronchiectasis are the most common causes of hemoptysis in the developed world

HISTORY OF COMPLAINT

Symptomatology

Ask about the following characteristics of each symptom using open-ended questions:

- Onset
- Severity
- Description of emesis
- Timing and duration
- Previous diagnosis of similar episodes
- Associated symptoms
- Precipitating factors
- Previous or current illness

Directed Questions to Ask

- When did you start coughing up blood?
- Is the blood mixed with sputum or phlegm?
- How often are you coughing up blood?
- Is this new or has it happened before?
- Are you having any shortness of breath?
- Are you having fevers, chills, sweats?
- Do you have any rashes, bloody urine, joint pain, or leg swelling?
- What were you doing when this started?
- Were you feeling ill before you started vomiting?
- Are you having pain anywhere?
- Did you take any supplements or illegal drugs recently?
- Any chance you are pregnant?

Assessment: Cardinal Signs and Symptoms

General
- Distress level
- Fever
- Chills
- Fatigue

Head, Eyes, Ears, Nose, Throat (HEENT)
- Vision changes
- Epistaxis
- Pharyngeal injury
- Headache

Cardiovascular
- Chest pain
- Chest tightness
- Hypertension
- Peripheral edema

Respiratory
- Shortness of breath
- Sputum
- Cough
- Hypoxia
- Blood

GI
- Vomiting
- Nausea
- Abdominal pain Genitourinary (GU): hematuria
- Costovertebral (CVA) tenderness

Musculoskeletal
- Joint pain

Skin
- Pale
- Diaphoresis
- Flushed

Medical History

- Medical conditions: denies past medical history
- Surgical history: appendectomy
- Allergies: seasonal
- Medication use: vitamin D, vitamin C, fish oil, magnesium, vitamin E (all one pill daily, unsure of dosages)
- Family history: mother—CVA, father—unsure
- Social history: denies smoking, alcohol, and drug use. Works full time in sedentary job. Has not been to the doctor in a couple of years.
- Psychiatric history: none
- Exercise and diet: patient recently started low-fat diet and exercise program, four times a week doing zumba

PHYSICAL EXAMINATION

Vital Signs

- Temperature
- Pulse
- Blood pressure (BP)
- Oxygen saturation (SpO$_2$)
- Respiration
- Body mass index (BMI)

General Appearance

- Weight
- Orientation
- Level of consciousness

HEENT
- Pupil reactivity
- Visual fields
- Epistaxis
- Oropharyngeal membranes intact
- Dental abscess
- Stridor

Cardiovascular
- Jugular venous distention (JVD)
- Cardiac rate and rhythm
- Carotid bruit
- Peripheral edema
- Capillary refill
- Peripheral pulses

Respiratory
- Lung sounds
- Chest expansion
- Cough
- Sputum
- Respiratory effort
- Hypoxia
- Blood

GI
- Vomiting
- Abdominal pain
- Organomegaly

GU
- CVA tenderness
- Urine characteristics

Musculoskeletal
- Joint swelling
- Tenderness

Skin
- Bruising
- Diaphoresis
- Pallor
- Nail color

CASE STUDY

History

Directed Question	Response
When did you start coughing up blood?	Last night.
Is the blood mixed with sputum or phlegm?	Sometimes I'm coughing up a pink, bubbly sputum.
How often are you coughing up blood?	It's kind of a mix of coughing and vomiting. But I'd say it's happening every 15 or 20 minutes.
Is this new or has it happened before?	It's never happened before.
Are you having any shortness of breath?	Not really.
Are you having fevers, chills, sweating?	No.
Do you have any rashes, bloody urine, joint pain, or leg swelling?	No.
What were you doing when this started?	I did a late night zumba class with my friends. I went home and went to bed. Then I woke up around 4 a.m. and felt really bad and starting coughing up blood.
Were you feeling ill before you started vomiting blood?	No. I was actually feeling really good and worked out. It woke me up when it happened.
Are you having pain anywhere?	My head and my chest.
Did you take any supplements or illegal drugs recently?	Just vitamins. I'm trying to get healthier.
Any chance you are pregnant?	No.

Physical Examination Findings

- VITAL SIGNS: temperature 98.9°F; RR 20; pulse 117; BP 217/120; SpO$_2$ 98% on 15 L non-rebreather; BMI 38
- GENERAL APPEARANCE: patient appears in good spirits; moderate distress, alert and oriented x 4; obese
- HEENT: head atraumatic; pupils equal, round, and reactive to light and accommodation (PERRLA); pupils 3 mm bilaterally; nasal passages clear, pink membranes, mouth bloody, good dentition; trachea midline, no stridor
- CARDIOVASCULAR: tachycardia, regular, no murmurs, gallops, or rubs; radial and dorsalis pedis pulses 3+ bilaterally; capillary refill <2 seconds; pitting edema to bilateral legs, 1+; no JVD or carotid bruit noted
- RESPIRATORY: + bloody sputum, crackles to bilateral lung bases, diminished throughout; + cough, per patient started with emesis; symmetric chest expansion; no increased work of breathing
- GASTROINTESTINAL: bowel sounds positive for all four quadrants, abdomen soft, nontender, rounded; no organomegaly
- GENITOURINARY: CVA nontender to palpation; urine yellow, clear
- SKIN: warm, dry, intact; nail beds pink

DIFFERENTIAL DIAGNOSIS

Clinical Observations	Bronchitis	Lung Cancer	Goodpasture's Syndrome	Hypertensive Crisis
Onset	Gradual, blood after long cough	Gradual	Symptoms gradual, blood sudden	Sudden
Hemoptysis appearance	Thick sputum with bloody streaks	Possible phlegm, rust-colored blood	Bright blood	Bright blood or bloody frothy sputum
BP changes	Possibly elevated, especially if chronic	No	Elevated	Elevated
Weight changes	No	Weight loss	Weight loss	No
Weakness, fatigue	Yes	Yes	Yes	Yes/No
Cough	Yes	Yes	Yes	No
Shortness of breath	Yes	Yes	Yes	Yes/No
Other possible symptoms	Fever, sore throat	Swollen lymph nodes, anorexia	Joint aches and pains, swelling of limbs	Chest pain, headache, vision changes, syncope

BP, blood pressure.

DIAGNOSTIC EXAMINATION

Exam	Code	Cost	Results
Chest x-ray	91.8	$67	A chest x-ray can demonstrate pleural effusions, opacities, masses, and possibly the site of the bleeding. The x-ray can help determine where in the lung the fluid is situated and can rule in or out several conditions, such as lung cancer, pulmonary artery congestion, tuberculosis, pneumonia, and cardiomegaly. A chest x-ray can help determine the course of further testing.
CBC with differential	R68.89	$21	An elevated white blood cell count can indicate infection. Hemoglobin and hematocrit should be evaluated to determine the magnitude and severity of blood loss. Platelet count can be used to exclude thrombocytopenia or coagulation disorders.
Urinalysis	R82.90	$6	A urinalysis allows you to determine if there is kidney dysfunction. Kidney dysfunction could be present in immune disorders, such as Goodpasture's or granulomatosis, or as target organ damage related to a hypertensive emergency. A BMP would show you the creatinine and BUN, but this alone would not demonstrate the damage to the kidney. A urinalysis with protein present would demonstrate this at a cheaper price.
BNP	402.11	$88	BNP is a hormone produced in the cardiac ventricles. The ventricles release BNP in response to stretch on the ventricle walls in an effort to reduce systemic vascular resistance. An elevated BNP indicates heart strain and possible heart failure.
Echocardiogram	R93.1	$547	An echocardiogram allows the practitioner to visualize the heart structure and functionality. It can show blood flow and turbulence to determine ejection fraction, valve insufficiency, stenosis, and muscle wall damage. Due to the cost, this should only be performed if other diagnostic testing indicates cardiac dysfunction and the degree needs to be assessed.

BMP, basic metabolic panel; BNP, brain natriuretic peptide; BUN, blood urea nitrogen; CBC, complete blood count.

CLINICAL DECISION MAKING

Case Study Analysis

The history and physical assessment led to a chest x-ray and blood work. This demonstrated:

- Chest x-ray: bilateral pleural effusions, cardiomegaly, pulmonary artery dilation
- Complete blood count (CBC): white blood cell (WBC) 6.3, Hgb 11.0 gm/dL, Hct 34%, platelets 337,000
- Urinalysis: 1+ proteinuria, otherwise normal
- Brain natriuretic peptide (BNP): 2178
- Echocardiogram: EF 40%–45%, left ventricular hypertrophy, cardiomegaly, elevated pulmonary artery pressures

Diagnosis: *Hypertensive emergency*

The patient has severely elevated blood pressures and evidence of heart damage. Placed on a nitroglycerin drip, titrated up to 100 mcg/min with minimal BP effect. Given 5 mg intravenous push of metoprolol with improvement of heart rate and BP. Oxygen changed to high flow nasal cannula 8 L. Through a chart review it was discovered that the patient had elevated BPs 2 years earlier during a hospital admission for pneumonia but did not follow up with primary care provider (PCP) after discharge. Patient educated on the importance of controlling BPs and discussed echocardiogram results. Patient will be started on oral antihypertensives, including amlodipine and lisinopril and weaned off nitroglycerin. Metoprolol intravenous push prn is prescribed to maintain systolic blood pressure (SBP) <180 mmHg.

Notified PCP with the findings of this current admission and recommendations for follow-up. Appointment scheduled for 1 week postdischarge.

DEPRESSED MOOD

> **Case Presentation:** A retired 73-year-old Caucasian female presents to the acute care practice complaining she has been unable to sleep for the previous 3 months.

INTRODUCTION TO COMPLAINT

The chief complaint of insomnia is nonspecific. Many conditions affect the sleep cycle of the patient. The cause of primary insomnia is unknown; secondary insomnia has a known cause. It is important to assess the patient's nighttime environment and rituals to assess modifiable lifestyle items that may be impairing the patient from falling or staying asleep. Additionally, the provider should assess the pharmacological regimen of the patient. Many medications such as beta-blockers can have an effect on the patient's health and can cause insomnia. Lastly, the patient may be suffering from insomnia due to a secondary disease process. This could include orthopnea secondary to congestive heart failure or restless legs secondary to anemia.

HISTORY OF COMPLAINT

Symptomatology

Ask about the following characteristics of each symptom using open-ended questions:

- Determine timing of the complaint
- Ask patient what events precipitate the situation
- Ask patient what aggravates the symptom and what relieves it
- Ask if the symptom prevents him from doing his daily activities

Directed Questions to Ask

- What time do you go to bed at night?
- Do you eat or drink directly before going to bed?
- Do you bring work to bed with you?
- Do you and your husband share a bed?
- Do you consume alcohol, tobacco, or caffeine in the hours leading up to bedtime?
- Once you are in bed do you try to fall asleep immediately or do you do other activities (reading, prayer, meditation)?
- Are you comfortable in bed?
- How long does it take for you to fall asleep?
- Once you are asleep, do you have trouble staying asleep?
- Do you have to get up during the night?
- What time do you awake in the morning?
- Do you feel rested?

- Do you drink caffeine throughout the day? How much?
- Do you feel sleepy or tired throughout the day?
- Do you nap throughout the day?
- Do you find yourself stressed out?
- What things are causing you stress?
- Are you a caregiver?
- How do you feel about being a caregiver?
- What emotional support do you have?
- How do you cope with your stress?

Assessment: Cardinal Signs and Symptoms

- Fatigue
- Restlessness
- Difficulty falling asleep
- Difficulty staying asleep
- Depressed mood

Medical History

Past Medical History

- Allergies: penicillin
- Medical: hypertension (HTN)
- Surgical: knee replacement at 55 years
- OB: two pregancies, two live births
- Psychological: no previous history
- Current medications: ibuprofen 400 mg as needed, Benadryl 50 mg orally, nightly as needed, hydrochloric thiazide 25 mg orally

Family History

- Unknown
- Patient states parents died of old age

Social History

- Tobacco: patient denies smoking
- Ethanol (ETOH): patient states she consumes the occasional glass of wine with dinner
- Sexual: patient not sexually active with her husband
- Illicit drugs: patient denies
- Diet: patient states she does not follow a specific diet
- Emotional support: patient lives with her husband; children live 8 hours away
- Occupation: secretary; patient states fatigue has affected her work performance
- Health maintenance: patient states she does not participate in exercise
- Socioeconomics: retired; patient cares for husband who has Alzheimer's disease

PHYSICAL EXAMINATION

Vital Signs

- Temperature
- Pulse
- Respiration
- Oxygen saturation (SpO_2)
- Blood pressure (BP)

General Appearance

- Apparent state of health: well-developed, elderly female
- Appearance of comfort or distress: patient tearful, and appears troubled
- Color: no signs of jaundice or hypoxia
- Nutritional status: patient appears to be undernourished
- State of hydration: no signs of dehydration or fluid overload
- Hygiene: patient well kept
- Match between appearance and stated age: pt appears to be her stated age
- Difficulty with gait or balance: no difficulty with gait

Neurologic Assessment

- Alert, oriented, tearful, emotionally distressed, and cooperative
- Thought process coherent
- Romberg: maintains balance with eyes closed
- No pronator drift; gait with normal base
- Good muscle build and tone
- Strength 5/5 throughout
- Rapid alternating movements (RAMs): finger to nose
- Hand flip flop and serial finger opposition intact
- Cranial nerves (CN) II through XII intact
- Deep tendon reflex (DTR): brachioradialis, biceps, triceps, patellar, Achilles all 2+ bilaterally
- Negative Babinski reflex

Mental Assessment

- Patient appears sad and fatigued, speech slowed and words mumbled, does not maintain eye contact, thought process coherent, digital 7s, and calculations accurate, three-item recall and clock drawing negative for demented processes.

Head, Eyes, Ears, Nose, Throat (HEENT)

- No thyroid enlargement
- Neck supple
- No tonsillar enlargement
- Mallampati airway score 2
- Soft pallet low lying

Respiratory

- Chest expansion even
- No cyanosis or pallor
- Lung sounds clear throughout, no crackles, rhonchi, wheezes, or rales
- No cough, productive sputum, or hemoptysis
- Trachea midline

Cardiovascular

- Regular rate and rhythm, +2 radial pulses bilaterally
- Point of maximum impulse (PMI) dime-sized
- Fifth intercostal space
- Midclavicular line
- No murmurs, rubs, or gallops
- S1 and S2 clearly auscultated
- No edema

CASE STUDY
History

Directed Question	Response
What time do you go to bed at night?	9:30 to 10:00.
Do you eat or drink directly before going to bed?	No.
Do you bring work to bed with you?	No.
Do you and your husband share a bed?	Yes.
Do you consume alcohol, tobacco, or caffeine in the hours leading up to bedtime?	No.
Once you are in bed do you try to fall asleep immediately or do you do other activities (reading, prayer, meditation)?	I occasionally read the paper.
Are you comfortable in bed?	Yes.
How long does it take you to fall asleep?	7 to 8 hours.
Once you are asleep, do you have trouble staying asleep?	Yes.
Do you have to get up during the night?	No.
What time do you awake in the morning?	7:30.
Do you feel rested?	No.
Do you drink caffeine throughout the day? How much?	Yes. One cup of coffee with breakfast.
Do you feel sleepy or tired throughout the day?	Yes.
Do you nap throughout the day?	No.
Do you find yourself stressed out?	Yes.
What things are causing you the most stress?	Caring for my husband.
How do you feel about being a caregiver?	I am tired of it, I am very lonely, I am unable to do the things I enjoy anymore.
What emotional support do you have?	I used to gripe to my husband but he doesn't understand and I am unable to visit with my friends like I used to.
How do you cope with your stress?	I don't have time for anything like that.

DIFFERENTIAL DIAGNOSIS

Clinical Observations	Primary Insomnia	GAD	MDD	OSA	Thyroid Disease
Depressed mood	No	No	Yes	No	No
Diminished interests	No	No	Yes	No	No
Weight change	No	No	Yes	No	Yes
Insomnia or hypersomnia	Yes	Yes	Yes	Yes	Yes
Psychomotor agitation	No	No	Yes	No	Yes
Fatigue	Yes	No	Yes	Yes	Yes
Self-guilt	No	Yes	Yes	No	No
Loss of concentration	No	Yes	Yes	No	No
Suicidal thoughts	No	No	Yes	No	No
Restlessness	Yes	Yes	Yes	No	Yes

GAD, generalized anxiety disorder; MDD, major depressive disorder; OSA, obstructive sleep apnea.

DIAGNOSTIC EXAMINATION

Exam	Code	Cost	Results
Beck's Depression Inventory	NA	$83 for manual	A combination of insomnia, psychomotor agitation, and fatigue would trigger a depression screening. 0–13 minimal depression 14–19 mild depression 20–28 moderate depression 29–63 maximum depression Maximum score is 63
TSH	R94.6	$95.68	Thyroid disease especially, hyperthyroidism can present as psychomotor agitation insomnia. 0.34–5.6 milliunits per liter (mU/L), depressed in hyperthyroidism
Serum T4			5–12 mcg/dL, elevated in hyperthyroidism

NA, not applicable; TSH, thyroid-stimulating hormone.

CLINICAL DECISION MAKING

Case Study Analysis

A major depressive disorder (MDD) was diagnosed due to the presence of a depressed mood, diminished interests in activities, insomnia, psychomotor agitation, and self-guilt, all for a period longer than 2 weeks.

The patient's chief complaint of insomnia must be thoroughly investigated. A diagnosis of generalized anxiety disorder (GAD) was not further examined because of the patient's depressed mood. Obstructive sleep apnea (OSA) was not further pursued because the patient did not have an obstructive airway as evidenced by a Mallampati airway score 2. Furthermore, thyroid disease could be ruled out by the thyroid test results.

This leaves primary insomnia and MDD. Even though primary insomnia is a possibility, further investigation revealed extensive social stressors that have the potential to cause MDD and further depression. Beck's depression inventory would confirm this diagnosis.

The patient's need to provide ongoing care to a spouse is significantly contributing to depression. To help this patient, it is recommended to refer to the Agency for Aging within the patient's geographic region. Respite care, home care, and other resources would be helpful to improve this patient's mood and reduce the symptoms. A follow-up in 1 month is suggested to determine actions taken to help with the home situation and reevaluate the patient's level and extent of depression.

Diagnosis: Major depressive disorder

DIARRHEA

Case Presentation: *A 37-year-old European American female presents to your practice with "loose stools."*

INTRODUCTION TO COMPLAINT

Diarrhea is a common manifestation of a number of gastrointestinal (GI) diseases. The definition is based on the frequency, *volume*, and consistency of stools. The patient's perception of the stool and the components of a definition of diarrhea often are variable.

- Acute: lasting less than 14 days in duration
- Persistent: more than 14 days in duration
- Chronic: more than 30 days in duration (chronic diarrhea involves a decrease in stool consistency of more than 1-month duration)

Etiology for Acute Diarrhea

- VIRAL: most common; examples of viruses are norovirus, adenovirus, rotavirus
- BACTERIAL: usually severe but self-limiting; examples of bacteria are *Salmonella, Shigella, Staphylococcus aureus, Clostridium difficile, Campylobacter*
- PROTOZOAL: not usually identified as a cause of diarrhea in the developed world; examples of protozoa are *Giardia lamblia, Cryptosporidium, Entamoeba histolytica*

Etiology for Chronic Diarrhea

- IRRITABLE BOWEL SYNDROME (IBS): defined as a symptom complex of chronic lower abdominal pain; altered bowel habits are the primary characteristic of IBS
- FUNCTIONAL DIARRHEA: defined as continuous or recurrent passage of loose (mushy) or watery stools with abdominal pain or discomfort
- INFLAMMATORY BOWEL DISEASE (IBD): refers primarily to Crohn's disease and ulcerative colitis; Crohn's disease may involve the entire GI tract; ulcerative colitis is often defined as mild, moderate, or severe and often presents in a variable manner with diarrhea as its main symptom
- MICROSCOPIC COLITIS: seen as chronic watery (secretory) diarrhea without bleeding; usually occurs in middle-aged patients but can affect children
- MALABSORPTION SYNDROME: is defined as impaired absorption of nutrients; it occurs as a result of congenital defects in the transport system, acquired defects, such as celiac disease, extensive surgical resection (gastric bypass)
- CHOLECYSTECTOMY: diarrhea occurs in 5% to 12% of patients; it will resolve or improve over the course of weeks to months and is related to excessive bile acids entering the colon

- CHRONIC INFECTIONS: persistent bacterial and protozoal infections can be seen in patients with chronic diarrhea; specific risk factors should be assessed such as travel, HIV infection, use of antibiotics, and consumption of contaminated drinking water

HISTORY OF COMPLAINT

Symptomatology

Ask about the following characteristics of each symptom using open-ended questions:

- Onset (sudden or gradual)
- Chronology
- Current situation (improving or deteriorating)
- Location
- Radiation
- Quality
- Timing (frequency, duration)
- Severity
- Precipitating and aggravating factors
- Relieving factors
- Associated symptoms
- Effects on daily activities
- Previous diagnosis of similar episodes
- Previous treatments
- Efficacy of previous treatments

Directed Questions to Ask

- How long have you had diarrhea?
- How frequently have you had diarrhea?
- Can you describe the color and consistency?
- Any associated symptoms? Fever? Abdominal pain? Nausea/vomiting?
- Where do you live/reside? Facility?
- What is your occupation?
- Any particular hobbies?
- Have you traveled anywhere recently?
- Have you traveled anywhere in the past year?
- What have you eaten in the past 24 hours, past 48 hours?
- Have you been on antibiotics recently?

Assessment: Cardinal Signs and Symptoms

In addition to the general characteristics outlined previously, additional characteristics of specific symptoms should be elicited.

General
- Fever, chills, malaise
- Fatigue
- Night sweats
- Weight, diet

Throat and Mouth
- Hoarseness
- Sore throat

- Ulcers
- Bleeding
- Teeth
- Taste

Gastrointestinal
- Heartburn
- Constipation
- Pain
- Appetite
- Blood
- Flatulence
- Hemorrhoids
- Jaundice
- Normal stool color

Medical History: General

- Medical conditions and surgeries
- Allergies (seasonal and others)
- Medication currently used (prescription, birth control pill [BCP] and over the counter [OTC])
- Herbal preparations and traditional therapies

Medical History: Specific to Complaint

- Risk factor for HIV infection
- Recent weight loss
- Fecal incontinence
- Fevers, joint pains, mouth ulcers, eye redness
- Family history specific to IBD
- Medications

Medical History: Specific to GI System

- Chronic GI disorders
- GI surgeries
- Trauma
- For other specific questions related to chronic diarrhea, see the preceding

PHYSICAL EXAMINATION

Vital Signs

- Temperature
- Pulse
- Respiration
- Oxygen saturation (SpO_2)
- Blood pressure (BP): assess orthostatic
- Weight

General Appearance

- Apparent state of health
- Appearance of comfort or distress
- Color/turgor of skin (check for dehydration caused by severe diarrhea)

Mouth and Throat
- Inspect for any mouth lesions (chronic diarrhea concern regarding IBD)

Eyes
- Inspect for any redness in eyes
- Inspect for exophthalmos and lid retraction

Neck
- Inspect for thyroid enlargement
- Palpate thyroid: size, consistency, contour, position, tenderness

Abdomen
- Inspect for contour, bruits, heaves, previous abdominal scars
- Auscultate for bowel sounds (BS)
- Palpate for masses, pain

Rectum
- Inspect for fissure, fistula
- Palpate for sphincter tone (fecal incontinence), visible or occult blood

CASE STUDY
History

Directed Question	Response
How long have you had "loose stools?"	3 days.
Is it getting better or worse or staying the same?	The same.
How frequently have you had the "loose stools?"	Every 2 to 3 hours.
What does the stool look like?	Semiformed to liquid consistency and brown.
Do you have any associated symptoms? Fever? Abdominal pain? Nausea/vomiting?	No fever, some abdominal cramping especially when I'm having a bowel movement; some nausea. No vomiting.
Where do you live/reside? Facility?	I live at home with my husband and three children.
What is your occupation?	Home day-care provider.
Do you have any particular hobbies?	No particular hobbies.
Have you traveled anywhere recently?	No recent travel.
Have you traveled anywhere in the past year?	Only to the mountains 2 hours away last summer.
What have you eaten in the past 24 hours, past 48 hours?	I have been trying to eat bland foods. Yesterday I had a piece of pizza, which caused an increase in diarrhea and cramping.

Directed Question	Response
Have you regularly ingested any sugar-free foods (foods containing sorbitol)?	*No.*
What recent medications are you taking?	*Only a women's multivitamin and vitamin D from Costco.*

Physical Examination Findings

- VITAL SIGNS: temperature 99°F; respiratory rate (RR) 16; heart rate (HR) 90; BP 110/78; no orthostatic changes noted
- GENERAL APPEARANCE: well-developed female in no acute distress, appears slightly fatigued
- SKIN: good skin turgor noted, moist mucous membranes
- EYES: pupils equal, round, and reactive to light and accommodation (PERRLA), no injection, anicteric
- MOUTH: no oral lesions, teeth and gums in good repair
- NECK: no palpable lymph nodes noted, thyroid not enlarged
- ABDOMEN: positive BS in all four quadrants; no masses; no organomegaly noted; diffuse, mild, bilateral lower quadrant pain noted
- RECTUM: good sphincter tone; stool occult blood negative, no hemorrhoids, fissures noted

DIFFERENTIAL DIAGNOSIS

Clinical Observations	Viral	Bacterial	Protozoal
Duration of symptoms	<2 to 3 days >2 to 3 days	>2 to 3 days	
Frequency	Every 2 to 3 hours	Profuse	Variable
Fever	Low or none	High	Low or none
Abdominal pain, cramping	Mild	Severe	Moderate
Pus in stool	No	Yes	Yes/No
Blood in stool	No	Yes	No
Previous antibiotics	No	Yes	No
Dehydration	Rare	More likely	Rare
Hours of overseas travel	Rare	More common	Common

DIAGNOSTIC EXAMINATION

Exam	Code	Cost	Results
Hemoccult stool for occult blood	82270	$10–$25	Testing for occult (hidden) blood is stool based. The best method for obtaining stool—digital examination of the rectum versus patient-submitted stool—is controversial. **Guaiac-based fecal occult blood test** • Test identifies hemoglobin by the presence of a peroxidase reaction, turns guaiac-impregnated paper blue • A positive test is more likely with more blood in the GI tract • Dietary factors may influence the test results, though a restrictive diet may not be needed • High rate of false positives in healthy populations (80% of positive tests are felt to be false positives) • Positives in diarrhea need to look for causes of GI bleeding, such as infections in acute diarrhea, in chronic diarrhea concerns regarding IBD
Fecal leukocytes	89055	$35	The presence of leukocytes is an indicator of inflammation. Generally, the inflammation is a product of a bacteria–host interaction. Leukocytes are found in stools in the presence of infection with bacteria that invade the colonic mucosa (i.e., *Salmonella, Shigella, Yersinia,* and invasive *Escherichia coli*). Other disorders that may be associated with fecal leukocytes are ulcerative colitis and antibiotic-associated colitis. Fecal leukocytes are usually absent in diarrhea secondary to toxigenic bacteria, parasites, or virus • Meta-analysis of diagnostic test accuracy estimates that for a peak sensitivity of 70% the specificity of fecal leukocytes was only 50% • There have been a number of studies showing variability of test performance • The presence of occult blood and fecal leukocytes supports a diagnosis of bacterial diarrhea in the context of the medical history and other diagnostic evaluations
Stool culture	87045	$70–$294	• Stool cultures are useful in determining a bacterial cause for diarrhea Low rate of positive stool cultures in most reports (2%–5%). Most episodes of diarrhea are self-limiting and the infection clears • Useful after several days of supportive therapy if diarrhea does not resolve. Determining a bacterial cause is useful in patients with severe disease • The following patients should have stool cultures on initial presentation: a. Immunocompromised patients (HIV) b. Patients with comorbidities that increase the risk for complications c. Patients with more severe, inflammatory diarrhea d. Patients with underlying IBD e. Food handlers who may need negative cultures to return to work

(continued)

Exam	Code	Cost	Results
Stool for O and P	870177	$70–$112	• Routine stool cultures identify *Salmonella, Campylobacter,* and *Shigella* • Other organisms need to be specified, such as: *Clostridium difficile, Staphylococcus aureus* • Stool testing for O and P should be done if the patient is at risk for parasitic infection. Multiple stool samples should be collected at different times because shedding of parasites may be intermittent Usually stool is collected at three different intervals or days. • Indications for O and P studies are: 　a. Persistent diarrhea (acute to chronic) 　b. Persistent diarrhea following travel to the developing world 　c. Persistent diarrhea with exposure to infants in day-care centers 　d. Diarrhea in MSM or patients with AIDS 　e. A community waterborne outbreak 　f. Bloody diarrhea with few or no fecal leukocytes

GI, gastrointestinal; IBD, inflammatory bowel disease; MSM, men who have sex with men; O and P, ova and parasites.

CLINICAL DECISION MAKING

Case Study Analysis

The advanced practice provider performs a detailed history and physical examination on the patient and finds the following data: diarrhea for the past 3 days with no fever, mild nausea, and no vomiting. Frequency is every 3 to 4 hours with liquid to soft light brown stools. Pertinent negatives include absence of fever, severe abdominal pain, vomiting, bloody stools, or weight loss, which rules out a bacterial infection. The absence of pus in the stool and no recent travel rules out a protozoan infection. The patient has no chronic health problems and the only risk factor for a persistent diarrhea is that she is a home child care provider. The diagnosis at this time is viral gastroenteritis.

> ***Diagnosis:*** *Acute diarrhea of a viral etiology*

Recommend returning for a follow-up examination in 1 week if cramping and diarrhea do not subside. At that time, a stool culture and sample for ova and parasites should be collected. Depending upon the results, medication may be prescribed. The patient was counseled on the importance of thorough and frequent handwashing considering the patient's occupation. Additionally, the patient was asked to identify any clients who might have the same symptoms. If so, all work surfaces/baby changing areas need to be thoroughly disinfected to prevent a widespread outbreak of the disorder.

DIFFICULTY ACHIEVING BOWEL MOVEMENT

> *Case Presentation:* A 27-year-old male reports to the clinic for a wellness evaluation. During history taking you discover that the patient is only having a bowel movement on average once a week. The patient does not consider that he is constipated, stating "that is normal for me."

INTRODUCTION TO COMPLAINT

- Constipation is defined as less than three bowel movements in a week
- Primary constipation results from altered colon or anorectal function
- Secondary constipation can be the result of organic or systemic disease, or from use of pharmacologic agents
- Functional constipation, also known as "normal transit" constipation, is the most common form of constipation seen by clinicians
- In constipation, patients report symptoms they believe are consistent with constipation such as the presence of hard stools or a perceived difficulty with evacuation
- The Rome III criteria are applied in defining functional constipation

HISTORY OF COMPLAINT

Symptomatology

Ask about the following characteristics of each symptom using open-ended questions:

- Onset (sudden or gradual)
- Chronology
- Current situation (improving or deteriorating)
- Location
- Radiation
- Quality
- Timing (frequency, duration)
- Severity
- Precipitating and aggravating factors
- Relieving factors
- Associated symptoms
- Effects on daily activities
- Previous diagnosis of similar episodes
- Previous treatments
- Efficacy of previous treatments

Directed Questions to Ask

- What has been your pattern of bowel movements over your lifetime?
- What are the characteristics of your bowel movements?
- What is your typical daily dietary intake?
- How much fluid intake do you typically have in a day?
- Are you on any medications? If yes, what are they?
- Do you ever use the assistance of any ingested substance to facilitate a bowel movement?
- If you use the assistance of an ingested substance, what is the substance and your response to it?
- Do you ever use the assistance of a mechanical or positional aid to facilitate a bowel movement?
- If you use a mechanical or positional aid, what do you do and what is your response to it?

Assessment: Cardinal Signs and Symptoms

- Infrequent bowel movements
- Straining to have a bowel movement
- Small and/or hard, dry bowel movement
- Lower abdominal discomfort
- If hard, dry bowel movements may have rectal bleeding and/or anal fissure development

Medical History: General

- Medical conditions and surgeries
- Allergies (seasonal as well as others)
- Medication currently used (prescription and over the counter [OTC])
- Herbal preparations and traditional therapies

Medical History: Specific to Complaint

- Constipation
- Use of laxatives or other ingested substances for facilitating bowel movements
- Dietary lifestyle
- Digestion problems, and/or food intolerances
- Hard, dry stools
- Hemorrhoids
- Rectal bleeding
- Pain with defecation

PHYSICAL EXAMINATION

Vital Signs

- Temperature
- Pulse
- Respiration
- Oxygen saturation (SpO_2)
- Blood pressure (BP)

General Appearance

- Apparent state of health
- Appearance of comfort or distress

- Color
- State of hydration

Neck
- Inspect for symmetry, swelling, masses
- Palpate for tenderness, thyroid enlargement

Abdomen
- Inspect for contour, heaves, masses, scars
- Auscultate for bowel sounds
- Palpate for pain, masses

Rectal
- Inspect for presence of tears, fissures, hemorrhoids
- Palpate for integrity of anal sphincter

CASE STUDY
History

Directed Question	Response
What has been your pattern of bowel movements over your lifetime?	*Oh, I would say I have one to two bowel movements per week.*
What are the characteristics of your bowel movements?	*Sometimes it might be a little hard to get a bowel movement going, but for the most part that really isn't a problem. I don't poop out hard rocks or anything. The poops are large but not overly hard or dry.*
What is your typical daily dietary intake?	*Breakfast might be nothing or maybe a toasted bagel with coffee, lunch is usually a sandwich with chips, and for dinner I have some sort of meat with a vegetable.*
How much fluid intake do you typically have in a day?	*I have a cup of coffee in the morning, maybe a glass of water with lunch, and maybe a glass of water or milk with dinner. I don't really drink between meals.*
Are you on any medications? If yes, what are they?	*I took an anti-depressant medication for a few months but that was about three years ago. I am not on any medications now.*
Do you ever use the assistance of any ingested substance to facilitate a bowel movement?	*Yes.*
If you use the assistance of an ingested substance, what is the substance and your response to it?	*I tried using some probiotics a few times but I wasn't really consistent with it. And I tried taking 250 mg of magnesium taurate at bedtime for a bit but I wasn't really consistent with that either. Best as I can recollect, they didn't really help this problem anyway.*

Directed Question	*Response*
Do you ever use the assistance of a mechanical or positional aid to facilitate a bowel movement	*Yes.*
If you use a mechanical or positional aid, what do you do and what is your response to it?	*I did try a "poop stool" for a while. Not sure I noticed a big difference in my bowel movement frequency by using the stool but I did notice that use of the stool eased the evacuation process.*

PHYSICAL EXAMINATION FINDINGS

- VITAL SIGNS: temperature 98.2°F; respiratory rate (RR) 16; heart rate (HR) 68, regular; BP 122/70; SpO_2 99%
- GENERAL APPEARANCE: well-developed; healthy-appearing male
- NECK: nontender; no masses; no thyromegaly noted
- ABDOMEN: soft, nontender without mass or organomegaly
- RECTAL: no fissure or tear noted; no hemorrhoids noted; anal sphincter tone intact with appropriate response to digital stimulation

DIFFERENTIAL DIAGNOSIS

Clinical Observations	Functional Constipation	Altered Physiologic Function	Organic/Systemic Disease	Medication Induced
Abdominal x-ray	Possible stool noted in colon	Possible stool noted in colon	Possible stool noted in colon	Possible stool noted in colon
Barium enema	Should demonstrate normal findings	May demonstrate abnormal function of colon or rectum	May demonstrate abnormal function of colon or rectum	May demonstrate abnormal function of colon or rectum
Colon transit time	Normal transit time	Will be abnormal in transit disorders	May be normal	May be normal
Defecography	Would likely not be utilized for this condition as transit time has been established to be "normal"	Function of the rectum and anal canal can be evaluated	Function of the rectum and anal canal can be evaluated	Function of the rectum and anal canal can be evaluated

DIAGNOSTIC EXAMINATION

If the constipation is sudden onset, worsening, or associated with a weight loss the following exams can be considered as a part of a workup.

Exam	Code	Cost	Results
TSH	84443	$49	If results indicate hypothyroidism, consider this as a possible etiology of the constipation
Abdominal x-ray	74000, single view 74020, complete series	$280, national average	May reveal the presence of stool in the intestines
Barium enema	74270	$618, national average	May reveal abnormal function of the colon or rectum
Colonic transit study	99070	Varies depending on facility	Allows for the evaluation of transit time of "material" through the intestines
Defecography	74270	Varies by wide range, depending on technique and facility	Allows for evaluation of the shape and function of the rectum during evacuation

TSH, thyroid-stimulating hormone.

CLINICAL DECISION MAKING

Case Study Analysis

The advanced practice provider performs the assessment and physical examination on the patient and finds the following data: no abnormal exam or lab findings.

History reveals that the patient's diet is low in both dietary fiber and fluid intake. The recommended fiber intake is 30 grams per day. The recommended fluid intake is 2 to 3 liters per day. Since the patient falls way below both of these recommendations, the sources of soluble and insoluble fiber were reviewed and he was instructed to ingest 6 to 8 ounces of water for every waking hour to ensure an adequate fluid intake.

Given that the patient reports a trial of taking probiotics and magnesium taurate for increasing the frequency of bowel movement, the APP recommends to the patient that he consider resuming one or both of these. The patient was reminded that it may take a couple weeks to notice an appreciable improvement in bowel frequency with these supplements and to take them consistently to see if a more regular pattern of bowel evacuation occurs. Since use of the "poop stool" did facilitate ease of stool evacuation it is advisable that he use this mechanical tool.

Depending on the success of dietary and fluid changes, the use of supplements, and the "poop stool," the patient may want to make a follow-up examination in 2 months. Should symptoms continue, further testing and interventions may be required to include abdominal x-ray, barium enema, and possibly colon transit time, and defecography.

Diagnosis: *Constipation*

DIFFICULTY SPEAKING

Case Presentation: *A 57-year-old Caucasian male presents with difficulty speaking and trouble forming words.*

INTRODUCTION TO COMPLAINT

- Cardiovascular accident (CVA)
- Medication induced
- Conversion disorders
- Anxiety
- Traumatic brain injury
- Myasthenia gravis
- Amyotrophic lateral sclerosis (ALS)
- Brain tumor
- Dementia
- Multiple sclerosis
- Dystonia
- Huntington's disease
- Alcohol withdrawal
- Illegal drug use
- Parkinson's disease (PD)
- Frontotemporal disorders
- Bell's palsy
- Poor fitting dentures

HISTORY OF COMPLAINT

Symptomatology

Ask about the following characteristics of each symptom using open-ended questions:

- Onset
- Chronology
- Current situation
- Timing
- Severity
- Precipitating and aggravating factors
- Relieving factors
- Associated symptoms
- Effects on daily activities
- Previous diagnosis of similar episodes
- Previous treatments

Directed Questions to Ask

- When did the speaking difficulty begin?
- Can you describe what happens when you try to speak?
- Do you have any difficulty swallowing?
- Have you had a sore throat?
- Have you had any recent weight loss without trying?
- Do you have any difficulty with weakness or numbness to any parts of your body?
- Do you have symptoms all the time or do they come and go?
- How has your daily activity been affected by this?
- Have you had any pain or headaches?
- Are you on any new medication?
- Have you had falls or recent trauma?
- Do you use any illicit drugs or drink alcohol?
- Do you have trouble moving or walking?
- Do you have any other symptoms you are concerned with?

Assessment: Cardinal Signs and Symptoms

General
- Soft spoken voice

Head, Eyes, Ears, Nose, Throat (HEENT)
- Excessive saliva
- Decreased sense of smell
- Facial bradykinesia
- Difficulty articulating words
- Reduced volume of speech
- Hoarse unsteady voice

Neurologic
- Forgetfulness
- Decreased facial expression
- Weakness
- Slurred speech

Cardiac
- Orthostatic hypotension

Respiratory
- Shortness of breath

Gastrointestinal
- Constipation

Genitourinary
- Urinary urgency

Musculoskeletal
- Tremors
- Sudden deceased dexterity
- Decreased arm swing on first involved side
- Bradykinesia
- Dystonia
- Akinesia

Integumentary
- Sweating abnormalities

Other Associated Symptoms
- Sleep disturbances
- General feeling of malaise
- Excessive daytime sleepiness

Medical History

Medical
- Hypertension (HTN)

Surgical
- Cholecystectomy

Allergies
- Penicillin (PCN)

Medication
- Hydrochlorothiazide (HCTZ) 25 mg daily
- Aspirin 81 mg daily

Family History
- Mother: HTN
- Father: dementia
- Grandfather: dementia, "shakes"

Psychosocial
- Denies tobacco use
- No drugs/drinks alcohol occasionally

Health Maintenance/Immunization
- Did receive influenza or pneumococcal vaccines

PHYSICAL EXAMINATION

Vital Signs
- Temperature
- Heart rate (HR)
- Respiration
- Blood pressure (BP)
- Oxygen saturation (SpO_2)

General Appearance
- No apparent distress
- Normal physique

HEENT
- No swelling, tenderness, or drainage noted.
- No adenopathy
- Monotone speech that varies in speed and volume

Cardiac
- Regular rate and rhythm (RRR)

Respiratory
- Lung sounds are clear bilaterally

Gastrointestinal
- Soft and nontender
- Constipation

Genitourinary
- No pain with palpation

Musculoskeletal
- No edema, redness, heat, crepitus or pain of joints. Resting tremor in right upper extremity

Integumentary
- No rash, swelling, or trauma noted
- Pink and warm

CASE STUDY

History

Directed Question	Response
When did the speaking difficulty begin?	*I noticed my speech problem 2 months ago.*
Can you describe what happens when you try to speak?	*I feel as though I have to strain my voice for people to hear me and the clarity in my voice is unpredictable. Sometimes my speech is slurred.*
Do you have any difficulty swallowing?	*I can swallow but sometimes I get the sensation of food being stuck in my throat.*
Have you had any recent weight loss?	*Yes, I have lost 15 pounds in the past month because I'm afraid to eat.*
Have you had a sore throat?	*No.*
Do you have any difficulty with weakness or numbness to any parts of your body?	*I don't have any numbness. Sometimes I feel weak all over. Sometimes I have difficulty writing because I get tremors.*
Has your handwriting gotten smaller?	*Yes, and I can't always write in a straight line because of the tremors.*
Do you have symptoms all the time or do they come and go?	*I always have a problem speaking loud. My speech is not always slurred.*
Have you had any pain or headaches?	*No.*
Did you take any medication to make it better?	*No.*

Directed Question	Response
How has your daily activity been affected by this?	I work as a teacher. My students have difficulty understanding me especially in a noisy room. My voice problems have caused me to lose income because I can't work when my voice is hoarse.
Are you on any new medication?	No.
Have you had falls or recent trauma?	No, but I do lose my balance occasionally.
Do you use any illicit drugs or drink alcohol?	I rarely drink.
Do you have trouble moving or walking?	No, but I occasionally lose my balance.
Do you have any other symptoms you are concerned with?	Sometimes I have a hard time remembering things and have difficulty sleeping at night. I'm afraid I'm getting dementia like my father and grandfather.

Physical Examination Findings

- VITAL SIGNS: temperature 98.1°F; RR 18; HR 74; BP 138/62; SpO$_2$ 100% on RA
- GENERAL APPEARANCE: Caucasian male in no acute distress; affect flat; soft spoken with occasional slurred speech and hoarseness
- NEUROLOGIC: cranial nerves II to XII intact; motor 5/5 upper extremities
- HEENT: head symmetric round; pupils equal, round, and reactive to light and accommodation (PERRLA) 3 mm; eye, ears, with no drainage, redness, tenderness, or trauma; tympanic membrane visualized, intact, and opaque; mucous membrane moist, pink, and intact; no lesion or sores; monotone speech that varies in speed and volume
- NECK: supple with full range of motion (ROM); no thyromegaly; no carotid bruits; no masses palpated; no adenopathy
- CHEST/CARDIOVASCULAR: RRR; no murmurs, gallops, or rubs; capillary refills <2 seconds
- RESPIRATORY: lung sounds clear through all lung fields, no adventitious sounds; symmetrical; no cough
- ABDOMEN: soft, nontender without mass or organomegaly; bowel sounds in all four quadrants
- SKIN: intact with no rashes, lesions, or ulcerations
- EXTREMITIES: no crepitus; swelling noted to lateral part of lower thigh, diffuse with ill-defined border
- MUSCULOSKELETAL: full weight bearing; full ROM all extremities; normal muscle strength, tone; deep tendon reflexes 2+; tremor to right hand at rest; bradykinesia; gait with stride-length ambulation

DIFFERENTIAL DIAGNOSIS

Clinical Observations	CVA	Parkinson's	Huntington's Disease	Bell's Palsy
Onset	Sudden	Gradual	Sudden/gradual	Sudden
Facial paralysis	Yes	No	No	Yes

(continued)

Clinical Observations	CVA	Parkinson's	Huntington's Disease	Bell's Palsy
Balance difficulties	Yes/No	Yes	Yes	No
Drooling	Yes/No	Yes/No	Yes/No	Yes/No
Occasional slurred speech	No	Yes/No	Yes/No	No
Bradykinesia	Yes/No	Yes	Yes/No	No
Postural Tremors	No	No	Yes	No

CVA, cardiovascular accident.

DIAGNOSTIC EXAMINATION

Exam	Code	Cost	Results
CBC	68.89	$25–$100	WBC—Determines infectious or inflammatory source. Elevated WBC indicative of active infectious source.
Basic metabolic panel	BW28	$15–$45	A basic metabolic panel is a blood test that measures glucose level, and fluid and electrolyte balance, and kidney function.
CT		$1,200	Computer-processed combinations of many images taken from different angles to produce cross-sectional images (virtual "slices") of specific areas of a scanned object, allowing the user to see inside the object without cutting.
MRI	R94.6	$2,700–$4,000	Using radio waves and a strong magnetic field, MRI scans can produce exceptionally detailed images of bones and the soft tissues that surround them.
T4, TSH	R94.02	$145–$300	Blood test to measure the amount of thyroid hormones, proteins present in the blood.
PET scan	R94.02	$4,900–$6,800	PET scanning is extremely sensitive to changes in the number of dopamine cells and all patients with clinical signs of PD will have an abnormal fluorodopa PET scan. Over the course of the disease, as the number of surviving dopamine neurons decreases, the imaging staff can reduce the intensity of the PET scan, thereby permitting finer measurement of the speed at which the disease has progressed.

CBC, complete blood count; PD, Parkinson's disease; TSH, thyroid-stimulating hormone; WBC, white blood cell.

CLINICAL DECISION MAKING

Case Study Analysis

The patient presented with complaint of difficulty speaking, for the past 2 months. He reports he feels as if he has to strain his voice for people to hear him and the clarity in his voice is unpredictable. He denies sore throat, headaches, or pain but states he sometimes feels the sensation of food being stuck in his throat, which has caused him not to eat. He currently works as a teacher but has missed work due to his speaking difficulties. He denies any paralysis but reports occasional generalized weakness, memory loss, and loss of balance when walking. He also reports tremors at rest and insomnia.

On physical exam he has a flat affect with little facial expression, soft spoken monotone speech with occasional hoarseness, and tremors are noted at rest to the right hand. Bradykinesia is noted. No paralysis, trauma, or signs of infection are noted. This rules out a possible CVA, Huntington's disease, or Bell's palsy.

Diagnosis: *Parkinson's disease*

Parkinson's disease (PD) is a chronic and progressive movement disorder, meaning that symptoms continue and worsen over time. Nearly one million people in the United States are living with PD. The cause is unknown, and although there is presently no cure, there are treatment options such as medication and surgery to manage its symptoms.

PD involves the malfunction and death of vital nerve cells in the brain, called neurons. PD primarily affects neurons in an area of the brain called the substantia nigra. Some of these dying neurons produce dopamine, a chemical that sends messages to the part of the brain that controls movement and coordination. As PD progresses, the amount of dopamine produced in the brain decreases, leaving a person unable to control movement normally and results in speech disturbances. There is no diagnostic test to diagnose PD. Tests can be done to rule out certain disorders. CT/MRI to r/o CVA, electrolyte panel to r/o electrolyte disturbances, a complete blood count (CBC) to r/o infection, and T4 thyroid-stimulating hormone (TSH) to r/o hyperthyroidism. Patient history, a current physical and two or more symptoms aid in the diagnosis. The patient presented here has tremors, bradykinesia, cognitive and speech disturbances.

Recommendations include medications to replace depleted dopamine levels, and teaching to address nutrition and mobility. A 15 lb weight loss over the past month is significant and can contribute to symptoms of weakness and instability with ambulation. A mechanical soft diet is recommended to reduce the feelings of "choking" while maintaining an adequate caloric intake. Teaching on the importance of an adequate fluid intake was provided since this will help with the ongoing symptom of constipation. An outpatient physical therapy consult is recommended to evaluate ambulation and to help suggest assistive devices to ensure stabilization with walking to prevent falling. A follow-up appointment in 1 month to 6 weeks is recommended to evaluate changes after starting medication, altering consistency of diet, and attending physical therapy. A referral to a neurologist is also recommended for intensive medication structuring to minimize symptoms and allay progression of the disease.

DIFFICULTY SWALLOWING

Case Presentation: A 49-year-old woman complains of difficulty swallowing.

INTRODUCTION TO COMPLAINT

- Difficulty swallowing: oral, oropharyngeal, and esophageal
- All involve different nerves and muscles, and difficulties can happen in any of these stages
- Dysphagia is an organic abnormality in the passage of solids or liquids from the oral cavity to the stomach. Patients can complain of difficulty initiating a swallow or the sensation of foods or liquids being hindered along the passage from the esophagus to the stomach
- Oropharyngeal dysphagia generally is accompanied by coughing, choking, nasopharyngeal regurgitation, aspiration, and a sensation of food in the pharynx
- Esophageal dysphagia is usually described as a sensation of food being stuck in the esophagus several seconds after swallowing
- Esophageal dysphagia can be due to intraluminal causes, intrinsic esophageal causes, extrinsic compression of the esophagus, due to an underlying motility disorder, or functional dysphagia

HISTORY OF COMPLAINT

Symptomatology

Ask about the following characteristics of each symptom using open-ended questions:

- Onset
- Location of sensation
- Duration and progression of symptoms
- Timing
- Types of foods that produce symptoms
- Associated symptoms/pain
- Medication use
- Use of alcohol and/or drugs
- History of esophageal surgery or radiation

Directed Questions to Ask

- When did you first notice this difficulty with swallowing?
- Where in your throat does the feeling happen?
- Do you have trouble getting food down or does it feel like it gets stuck?
- Has it gotten worse over time?
- Does it occur when you try to swallow or after you swallow?
- Does this happen more with solids, liquids, or both?

- Do you have other symptoms at the same time or other times such as heartburn, regurgitation, or vomiting blood?
- Have you lost weight recently without trying?
- Have you had a cough?
- Do you use any nonprescribed drugs?
- Have you had any throat or stomach surgeries or radiation?

Assessment: Cardinal Signs and Symptoms

General
- Weight loss
- Fever
- Chills

Head, Eyes, Ears, Nose, Throat (HEENT)
- Acidic erosion of teeth
- Hoarseness
- Oropharyngeal irritation
- Excess saliva
- Excessive swallowing

Cardiac
- Murmur
- Chest pain
- Left or right arm pain

Respiratory
- Cough
- Shortness of breath
- Sputum production

Gastrointestinal (GI)
- Vomiting
- Regurgitation
- Abdominal pain
- Belching
- Diarrhea
- Constipation

Musculoskeletal
- Progressive weakness

Skin
- Pale due to anemia

Medical History

- Medical conditions: inappropriate sinus tachycardia; history of diabetes mellitus (DM); gastroesophageal reflux disease (GERD)
- Surgeries: ablation 2010; C-section 1995 and 1998; appendectomy
- Allergies: no known drug allergy (NKDA)
- Medication use, including illicit drugs: metformin 500 mg BID, omeprazole 20 mg daily
- Exercise and diet: no consistent exercise; patient works in financial services in high stress job; tries to maintain a low-sugar diet

Family History
- Mother—hypertension, DM; father—Crohn's disease, DM, colon cancer

Social History
- Patient denies tobacco and drug use
- Drinks glass of wine most nights

Sexual History
- Patient is married in a monogamous relationship

PHYSICAL EXAMINATION

Vital Signs
- Temperature
- Pulse
- Blood pressure (BP)
- Respiration
- Oxygen saturation (SpO_2)
- Body mass index (BMI)

General Appearance
- Coloring
- Nutritional status
- Orientation

HEENT
- Appearance of dentition
- Oral and oropharyngeal appearance

Respiratory
- Lung sounds
- Effort
- Depth of respirations

Cardiovascular
- Heart rate and rhythm
- Murmurs
- Gallops, or rubs
- Capillary refill
- Distal pulses

GI
- Distention
- Bowel sounds
- Tenderness/pain
- Nausea
- Vomiting
- Appetite
- Organomegaly

Musculoskeletal
- Extremity strength

Skin
- Color
- Turgor

CASE STUDY
History

Directed Question	Response
When did you first notice this difficulty swallowing?	*It seems like it's been developing over the past few months.*
Where in your throat does the feeling happen?	*It's lower, under my breastbone.*
Do you have trouble getting food down or does it feel like it gets stuck?	*It feels more stuck.*
Has it gotten worse over time?	*Yes.*
Does it occur when you try to swallow or after you swallow?	*After I swallow.*
Does this happen more with solids, liquids, or both?	*Just with solids.*
Do you have other symptoms at the same time or other times such as heartburn, regurgitation, or vomiting blood?	*I've had heartburn for a long time, but sometimes I can't keep the food down now.*
Have you lost weight recently without trying?	*Yes, because I'm scared to eat something that's too solid because it gets stuck.*
Have you had a cough?	*Sometimes in the morning.*
Do you use any nonprescribed drugs?	*No.*
Have you had any throat or stomach surgeries or radiation?	*No.*

Physical Examination Findings

- VITAL SIGNS: temperature 97.9°F; RR 16; pulse 88; BP 110/76; SpO$_2$ 97% on RA; BMI 22
- GENERAL APPEARANCE: patient appears in no acute distress, alert and oriented x 4
- HEENT: PERRLA; mucous membranes pink and moist; minor erosion of teeth; trachea midline
- RESPIRATORY: lungs clear to auscultation bilaterally; symmetric chest rise
- CARDIAC: regular rate and rhythm; no murmurs, gallops, or rubs; capillary refill <2 seconds; radial and dorsalis pedis pulses 2+ bilaterally
- GASTROINTESTINAL: bowel sounds present in four quadrants; abdomen soft and nontender; no organomegaly noted
- SKIN: skin warm, dry, intact; no lesions or masses noted; normal coloring

DIFFERENTIAL DIAGNOSIS

Clinical Observations	Obstruction From Enlarged Left Atrium	Esophageal Stricture	Carcinoma of Esophagus
Onset	Gradual	Gradual	Gradual
Progressive	Yes	Yes	Yes
Burping	No	Yes	No
Regurgitation	No	Yes	Possible
Cough	Possible	In the mornings or after eating	Yes
Weight loss	If not eating well	If not eating well	Yes
Hoarseness	No	Yes	Yes
Possible symptoms	Sputum production, murmur	Heartburn (possibly described as chest pain), GI bleed	Hiccups, pneumonia, bone pain, GI bleed

GI, gastrointestinal.

DIAGNOSTIC EXAMINATION

Exam	Code	Cost	Results
Upper endoscopy	Z12.9	$1,832 ($1,966 with biopsy)	Performed under sedation, a camera is inserted into the esophagus. Ability to see into the esophagus to determine if there are erosions or hyperplasia of the esophageal lining or stricture or rings narrowing the passage. It also gives the ability to obtain tissue samples through biopsy or therapeutic interventions such as dilation of narrowing. Ultrasound can be used internally with this procedure to view tumors, lymph nodes, or heart enlargement.
Barium swallow	Z13.9	$305	Uses x-rays to track swallowed food or liquid through the upper GI tract. Less invasive, can be helpful in assessing the location of dysfunction, outpouchings, mechanical obstruction, or for those in whom sedation or introduction of a scope could be dangerous with known conditions. It is less helpful in determining the cause of dysfunction.

(*continued*)

Exam	Code	Cost	Results
Motility testing (esophageal manometry)	Z13.818	$1,535	Performed with a catheter inserted through the nose and down the esophagus. It allows the clinician to view the muscle contractions of the esophagus to determine if there are defects in the musculature or esophageal sphincter.
CBC	R68.89	$17	With this test you can see if there is an increase in WBCs, which may point to infection; a decrease in hemoglobin or hematocrit, which could signal anemia or blood loss; or a decrease in platelet counts, which could indicate a risk for bleeding.

CBC, complete blood count; GI, gastrointestinal; WBC, white blood cell.

CLINICAL DECISION MAKING

Case Study Analysis

Based on the history of GERD, morning coughing, progressive dysfunction, and heartburn this was thought to be an esophageal stricture, which can be a complication of GERD due to repeated exposure to stomach acid, which causes changes to the esophageal lining. An upper endoscopy was performed, which showed inflammation and narrowing of the esophagus, confirming this diagnosis. A barium swallow was not performed as this would not show a cause for narrowing; motility testing was not used as this was not suspected to be a nerve problem, and labs were not needed as there was no evidence of bleeding.

Diagnosis: *Esophageal stricture related to long-term GERD*

Dilation was performed during the endoscopy and the patient was instructed to take 20 mg omeprazole twice a day until follow-up at 1 month. The patient was also instructed to engage in mindful eating—to chew food thoroughly, not to rush during meals, and take frequent sips of water between bites of food. Additionally, it was reinforced that the patient should remain in an upright position for at least 1 hour after eating, to avoid eating at least for 4 hours before going to sleep, and to sleep on several pillows to prevent reflux. Food and beverages to be avoided or taken in extremely limited quantities include chocolate, cola beverages, caffeine, highly spiced foods, and alcohol since these items are known to irrigate gastric and esophageal mucosa. Depending upon the results of the 1-month follow-up examination, further interventions may be required.

DIZZINESS

Case Presentation: A 58-year-old female presents with a complaint of dizziness.

INTRODUCTION TO COMPLAINT

- The sensation of movement, either of the patient in relation to his or her environment or environment in relation to the patient, which often has a spinning or rotational component
- It is not a lightheaded or faint-like disorientation
- Balance is the sense of continuity that a person has with his or her environment
- It is the accurate sensory information from the eyes, proprioceptive receptors (in the joints), and the balance organs of the inner ear (vestibular labyrinth); accurate coordination of sensory input by the brain and functioning motor output from the central nervous system to a normal musculoskeletal system
- If one or more of these functions is not working properly, then a sense of imbalance or dizziness will result
- Dizziness is caused by disturbance of the input or central processing of sensory signals from the vestibular apparatus that provide information regarding the position of the body in space
- It is caused either by asymmetric disruption of sensory input from the vestibular organs or asymmetric integration of vestibular input into the central nervous system
- Vertigo is readily differentiated from other causes of dizziness by a sensation of motion

HISTORY OF COMPLAINT

Symptomatology

Ask about the following characteristics of each symptom using open-ended questions:

- Onset
- Chronology
- Current situation
- Timing (frequency, duration)
- Severity
- Precipitating/aggravating factors
- Alleviating factors
- Associated symptoms
- Effects on daily activities
- Previous diagnosis of similar episodes
- Previous treatments and their effectiveness in symptom relief

Directed Questions to Ask

- Describe how you feel when it happens.
- Did it start suddenly or progressively got worse until you noticed it?
- Which activities are you doing when it happens?
- How does it resolve itself? Does it resolve quickly or slowly?
- How frequently does it happen?
- Do you notice any limb-specific weakness or numbness; is it on one side of your body?
- Are you able to stand upright when it happens; do you need to sit or grab onto furniture to stay on your feet?
- Can you describe any hearing or vision changes you experience while it's happening?
- Have you sustained any injuries from falling?
- What medications do you take? Do any of them make you sleepy or dizzy?
- Does anyone in your family have a history of heart attack or stroke?
- Have you ever had a heart attack or stroke?
- Tell me about your headaches. Do you get them frequently; have you ever had migraines or been diagnosed with migraines?
- Describe any illnesses you've had lately.
- Tell me about any blood clots or seizures you've been diagnosed with.
- How have these episodes kept you from doing your normal routine?

Assessment: Cardinal Signs and Symptoms

General
- Anxiety
- Dizziness
- Sense of imbalance

Gastrointestinal (GI)
- Nausea
- Vomiting

Neurologic
- Spinning or rocking sensation

Head, Eyes, Ears, Nose, Throat (HEENT)
- Hearing loss
- Tinnitus
- Vision changes
- Nystagmus

Musculoskeletal
- Weakness
- Impaired gait

Medical History

- MEDICAL CONDITIONS: osteoarthritis, diabetes mellitus type 2, hyperlipidemia, seasonal allergies
- SURGICAL HISTORY: none
- Patient denies history of heart attack, arrhythmia or stroke, no significant family history for heart attack, stroke, migraine headaches or vertigo
- PSYCHIATRIC: denies depression, anxiety, suicidal ideation or domestic violence

- MEDICATIONS: metformin 500 mg twice a day with meals, simvastatin 40 mg HS, loratadine 10 mg daily as needed for allergies, ibuprofen 400 mg every 6 hours as needed for arthritis pain. Patient completed a recent Augmentin 875 mg orally, twice a day prescription for sinus infection
- ALLERGIES: no known drug allergies (NKDA)
- Patient denies illicit drugs, denies ever having smoked, drinks one 8 oz. glass of red wine every evening with dinner
- DIET/EXERCISE: she states she walks her dog 0.5 miles around her subdivision twice a day; she engages in water aerobics for 45 minutes three times a week

PHYSICAL EXAMINATION

Vital Signs

- Temperature
- Pulse
- Respiration
- SpO2
- Blood pressure (BP)

General Appearance

- Apparent state of health
- Appearance of comfort or distress
- Color
- Nutritional status
- State of hydration
- Hygiene
- Match between appearance and stated age
- Difficulty with gait or balance

Mouth and HEENT

- Lips: color, lesions, symmetry
- Oral cavity: breath odor, color, lesions of buccal mucosa
- Teeth and gums: redness, swelling, caries, bleeding
- Tongue: color, texture, lesions, tenderness of floor of mouth
- Throat and pharynx: color, exudates, uvula, tonsillar symmetry and enlargement
- Ears: color, texture, lesions, tenderness

Neck

- Symmetry
- Swelling
- Masses
- Active range of motion
- Thyroid enlargement

Palpation

- Tenderness, enlargement, mobility, contour and consistency of nodes and masses
- Nodes: pre- and postauricular, occipital, tonsillar, submandibular, submental, anterior, and posterior cervical; supraclavicular
- Thyroid: size, consistency, contour, position, tenderness

Associated Systems for Assessment

- A complete assessment should include the respiratory and cardiovascular system

CASE STUDY
History

Directed Question	Response
Describe how you feel when it happens	*I feel like the room is spinning around me and like I will fall over sometimes. But if I stand still it gets a little better.*
Did it start suddenly or progressively got worse until you noticed it?	*It actually seemed to start as soon as I woke up and progressively got worse throughout my day yesterday, and today when I woke up everything was still spinning!*
Which activities are you doing when it happens?	*It hung on no matter what I was doing. Even when I laid down to go to sleep I felt like the bed was spinning slowly.*
How does it resolve itself? Does it resolve quickly or slowly?	*It gets a little better sometimes by itself but it's been very consistent, it hasn't gotten any better.*
How frequently does it happen?	*It's been going on since yesterday, but I've never experienced this before. It's almost like a terrible hangover.*
Are you able to stand upright when it happens; do you need to sit or grab onto furniture to stay on your feet?	*It's been getting worse and worse as the day goes on; my husband had to drive me here because I felt so dizzy. But I can stand upright, sometimes I feel like I lean to one side or the other a little bit.*
Can you describe any hearing (decrease, ringing or muffled) or vision changes you experience while it's happening?	*I haven't noticed any ringing or muffled noises, I think my hearing has stayed the same as it always is and I haven't had any changes to my vision since I started wearing reading glasses 5 years ago.*
Have you sustained any injuries from falling?	*No, thankfully I haven't fallen. My husband has had to drive me everywhere and my neighbor has been walking my dog because he pulls me around sometimes. I don't think I could stay on my feet with him pulling and me feeling so dizzy.*
What medications do you take? Do any of them make you sleepy or dizzy?	*I take my sugar pills with breakfast and supper, my cholesterol medicine at night and my Claritin every morning during the summer and fall.*
Does anyone in your family have a history of heart attack or stroke?	*No, none of my family have ever had a stroke or heart attack.*
Have you ever had a heart attack or stroke?	*No, but my doctor told me I have high cholesterol and it could lead to a heart attack. That's why I take my cholesterol pills and exercise; do you think this is a heart attack?*

Directed Question	Response
Tell me about your headaches: do you get them frequently; have you ever had migraines or been diagnosed with migraines?	*I had a terrible dull headache every day for a week last week, otherwise I sometimes get a little nagging headache in my temples when I read for too long.*
Describe any illnesses you've had lately	*My doctor said I had a sinus infection and gave me some antibiotics that I just finished the other day. But I get those at least twice a year and I've never had this happen before.*
Tell me about any blood clots or seizures you've been diagnosed with.	*I've never had a blood clot and I don't think I have ever had a seizure.*
How have these episodes kept you from doing your normal routine?	*The dizziness is keeping me from exercising like normal. I don't feel comfortable driving and I'm having a hard time doing housework and cooking.*

Physical Examination Findings

- VITAL SIGNS: temperature 98.5°F; 20 R/min; 72 bpm; BP 130/72; 96% on room air
- GENERAL APPEARANCE: patient is well-groomed, age-appropriate in appearance and anxious; she appears in mild distress
- HEENT: face symmetrical, no ptosis or droop noted, pupils equal, round, and reactive to light and accommodation (PERRLA); saccadic nystagmus movements to the left during head thrust test, but no prolonged nystagmus noted
- NECK: no lymphadenopathy noted, no carotid bruit, no jugular venous distention (JVD) noted
- CARDIOVASCULAR: S1, S2; no murmur, capillary refill in less than 2 seconds
- NEUROLOGIC: no vision changes, denies tinnitus or hearing loss, consistent dizzy feeling
- GASTROINTESTINAL: mild nausea, denies vomiting
- MUSCULOSKELETAL: normal, active range of motion (ROM) in all extremities, 5/5 strength in all extremities; slight lean to the left when moving to stand upright, which is self-corrected

DIFFERENTIAL DIAGNOSIS

Clinical Observations	Benign Paroxysmal Positional Vertigo	Cerebellar Stroke	Vestibular neuronitis (labyrinthitis)	Ménière's Disease
Onset	Sudden	Sudden	Slow	Sudden
Acute episode duration	Few minutes	Until treatment	Days to weeks	Minutes to hours
Symptom resolution	1–6 months	Ongoing until treatment	Within 2 months	Ongoing

(continued)

Clinical Observations	Benign Paroxysmal Positional Vertigo	Cerebellar Stroke	Vestibular neuronitis (labyrinthitis)	Ménière's Disease
Tinnitus	No	No	No	Yes
Hearing loss	No	No	No	Yes
Vision changes	No	Yes	No	No
Ataxia	No	Yes (severe)	Yes (mild)	Yes (mild)
Nystagmus	Yes (rotational, only during vertigo)	Yes (bidirectional, persistent)	Yes (unilateral toward affected ear with head thrust test, resolves within 48 hr)	No
Headaches	No	Yes	No	No
Worse with position change	Yes	No	Yes	Yes
Nausea/vomiting	No	Yes/No	Yes/No	Yes
Head thrust test	No	Yes/No	Yes	No

DIAGNOSTIC EXAMINATION

Exam	Code	Cost	Results
Brain CT (no contrast)	B0270ZZ	$624	Normal results: all tissue and sulci of the brain are intact and without swelling. No lesions, hemorrhages, plaques, or inflammation is noted. No ischemic areas are noted. Abnormal: Areas of compression by inflammation or hemorrhage within the skull will inhibit brain function and possibly cause herniation. Lesions, plaques, or inflammation can be a sign of auto-immune disorders or other disease processes. Masses within the brain can cause compression as well as inhibit normal electrical activity and conduction within the brain tissue.
Otoscopy	Z01.10	$0, included in physical examination by provider	Normal results: All organs of middle ear are visualized and no extra fluid, obstructive, purulent discharge, or excessive wax is seen. Abnormal: Purulent fluid within the ear drum can indicate otitis media; excessive wax can impair sensory information being processed correctly by the fine bones within the inner ear.

(*continued*)

Exam	Code	Cost	Results
Head thrust test	T 14.90	$0, included in physical examination by provider	Normal results: test of the vestibulo-ocular reflex; patient is able to keep gaze fixed on provider's nose despite swift rotational movements of the patient's head (15–20 degrees), or the smooth movement of eyes to refocus on fixation point. Abnormal: nystagmus persistent despite movements, jumping of one or both eyes in maintaining fixation point indicates a vestibular defect on the "jumping" side.
CMP	I10	$28	Normal results: Glucose 70–99 mg/dL (fasting), 70–125 mg/dL (nonfasting) Sodium 136–144 mEq/L Potassium 3.7–5.2 mEq/L Chloride 96–106 mmol/L CO_2 20–29 mmol/L BUN 7–20 mg/dL Creatinine 0.8–1.4 mg/dL BUN/creatinine ratio 10:1–20:1 Calcium 8.5–10.9 mg/dL Magnesium 1.8–2.6 mEq/L Protein 6.3–7.9 g/dL Albumin 3.9–5.0 d/dL Globulin 2.0–3.5 g/dL Albumin/globulin ratio 1.7–2.2 Bilirubin 0.3–1.9 mg/dL ALP 44–147 IU/L ALT 8–37 IU/L AST 10–34 IU/L Glomerular filtration rate 90–120 mL/min/1.73 m^2 Abnormal results: values outside of normal range can be indications of dehydration, kidney/liver dysfunction, malnutrition or malignant disease process
CBC	D64.9	$29	Measures the different blood cell components and assists in diagnosis of nutrient/oxygen delivery dysfunction, infective process, and further blood cell production. Hemoglobin is responsible for delivering oxygen to cells; normal level in females ranges from 13.5 to 17.5 g/dL. A decrease in this number is indicative of anemia and can result in impaired oxygen delivery to tissues. Hematocrit is the total percentage of blood composed of red blood cells; normal level in females ranges from 40% to 55%. A decrease in this number can indicate anemia or dilution of blood with fluid. WBCs attach themselves to foreign cells, infected tissues and wounds to promote phagocytosis and removal of dangerous products. A decrease in WBCs can be a sign of bone marrow damage, dysfunctional cell production, or leukemia; an elevated WBC count is a sign of an active infection process within the body. Normal 5,000–10,000/mL Platelets are the cells that aid in clotting, whether it be helpful (tissue damage and cuts) or malignant (thrombi formation). Decreased platelets indicate the potential to have uncontrolled bleeding in response to an assault, while an increase can indicate the patient is at increased risk for DVT/PE/clots. Normal 150k–400k/mL

ALP, alkaline phosphatase; ALT, alanine amino transferase; AST, aspartate amino transferase; BUN, blood urea nitrogen; CBC, complete blood count; CMP, complete metabolic panel; DVT, deep vein thrombosis; PE, pulmonary embolism; WBC, white blood cell.

CLINICAL DECISION MAKING

Case Study Analysis

After detailed history of onset, the patient was sent for a brain CT with contrast to rule out ischemic or hemorrhagic stroke in the cerebellum, which can also cause vertigo. When no significant findings were presented, physical assessment continued with testing of the vestibulo-ocular reflex (head thrust test) and vestibulo-spinal reflex (patient moving to stand unassisted). The patient demonstrated left-sided saccadic nystagmus during the head thrust test, indicative of unilateral vestibular deficit. Otoscopic examination was conducted to rule out inner ear involvement in vertigo, with no signs or symptoms of otitis media infection or trauma. The patient's blood work was all within normal limits. Given the gradual onset, with persistent symptoms, presence of mild ataxia, left saccadic movements during head thrust test, and prior history of recent upper respiratory infection (URI)—left vestibular neuritis is the diagnosis.

The patient was prescribed prochlorperazine 5 mg three times a day as needed for 7 days, for relief of nausea. Prochlorperazine acts as a vestibular sedative, which aids with symptoms in the short term, but if used too long can prevent cerebral recalibration; therefore it is recommended to be used for 7 days or less. She was educated on the dystonic effects that can occur with prochlorperazine and to contact her primary care provider and stop taking the medication if these occurred. She was also educated on the importance of reporting any hearing changes immediately for an ear, nose, and throat (ENT) referral. The acute and resolvable nature of her affliction was explained to her, with the expected resolution of her symptoms expected within 2 to 3 weeks, as well as instructions to avoid driving until her symptoms improve.

> **Diagnosis:** *Left vestibular neuritis*

- No specific imaging tests (CT/MRI) are recommended for the differentiation of vertigo inducing disorders, aside from ruling out stroke. Distinguishing between the various disorders (Ménière's vestibular neuronitis/labyrinthitis/neuritis, benign positional paroxysmal vertigo) is done with careful physical assessment and examination of symptoms.
- Vestibular neuritis often is preceded by a viral illness or URI such as a sinus infection. The patient just ended a course of antibiotics for a diagnosed sinus infection.
- Labyrinthitis, a subcategory of vestibular neuronitis, is differentiated by its positive hearing changes including tinnitus whereas neuritis has no hearing changes.
- Evaluation of onset, hearing changes, duration of symptoms, ataxia, and preceding illnesses or previous vertigo episodes is very important in distinguishing between the different disorders that cause vertigo.
- If patients diagnosed with vestibular neuritis develop hearing changes, it is very important they receive steroids and an urgent referral to ENT for a formal hearing test to identify acoustic neuroma and/or evolving neural inflammation and damage.

DOUBLE VISION

> **Case Presentation:** *A 31-year-old female reports to the emergency department (ED) with acute onset of double vision in her right eye while she was at church this morning.*

INTRODUCTION TO COMPLAINT

- When a person sees two images of a single object, he or she is experiencing double vision
- Double vision, also known as diplopia, can present as monocular or binocular
- Causes of monocular diplopia include:
  - Astigmatism
  - Keratoconus
  - Pterygium
  - Cataracts
  - Dislocated lens
  - Swelling of the eyelid
  - Dry eye
  - Retinal problems
- Causes of binocular diplopia include:
  - Strabismus
  - Extraocular muscle damage
  - Diabetes
  - Grave's disease
  - Myasthenia gravis
  - Eye muscle trauma

HISTORY OF COMPLAINT

Symptomatology

Ask about the following characteristics of each symptom using open-ended questions:

- Onset (sudden or gradual)
- Chronology
- Current situation (improving or deteriorating)
- Location
- Radiation
- Quality
- Timing (frequency, duration)
- Severity
- Precipitating and aggravating factors
- Relieving factors

- Associated symptoms
- Effects on daily activities
- Previous diagnosis of similar episodes
- Previous treatments
- Efficacy of previous treatments

Directed Questions to Ask

- When did the double vision problem start?
- Is the double vision problem affecting one eye or both eyes?
- Have you had/do you have any other visual disturbances?
- Do you have any pre-existing eye problems that you have been seen/treated for?
- Have your eyes been very dry recently?
- Did you sustain an injury to your eye?
- Are you diabetic? If yes, what have your fasting a.m. blood sugars been?
- Have you been diagnosed with Grave's disease?
- Have you been acutely ill recently?
- Do you have a history of any autoimmune problems?
- Is there a history of autoimmune problems in your family?

Assessment: Cardinal Signs and Symptoms

- Double vision in one or both eyes

Medical History: General

- Medical conditions and surgeries
- Allergies (seasonal as well as others)
- Medication currently used (prescription, birth control pill [BCP] and over the counter [OTC])
- Herbal preparations and traditional therapies

Medical History: Specific to Complaint

- Onset of the double vision
- Pre-existing vision problems
- Eye injury
- Diabetes
- Autoimmune disorders
- Graves' disease

PHYSICAL EXAMINATION

Vital Signs

- Temperature
- Pulse
- Respiration
- Oxygen saturation (SpO_2)
- Blood pressure (BP)

General Appearance

- Apparent state of health
- Appearance of comfort or distress

- Color
- State of hydration

Eyes
- Inspect for orbit/lids/lens for signs of injury or swelling; conjunctiva—color/characteristics; pupil reflexes and responses; lens for cloudiness or opacities; extraocular movements; condition of retinal tissues

Neck
- Inspect for symmetry, swelling, masses
- Palpate for tenderness; thyroid enlargement, masses/nodules; lymph node chain

Cardiovascular
- Inspect for capillary refill time
- Auscultate for heart sounds, check for murmurs, gallops, rubs
- Palpate for peripheral pulses

Respiratory
- Auscultate lungs for crackles, and wheezing

Abdomen
- Inspect for contour, heaves, scars, bruising, contusions
- Auscultate for bowel sounds, bruits
- Palpate for pain, masses, organomegaly

Neurologic Exam
- Test cranial nerves (CNs) II to XII
- Test fine and gross motor movements
- Test deep tendon reflexes
- Testing of extremity strength
- Testing of extremity sensory and motor function

CASE STUDY

History

Directed Question	Response
When did the double vision problem start?	A few hours ago while I was playing the keyboard at church.
Is the double vision problem affecting one eye or both eyes?	Just my right eye.
Have you had/do you have any other visual disturbances?	No.
Do you have any pre-existing eye problems that you have been seen/treated for?	I have worn glasses since I was in middle school for "eye strain."
Have your eyes been very dry recently?	Yes, especially my right eye. I have an appointment with my eye doctor this week to get that checked out.
Did you sustain an injury to your eye?	No.

Directed Question	*Response*
Are you diabetic? If yes, what have your fasting a.m. blood sugars been?	*No.*
Have you been diagnosed with Grave's disease?	*No.*
Have you been acutely ill recently?	*No.*
Do you have a history of any autoimmune problems?	*No.*
Is there a history of autoimmune problems in your family?	*No.*

Physical Examination Findings

- VITAL SIGNS: temperature 96.8°F; respiratory rate (RR) 16; heart rate (HR) 78, regular; BP 101/58; SpO$_2$ 99%
- GENERAL APPEARANCE: well-developed, healthy-appearing female in mild distress
- EYES: lids without erythema or edema; conjunctiva white without injection or redness; pupil reflexes and responses to light normal; extraocular eye movements normal; no opacities noted in lenses; retinal tissue pink, no hemorrhages or disruption of tissue noted
- NECK: nontender, no thyroid enlargement or masses/nodules
- CARDIOVASCULAR: regular rate/rhythm without murmur or gallop
- ABDOMEN: soft, nontender without mass or organomegaly
- NEUROLOGIC: CNs II to XII grossly intact; fine and gross motor movements intact; deep tendon reflexes normal; extremity strength WNL: no impaired motor or sensory function appreciated on exam

DIFFERENTIAL DIAGNOSIS

Clinical Observations	Eye Injury/ Muscle Problems	Conjunctival Problems	Lens/ Retinal Problems	Diabetes	Graves' Disease	Myasthenia Gravis
Monocular	Yes/No	Yes	No	No	No	No
Binocular	Yes/No	No	Yes	Yes	Yes	Yes
Lab evaluation helpful	No	Yes/No	Yes/No	Yes	Yes	Yes

DIAGNOSTIC EXAMINATION

Exam	Code	Cost	Results
Comprehensive metabolic panel	80053	$49	Fasting for evaluation of serum glucose level

(*continued*)

Exam	Code	Cost	Results
TSH	84443	$49	To evaluate for Grave's disease
Acetylcholine receptor antibodies	83519	Varies based on lab and market	To evaluate for Myasthenia Gravis

TSH, thyroid-stimulating hormone.

CLINICAL DECISION MAKING

Case Study Analysis

The advanced practice provider (APP) performs the assessment and physical examination on the patient and finds the following data: history of acute onset of monocular diplopia, right eye; recent history of dry eyes; no abnormal physical exam findings

Given that this patient has an appointment already scheduled with her eye doctor in a few days, the APP provides the patient with recommendation of OTC drops for the "dryness" of her eyes. The APP instructs the patient to keep her appointment with her eye doctor for further evaluation and management. Monocular diplopia is associated with an eye injury or muscle problem. The patient should be evaluated for eye strain given a history of wearing glasses for the disorder. A change in prescription may be required.

Diagnosis: *Monocular diplopia right eye, possibly related to eye dryness*

EAR DISCHARGE

Case Presentation: A 57-year-old man presents to the clinic with a complaint of left ear drainage.

INTRODUCTION TO COMPLAINT

Ear discharge can be caused by several conditions, including rupture of the tympanic membrane, infection or trauma of the external ear, or as a result of cerumen that has softened (i.e., due to increased temperature).

Bacterial Infections

Ear discharge can be related to a bacterial infection that has caused increased fluid accumulation and inflammation behind the tympanic membrane leading to rupture. Bacterial infections in the ear canal or external ear may have exudate present that drains from the ear.

Allergic Conditions

Allergic conditions (e.g., seasonal and environmental factors) or allergies to a specific irritant (e.g., animal dander) can cause inflammation in the upper respiratory tract, including the Eustachian tubes. This can cause fluid accumulation in the absence of bacterial infection. Although an infection may not be present, the pressure from the fluid accumulation can still cause pressure inside the middle ear. With excessive increase in pressure, the tympanic membrane can rupture, leading to drainage from the ear.

Trauma

Ear discharge can be caused by direct trauma to the ear. The drainage may be bloody and directly related to the trauma, or the trauma may lead to a point of entry for an infectious agent, resulting in drainage that is more exudative in appearance.

HISTORY OF COMPLAINT

Symptomatology

Ask about the following characteristics of each symptom using open-ended questions:

- Onset
- Contributing factors: history prior to drainage
- Exposure to illness
- Exposure to second- or third-hand smoke
- Associated symptoms
- Description of drainage
- Aggravating factors

- Alleviating factors
- Effect on hearing
- History of similar episodes
- Previous treatments tried

Directed Questions to Ask

- Was the onset sudden or gradual?
- Have you had any ear pain?
- Have you had sinus or nasal congestion?
- Have you had a sore throat?
- What does the ear drainage look like?
- Is the drainage from just one ear, or both?
- Have you been exposed to anyone who is sick?
- Do you or anyone in your household smoke?
- Has your hearing changed?
- Have you had a fever?
- Have you been coughing?
- Have you been short of breath?
- Has your appetite changed?
- Have you vomited?
- Have you ever had anything like this before?
- If yes, what treatment did you receive?

Assessment: Cardinal Signs and Symptoms

In addition to the directed questions listed previously, the following need to be included in the assessment.

Ears

- Drainage: color, consistency, odor, amount
- Edema
- Erythema
- Hearing change

Eyes

- Conjunctivitis
- Vision change
- Pain

Nose

- Congestion

Mouth and Throat

- Sore throat
- Cough
- Dental status
- Dysphagia
- Oral lesions

Neck

- Pain
- Decreased range of motion (ROM)
- Swelling
- Enlarged glands

Nervous System
- Dermatome involvement

Skin
- Rash

Other Associated Symptoms
- Fever
- Fatigue
- Headache

Medical History: General

- Medical conditions and surgeries
- Allergies (seasonal or other)
- Current medications

Medical History: Specific to Complaint

- Frequent ear infections
- Smoking history
- History of ear surgery
- Trauma to ear
- Recent history of swimming
- Recent history of travel

PHYSICAL EXAMINATION

Vital Signs

- Temperature
- Pulse
- Respiration
- Oxygen saturation (SpO_2)
- Blood pressure (BP)

General Appearance

- Apparent state of health
- Current level of comfort or distress
- Skin color and temperature
- Nutritional status
- Hydration status
- Hygiene
- Appearance in accordance with stated age
- Gait or balance difficulty

Ear Inspection
- EXTERNAL EAR: color, structure, swelling, presence of cerumen
- CANAL: redness, swelling; presence, character, and amount of exudate
- TYMPANIC MEMBRANE: intact, color, light reflex, landmarks, presence of effusion, injection, apparent pressure

Eye Inspection
- Drainage
- Color

Nose Inspection
- Congestion
- Drainage
- Pallor

Mouth and Throat Inspection
- Color
- Presence of lesions
- Symmetry
- Exudate

Neck Inspection and Palpation
- Symmetry
- Swelling
- Masses
- Active ROM
- Thyroid: size, symmetry, masses

Neurologic Examination
- Facial nerve assessment
- Hearing test

Associated Systems for Assessment

A complete assessment should include the respiratory system, abdominal assessment, general skin inspection, and general extremities assessment.

CASE STUDY
History

Directed Question	Response
Was the onset sudden or gradual?	*It came on gradually.*
Have you had any ear pain?	*Yes, but it has gotten a little better.*
What does the drainage look like?	*Clear, with some wax in it.*
Have you been exposed to anyone who is sick?	*Not that I know of.*
Do you or anyone in your household smoke?	*No.*
Is the pain just in the ear, or is there pain in other areas?	*A little in my throat, but mostly my ear.*
Are you able to describe the pain?	*It's a sharp ache.*
Is the pain interfering with activities?	*Some, it's hard to focus.*
Have you noticed a hearing change?	*My left ear feels muffled.*
Does anything make the pain better?	*Not that I've noticed.*
Does anything make the pain worse?	*When I take a shower.*
Have you had a fever?	*No.*
Have you had a runny nose?	*Yes.*

Directed Question	Response
Have you been coughing?	*Occasionally I have a dry cough.*
Have you been short of breath?	*No.*
Has your appetite changed?	*No.*
Have you vomited?	*No.*
Have you ever had anything like this before?	*No, I've had ear aches before, but not drainage.*
If yes, what treatment did you receive?	*Antibiotics and allergy pills.*
Have you ever had the chicken pox, cold sores, or shingles?	*No.*

Physical Examination Findings

- VITAL SIGNS: temperature 98.9°F; respiratory rate (RR) 14; heart rate (HR) 76; BP 126/84; SpO_2 96% room air
- GENERAL APPEARANCE: well-developed, healthy appearing male
- EAR INSPECTION: right ear—external ear normal, canal without erythema or exudate, small amount of cerumen, tympanic membrane pearly grey, intact with light reflex and bony landmarks present; left ear—external ear normal, canal with white exudate and crusting, no visualization of tympanic membrane or bony landmarks, no light reflex
- EYE INSPECTION: bilateral mild conjunctivitis, anicteric, pupils equal, round, and reactive to light and accommodation (PERRLA), extraocular movements intact
- NOSE INSPECTION: nares are patent with soft tissue edema, pale, with moderate clear rhinorrhea
- MOUTH AND THROAT INSPECTION: no oral lesions, teeth and gums in good repair, oropharynx moderately erythematous with postnasal drip
- NECK INSPECTION AND PALPATION: no cervical lymphadenopathy, soft, supple, fully active ROM, thyroid normal size without mass
- NEUROLOGIC: hearing grossly normal, sensation of face normal and symmetric, gait normal
- CHEST: lungs are clear in all fields, HR and rhythm are regular without murmur or rub
- ABDOMEN: soft, nontender without mass or organomegaly
- SKIN: no rashes
- EXTREMITIES: no joint pain or swelling

DIFFERENTIAL DIAGNOSIS

Clinical Observations	Bacterial	Allergic	Trauma
Onset	Abrupt	Gradual	Abrupt
Fever	Yes/No	No	No
Chills	Yes/No	No	No

(continued)

Clinical Observations	Bacterial	Allergic	Trauma
Ear pain	Common	Common	Common
Sore throat	Yes/No	Yes/No	No
Nasal congestion	Yes/No	Yes	No
Nasal discharge	Yes/No	Yes	No
Postnasal drip	No	Yes	No
Cough	Yes/No	Yes	No
Fatigue	Yes/No	Yes/No	No
Headache	Yes/No	Yes/No	Yes/No
Nodes in neck	Yes/No	Yes/No	No

DIAGNOSTIC EXAMINATION

Exam	Code	Cost	Results
Otoscopy	NA	Included in office visit	Visualization of the ear canal and tympanic membrane to assess for presence of foreign body, signs of trauma, erythema, effusion, or rupture

CLINICAL DECISION MAKING

Case Study Analysis

The advanced practice provider performs the assessment and physical examination on the patient and finds the following positives: gradual onset of left ear pain with eventual rupture and drainage of effusion, nasal congestion, mild sore throat with postnasal drip, and occasional dry cough. Pertinent negatives include lack of trauma to ear, no recent swimming, and lack of fever or loss of hearing.

> **Diagnosis:** *Otitis media with effusion and rupture*

The gradual onset indicates an allergic cause for the patient's symptoms. This is supported by the patient's bilateral mild conjunctivitis, which is seen with an allergic reaction along with nasal congestion and cough. Treatment will be symptomatic to include decongestants and over-the-counter analgesics. The patient should avoid getting water into the ears and place nothing in the ears. A follow-up examination is recommended in 2 weeks.

EAR PAIN

Case Presentation: A 3-year-old girl presents to the clinic with a complaint of left ear pain for 2 days. She arrives in the company of her mother.

INTRODUCTION TO COMPLAINT

Ear pain can range from mildly uncomfortable to very painful. It can resolve spontaneously or progress to more serious infections involving the surrounding tissue, even, though rare, the brain. Several conditions can cause ear pain.

Viral or Bacterial Infections

Often ear pain can be related to an infection that has caused increased fluid and inflammation behind the tympanic membrane (TM). Bacterial infections may also occur in the ear canal or external ear, causing inflammation and/or cellulitis of the soft tissue.

Allergic Conditions

Allergic conditions, such as seasonal and environmental conditions, or allergies to a specific irritant (i.e., animal dander) can cause inflammation in the upper respiratory tract, including the Eustachian tubes. This can cause fluid accumulation in the absence of bacterial infection. Although an infection may not be present, the pressure from the fluid accumulation can still cause pressure inside the middle ear, thereby causing sensation of pain.

Neuropathic Conditions

Sometimes pain that is caused by nerve root irritation can present as ear pain. This can be caused by impingement of a nerve (auricular or temporal nerves), or may be related to activation of a viral infection, such as herpes simplex virus (HSV) or herpes zoster.

Trauma/Foreign Body (FB)

Ear pain can be caused by direct trauma to the ear or by the presence of an FB. This is typically due to a specific event.

Referred Pain

Pain felt in the ear may have a point of origin that is in the surrounding anatomic structures and is referred and/or radiating to the ear. The site of origin may be the sinus cavities, the throat, the eye, the thyroid, cervical spine, or surrounding support muscles.

HISTORY OF COMPLAINT

Symptomatology

Ask about the following characteristics of each symptom using open-ended questions:

- Onset
- Exposure to illness
- Exposure to second-hand or third-hand smoke
- History of health conditions, specifically exposure to HSV or herpes zoster
- Location of pain
- Radiation
- Character of the pain
- Aggravating factors
- Alleviating factors
- Associated symptoms
- Effect on activity level
- Effect on hearing
- History of similar episodes
- Previous treatments tried

Directed Questions to Ask (to Mother)

- Was the onset sudden or gradual?
- Has she been exposed to anyone who is sick?
- Does she or anyone in your household smoke?
- Is the pain just in the ear, or is there pain in other areas?
- How does she describe the pain?
- Is the pain interfering with activities?
- Has her hearing changed?
- Does anything make the pain better?
- Does anything make the pain worse?
- Has she had a fever?
- Has she had a runny nose?
- Has she been coughing?
- Has she been short of breath?
- Has her appetite changed?
- Has she vomited?
- Has she ever had anything like this before?
- If yes, what treatment did she receive?
- Has she ever had the chicken pox, cold sores, or shingles?

Assessment: Cardinal Signs and Symptoms

In addition to the directed questions listed previously, the following need to be included in the assessment:

Ears
- Drainage
- Edema
- Erythema
- Hearing change

Eyes
- Conjunctivitis
- Vision change
- Pain

Nose
- Congestion

Mouth and Throat
- Sore throat
- Cough
- Dental status
- Dysphagia
- Oral lesions

Neck
- Pain
- Decreased range of motion (ROM)
- Swelling
- Enlarged glands

Nervous System
- Dermatome involvement

Skin
- Rash

Other Associated Symptoms
- Fever
- Fatigue
- Headache

Medical History: General
- Medial conditions and surgeries
- Allergies (seasonal or other)
- Current medications

Medical History: Specific to Complaint
- Frequent ear infections
- Smoking history
- History of ear surgery
- Trauma to ear
- Recent history of swimming
- Recent history of travel

PHYSICAL EXAMINATION
Vital Signs
- Temperature
- Pulse
- Respiration
- Oxygen saturation (SpO_2)
- Blood pressure (BP)

General Appearance

- Apparent state of health
- Current level of comfort or distress
- Skin color and temperature
- Nutritional status
- Hydration status
- Hygiene
- Appearance in accordance with stated age
- Gait or balance difficulty

Ear Inspection

- EXTERNAL EAR: color, structure, swelling, presence of cerumen
- CANAL: redness, swelling, presence of exudate
- TYMPANIC MEMBRANE: intact, color, light reflex, landmarks, presence of effusion, injection, apparent pressure

Eye Inspection

- Drainage
- Color

Nose Inspection

- Congestion
- Drainage
- Pallor

Mouth and Throat Inspection

- Color
- Presence of lesions
- Symmetry
- Exudate

Neck Inspection and Palpation

- Symmetry
- Swelling
- Masses
- Active ROM
- Thyroid: size, symmetry, masses

Neurologic Examination

- Facial nerve assessment
- Hearing test

Associated Systems for Assessment

A complete assessment should include the respiratory system, abdominal assessment, general skin inspection, and general extremities assessment.

CASE STUDY

History

Directed Question	Response
Was the onset sudden or gradual?	*It was sudden.*
Has the child been exposed to anyone who is sick?	*She goes to day care, so it's hard to tell.*

Directed Question	Response
Do you or anyone in your household smoke?	*No.*
Is the pain just in the ear, or is there pain in other areas?	*It just seems to be the ear.*
Is she able to describe the pain?	*No.*
Is the pain interfering with activities?	*No.*
Have you noticed a hearing change?	*No.*
Does anything make the pain better?	*No.*
Does anything make the pain worse?	*No.*
Has she had a fever?	*No.*
Has she had a runny nose?	*She did about a week ago, but it's getting better.*
Has she been coughing?	*Occasionally.*
Has she been short of breath?	*No.*
Has her appetite changed?	*No.*
Has she vomited?	*No.*
Has she ever had anything like this before?	*Yes, the same time last year.*
If yes, what treatment did she receive?	*Antibiotics.*
Has she ever had chicken pox, cold sores, or shingles?	*No.*

Physical Examination Findings

- VITAL SIGNS: temperature 98.5°F; respiratory rate (RR) 22; heart rate (HR) 110; BP 92/60; SpO$_2$ 96% room air
- GENERAL APPEARANCE: well-developed, healthy-appearing child; fussy, but active
- EAR INSPECTION: right ear—external ear normal, canal without erythema or exudate, small amount of cerumen, TM pearly grey, intact with light reflex and bony landmarks present; left ear—external ear normal, canal without erythema or exudate, small amount of cerumen, TM erythematous and bulging
- EYE INSPECTION: no injection; anicteric; pupils equal, round, and reactive to light and accommodation (PERRLA); extraocular movements intact
- NOSE INSPECTION: nares are patent, no edema, minimal clear rhinorrhea
- MOUTH AND THROAT INSPECTION: no oral lesions, teeth and gums in good repair
- NECK INSPECTION AND PALPATION: no cervical lymphadenopathy, soft, supple, fully active ROM, thyroid normal size without mass
- NEUROLOGIC: hearing grossly normal, sensation of face normal and symmetric, gait normal
- CHEST: lungs are clear in all fields, HR and rhythm are regular without murmur or rub
- ABDOMEN: soft, nontender without mass or organomegaly
- SKIN: no rashes
- EXTREMITIES: no joint pain or swelling

DIFFERENTIAL DIAGNOSIS

Clinical Observations	Bacterial	Allergic	Neuropathic	Trauma/FB	Referred
Onset	Abrupt	Gradual	Either	Abrupt	Either
Fever	Yes/No	No	No	No	Yes/No
Chills	Yes/No	No	No	No	Yes/No
Sore throat	Yes/No	Yes/No	No	No	Yes/No
Nasal congestion	Yes/No	Yes	No	No	Yes/No
Nasal discharge	Yes/No	Yes	No	No	Yes/No
Postnasal drip	No	Yes	No	No	No
Cough	Yes/No	Yes	No	No	Yes/No
Fatigue	Yes/No	Yes/No	Yes/No	No	Yes/No
Headache	Yes/No	Yes/No	Yes/No	Yes/No	Yes/No
Nodes in neck	Yes/No	Yes/No	Yes/No	No	Yes/No
Thyroid disease	No	No	No	No	Yes/No
History of neck injury	No	No	Yes/No	Yes/No	Yes/No
Muscle spasm	No	No	Yes/No	Yes/No	Yes/No
History of HSV	No	No	Yes/No	No	Yes/No
Dermatome involvement	No	No	Yes	No	Yes/No
History of TMJ disorders	No	No	No	No	Yes

FB, foreign body; HSV, herpes simplex virus; TMJ, temporomandibular joint.

DIAGNOSTIC EXAMINATION

Exam	Code	Cost	Results
Otoscopy	NA	Included in office visit	Visualization of the ear canal and TM to assess for presence of FB, signs of trauma, erythema, effusion, or rupture

(continued)

Exam	Code	Cost	Results
Tympanometry	92567	$41	The measurement of pressure behind the TM does not determine whether or not an infectious process is present. Normal pressure levels are between −150 and +25 daPa. An elevated pressure indicates increased pressure behind the TM. Further assessment is necessary to determine the cause of increased pressure
Herpes simplex IgG	86694 86695 86696	$13–$17	If ear pain is neuropathic in nature with presence or history of oral lesions, this test would help determine whether nerve root irritation is a causative factor If this test returns a positive result in the presence of additional examination findings consistent with neuropathic pain, antiviral therapy may be considered to assist with suppression of HSV. Additionally, use of steroidal agents may assist with pain reduction

FB, foreign body; HSV, herpes simplex virus; IgG, immunoglobulin G; TM, tympanic membrane.

CLINICAL DECISION MAKING

Case Study Analysis

The nurse practitioner performs the assessment and physical examination on the child and finds the following pertinent positives: day–care-attending child with sudden onset of left ear pain without radiation to other areas and without discharge, with a history of similar occurrence last year. Left TM injected with effusion. Pertinent negative is absence of fever. However, she is recovering from a "runny nose" and continues to have nasal drainage and a cough, both of which contribute to the diagnosis of acute otitis media. Since the problem appeared suddenly, an allergic cause can be ruled out. The otoscopic examination did not reveal the presence of an object or other trauma to the ear canal or TM. Cough and nasal drainage would not be present if the current problem had a neuropathic or referred cause.

> **Diagnosis:** *Acute otitis media (left ear)*

Treatment would include either a systemic or topical antibiotic, over-the-counter analgesics, and warm soaks to the external ear region. The child should refrain from attending day care until symptoms subside. If changes in hearing occur, the child should be scheduled for audiometry studies. A follow-up appointment should be made with an ear, nose, and throat (ENT) physician should symptoms persist beyond 10 days to 2 weeks.

ELBOW PAIN

Case Presentation: A 37-year-old male states, "My right elbow has been hurting for weeks."

INTRODUCTION TO COMPLAINT

Elbow pain results from one of the following:

- Repetitive or overuse syndromes
- Tendon and muscle pain due to work or sports activities
- Inflammation
- Joint capsule inflammation of the internal capsule due to arthritis, gout, or infection
- Swelling
- Bursitis or swelling of the olecranon bursa from direct pressure or trauma
- Trauma
- Bone pain due to fracture of the bone due to trauma or severe stress
- Nerve entrapment
- Nerve pain or numbness and tingling along the median or ulnar nerve due to compression
- Tendonitis

HISTORY OF COMPLAINT

Symptomatology

Ask about the following characteristics of each symptom using open-ended questions:

- Onset: gradual or abrupt
- Timing and duration: intermittent or constant
- Intensity: severity of pain on a scale of 0 to 10
- Character: Is the pain sharp, dull, aching, burning?
- Radiation: Does the pain radiate into the shoulder, forearm, or wrist?
- Triggering: What movements trigger the pain?
- Alleviating: What lessens or resolves the pain?
- Effect on daily activity or sport
- Previous injury or treatment

Directed Questions to Ask

- Can you describe the injury from beginning to end? (if there was an acute injury)
- Was there immediate pain or swelling or did that occur later?
- Specifically, where does the elbow hurt, can you put a finger on it?
- What types of movement makes the pain worse?

- Does the joint ever lock?
- Do you have weakness of your handgrip or difficulty lifting?
- Has anyone pulled on your elbow?
- Do you play a particular sport or have a hobby that uses your arms, elbows, wrist, or hand?
- Do you have any numbness or tingling?
- Do you have pain that wakes you up at night?
- Do you have any other joint pains? Have there been previous injuries?

Assessment: Cardinal Signs and Symptoms

- Pain over lateral elbow
- Pain over medial elbow
- Swelling over elbow
- Decreased range of motion

Medical History: General

- Medical history of gout, osteoarthritis, or rheumatoid arthritis
- Family history of gout, osteoarthritis, or rheumatoid arthritis
- Medications
- Allergies to medications
- Social history, including occupation, habits, and activities

Medical History: Specific to Complaint

- Medical history of gout, osteoarthritis, or rheumatoid arthritis
- Family history of gout, osteoarthritis, or rheumatoid arthritis

PHYSICAL EXAMINATION
Vital Signs

- Temperature
- Pulse
- Respiration
- SpO_2
- Blood pressure (BP)

General Appearance

- Apparent state of health
- Appearance of comfort or distress
- Color
- Nutritional status
- State of hydration
- Hygiene
- Match between appearance and stated age
- Difficulty with gait or balance

Extremeties

- Humerus: The medial and lateral epicondyles form prominent bony landmarks of the distal humerus
- Ulna: The proximal ulna articulates with the humerus; the olecranon process or point of the posterior elbow joint is part of the ulna

- Radius: The proximal radial head articulates with the lateral elbow joint and allows for pronation and supination of the forearm
- Olecranon bursa: This is an external bursa that lies over the olecranon or point of the elbow joint

Neuromuscular
- Triceps extends the forearm (C7)
- The biceps flexes the forearm (C5 and C6)
- The brachioradialis assists with pronation (C6)
- The extensor carpi radialis longus extends and abducts the hand and wrists (C6)
- The supinator turns palms forward or supinates the forearm (C6 and C7)
- Ulnar and collateral ligaments stabilize the elbow joint

Neurologic Anatomy
There are three nerves that innervate the elbow joint:

- Ulnar: medial side attaches to flexors
- Median: attached to pronators and passes through the carpal tunnel at the wrist
- Radial: provides sensation to the posterior forearm and moves extensor muscles
- Cervical nerves C5 and C6 may cause radicular pain and numbness in the elbow joint

Range of Motion of the Elbow
- Flexion, extension, supination, and pronation
- Musculoskeletal examinations should be performed in a systemic manner and include the following:
  - Inspection and palpation
  - Range of motion
  - Strength testing of muscles above and below the joint
  - Special test
  - Reflexes and nerve testing
  - Vascular status

Inspection and Palpation
- Starting with the anterior elbow in supination, observe and palpate the antecubital fossa for tenderness or masses
- The biceps tendon and muscle is located superior to the fossa and a biceps tendon rupture would cause a palpable mass above the fossa
- Observe and palpate the olecranon or the posterior elbow for tenderness or swelling
- Bursitis is a common cause of nontraumatic swelling here and may be tender or nontender
- Inspect and palpate the lateral elbow for tenderness, which may indicate "tennis elbow"
- If there has been trauma, tenderness over the radial head may indicate a fracture
- Inspect and palpate the medial elbow for tenderness, which may indicate "golfer's elbow"
- If there has been trauma to the elbow, there may be tenderness along the ulnar collateral ligament
- Asses the ulnar nerve by tapping or performing Tinel's sign posterior to the medial epicondyle
- If painful, this may indicate ulnar nerve injury

Range of Motion
- Flexion/extension: 0 to 145 degrees
- Pronation: 80 to 90 degrees
- Supination: 85 to 90 degrees

Strength Testing

Test muscles against resistance on a scale of 0 to 5 for:

- Flexion
- Extension
- Pronation
- Supination

Test Ligaments Against Resistance

Exert pressure on the medial (varus) side, then laterally (valgus side), and feel for an opening on the opposite side indicating a torn or weakened ligament.

Reflexes
- Biceps (C5)
- Triceps (C7)

Tinel's Sign

Evaluate the ulnar nerve by tapping above the medial epicondyle. If there is tingling, this may mean there is ulnar nerve entrapment or cubital tunnel syndrome.

Vascular Status

Brachial and radial pulse should document that there is a normal vascular supply, especially if there has been an acute injury.

CASE STUDY

History

The patient is a 37-year-old male who is usually healthy but has a nagging pain in the right elbow lasting for the past 2 weeks. He has tried taking ibuprofen and icing it, but it does not feel better. The pain is constant but worse when he picks up a heavy suitcase. He plays tennis for 2 hours three times a week, but a month ago he increased playing to 2 hours a day. He does not have any other joint pain, stiffness, fever, or fatigue.

Directed Question	Response
Did the pain start suddenly or gradually?	*Kinda gradual.*
Was there any trauma or injury?	*No.*
Is there any stiffness, heat, or swelling?	*No.*
Is it stiff or hard to move?	*No, I can do everything with it.*
Do you have any tingling or numbness?	*No.*
Have you changed your routine activities?	*Yes, I am playing tennis daily now.*
Have you ever injured the joint before?	*No, I'm pretty lucky.*
Do any other joints hurt?	*No, just the right elbow.*
Is there a family history of arthritis?	*No, just heart disease in my dad.*

Physical Examination Findings

- VITAL SIGNS: temperature 98.6°F; RR 20 regular; PR 72 regular; blood pressure 128/72
- GENERAL APPEARANCE: athletic male in no acute distress
- NECK: full range of motion; nontender C spine
- SHOULDER: no deformity; nontender; full range of motion
- LEFT ELBOW: no deformity; nontender; full range of motion
- RIGHT ELBOW: no deformity; tender over the lateral epicondyle; pain with extension of wrist against resistance; no pain with supination or pronation
- TINEL'S SIGN: negative
- STRENGTH: biceps, triceps, supination, and pronation 5/5; valgus and varus ligaments intact
- VASCULAR: brachial and radial pulse 2+ and equal
- NEUROLOGIC: sensation intact to C6, C7, C8 light touch and sharp; brachial and brachioradialis reflex 2+ and equal

Most common causes of elbow pain are as follows.

Lateral Epicondylitis	Medial Epicondylitis
History of playing tennis or racquet sport	History of golfing, or flexing the wrist
Pain over the lateral aspect of the elbow	Pain over the medial aspect of the elbow
Pain worse on lifting heavy objects	Pain worse on lifting heavy objects
Physical examination	Physical examination
Tender over the lateral epicondyle	Tender over the medial epicondyle
Pain worse on extending the wrist against resistance	Pain worse on flexing the wrist against resistance
No pain with full range of motion	No pain with full range of motion

DIFFERENTIAL DIAGNOSIS

Clinical Observations	Epicondylitis	Fracture	Gout	Arthritis
Pain	Yes, lateral or medial	Yes, diffuse over joint	Yes, red, warm, diffuse pain	Yes, over joint lines
Range of motion	Decreased	Decreased	Decreased	Decreased
Edema	No	Yes	Yes	Slight
Decreased strength	Mild, due to pain	Yes	Due to pain	Due to pain
Numbness	No	Possible	No	No

DIAGNOSTIC EXAMINATION

Exam	Code	Cost	Results
X-ray, plain film	733120	$200	Trauma, weakness, locking; may reveal calcification or fracture
MRI	74200	$850	Suspected tendon rupture or soft tissues pathology

CLINICAL DECISION MAKING

Case Study Analysis

The clinician performs a history and physical examination and finds the following data:

- The pertinent positives are history of pain in the lateral elbow after increasing the number of hours the patient plays tennis.
- The pain is worse when the patient lifts heavy objects, and is partially relieved with rest.
- There is no numbness, tingling, or weakness to suggest nerve involvement.
- The physical examination confirms tenderness over the lateral epicondyle with normal joint motion otherwise.
- In the presence of full range of motion without pain, arthritis or gout is less likely.
- The patient has no edema, redness, or warmth over the elbow joint, which rules out a fracture, gout, or arthritis.

Based on the findings it is recommended that the patient reduce the number of hours of playing tennis. Treatment consists of applying ice, as needed, for 20 minutes maximum, three to four times a day, and use over-the-counter analgesics for pain management. The patient was instructed to return for a follow-up appointment if the symptoms do not subside over the next 2 to 4 weeks.

> ***Diagnosis:*** *Lateral epicondylitis*

Lateral epicondylitis is the most common cause of tendonitis. It is a clinical diagnosis and rarely is any diagnostic study needed unless there is a history of injury or weakness or nerve deficits are noted on examination.

ENLARGED LYMPH NODES

Case Presentation: A 64-year-old female presents to urgent care with swelling of a mass in her neck for the past 4 weeks.

INTRODUCTION TO COMPLAINT

There are numerous lymph nodes throughout the body. A few areas are palpable, namely, the submandibular, axillary, and inguinal regions. Most enlarged nodes are benign. If a node is larger than 1 cm, it should be considered potentially abnormal and if it is 3 cm or greater, suspect neoplastic (cancer) disease.

Common causes of enlarged lymph nodes are infections and malignancies. When a node is enlarged due to an infection it is called a "reactive node."

Bacterial Infections

- AIDS or HIV infection
- Mononucleosis
- Toxoplasmosis
- Secondary syphilis
- AIDS-related complex

Malignancy

- Non-Hodgkin's lymphoma
- Hodgkin's disease in advanced stages
- Leukemia

HISTORY OF COMPLAINT

Symptomatology

Ask about the following characteristics of each symptom using open-ended questions:

- Chronology
- Current situation (improving or deteriorating)
- Location
- Radiation
- Quality
- Timing (frequency, duration)
- Severity
- Precipitating and aggravating factors
- Relieving factors
- Associated symptoms
- Effects on daily activities

- Previous diagnosis of similar episodes
- Previous treatments
- Efficacy of previous treatments

Directed Questions to Ask

- Can you remember how long this swelling of the node has been present?
- Can you describe the way it feels? Is it hard, rubbery, or soft?
- Has it changed in size, shape, or consistency over time?
- Has it been tender?
- Have you had any fever, chills, sweats, or weight loss?
- Have you felt more fatigued than usual?
- Have you had any bruising or abnormal bleeding?
- Have you had more than the usual number of illnesses lately?
- Have you had a sore throat, nasal congestion, or eye infection?
- Have you had any problems with your teeth or dental infections?
- Have you had sex with men, women, or both? Do you practice safe sex?
- Have you had any sexually transmitted infections such as herpes? Do you have any open sores?
- Do you have a cat or any other animals? Have they bitten or scratched you?

Assessment: Cardinal Signs and Symptoms

Location of the Node	Questions
Submandibular	Is there a sore throat or infection in the mouth?
Cervical anterior aspect	Head, neck, or throat infection? Do you have fever, chills, sweats, or weight loss?
Cervical posterior	Have you had any localized infections of the skin in the area of the enlarged node? Infection of the scalp, mononucleosis, toxoplasmosis? Any recent contact with others who are ill? Do you have a cat?
Right supraclavicular	Do you have difficulty swallowing? Have you been a smoker? Do you have a cough?
Left supraclavicular	Do you have heartburn, lack of appetite, change in bowel habits? Have you been screened for colon cancer? When was your last Pap smear?
Epitrochlear	Do you have sores anywhere? Have you injured your hand? Do you have a cat or has any animal scratched or bitten you?
Inguinal	Do you have any open sores on the genital area? Do you have any recent injury or infection to the leg or feet?
Preauricular	Do you have pain in the eyes, discharge? Do you have pain in the ears? Do you have nasal discharge or pain?

Medical History: General

- Medical history: acute and chronic illness
- Family history: any history of cancer, sarcoidosis, tuberculosis, or autoimmune disease
- Social history, including exposures to carcinogens, tobacco, and alcohol; any pets
- Medications especially Dilantin, which may cause a reactive node

Medical History: Specific to Complaint

- Previous history of enlarged lymph nodes
- Autoimmune disorders

PHYSICAL EXAMINATION

Vital Signs

- Temperature
- Pulse
- Respiration
- Blood pressure (BP)

General Appearance

- Overall appearance
- Any signs of obvious distress
- Color of skin
- Skin turgor
- Hygiene

Head, Eyes, Ears, Nose, Throat (HEENT)
- Examine HEENT to determine presence of infectious process especially noting dental, ears, and throat infection or abnormality

Neck
- Palpate all lymph nodes and describe size, shape, mobility, and texture

Cardiac
- Listen to heart for rate, rhythm, the presence of murmurs

Lungs
- Listen to all lobes
- Note any abnormality or diminished breath sounds that may indicate a pleural effusion

Abdomen
- Observe for enlarged abdominal girth indicating the presence of fluid
- Palpate for tenderness
- Evaluate the liver and spleen for any increase in size
- Palpate for abnormal masses

Genitourinary
- Perform a pelvic or genital examination if lesions are in the inguinal area

Rectal
- Perform a rectal examination if lesions are in the left supraclavicular or inguinal area

Skin
- Observe for jaundice, purpura, and petechial or abnormal rashes; observe for redness, scratches, or open wounds

Extremities
- Observe for edema of lower extremities, clubbing of nails, or deformity

CASE STUDY
History

Directed Question	Response
How long has swelling of the node been present?	At least 4 weeks, maybe more.
Did it occur all of the sudden?	Yes, just woke up with it.
Can you describe the way it feels?	It is just hard, no pain, just hard.
Has it changed at all?	Yes, it is twice the size it was the past month.
Have you had any fevers or chills?	No, never.
Have you had any sweats?	On occasion, I do sweat at night.
Have you lost any weight?	I wish, no, I eat well and my weight is good.
Have you been more fatigued?	A little bit, but I watch the grandbaby now.
Have you had any abnormal bruising?	No, have not noticed that.
Have you been sick a lot this year?	Yes, I watch the baby, so I am always sick.
Have you had a recent dental problem?	No, I have dentures now.
Have you had a sore throat?	Yes, about 2 months ago, with another cold.
Is it sore now?	No, it is fine.
Have you had any sinus pain?	No, nothing hurts.
Have you had nasal discharge?	Not now, that cleared up months ago.
Do you have problems swallowing?	No, I eat everything.
Do you have any cats or animals?	No, not now, our tabby died 6 months ago.
Have you had any scalp infections?	I do get dandruff now and then.
Is there anything else you would like to add?	No, you have been quite thorough.

Physical Examination Findings
- VITAL SIGNS: temperature 98.8°F; respiratory rate (RR) 20; heart rate (HR) 72; BP 124/72
- GENERAL APPEARANCE: well-developed, petite female in no distress
- EYES: no injection, anicteric, pupils equal, round, and reactive to light and accommodation (PERRLA), extraocular movements intact
- NOSE: nares are patent; no edema or exudate of turbinates
- MOUTH: teeth and gums are in good repair (gums are pink; teeth are without decay); no oral lesions
- PHARYNX: tonsils not enlarged; no redness, exudate

- NECK: right tonsillar node is 3 × 3 cm, hard, and fixed; no other anterior or posterior nodes are enlarged; neck is supple; thyroid is not enlarged
- LYMPH: axillary, epitrochlear, and inguinal nodes are not palpable
- CHEST: lungs are clear in all fields; heart S1 and S2, no murmur, gallop, or rub
- ABDOMEN: soft, obese, nontender without mass or organomegaly
- SKIN: no rashes

DIFFERENTIAL DIAGNOSIS

Clinical Observations	Oral or Pharyngeal Infection	Non-Hodgkin's Lymphoma	Mononucleosis
Onset	Gradual or sudden	Sudden	Gradual or sudden
Dental pain or sore throat	Yes	No	Yes/no
Fever	Yes	No	Yes
Weight loss	No	Later stages	No
Night sweats	If fever	Yes	If fever
Fatigue	Yes/No	Later stages	Yes
Exposed to cat	No	No	No
Node	Tender, rubbery mobile	Hard, tender, nonmobile	Tender, firm posterior and anterior

DIAGNOSTIC EXAMINATION

Exam	Code	Cost	Results

CBC	85025	$75	CBC
			The CBC typically has several parameters that are created from an automated cell counter. The most relevant are:
			• WBC count: WBCs protect the body against infection. When there is an infection present, the WBC count rises very quickly. WBC count includes a differential white count.
			• WBC differential:
			  ▪ Neutrophils: The most abundant of the WBCs increase rapidly to areas of injury and infection
			  ▪ Eosinophils: Are active during allergic or parasitic illnesses
			  ▪ Basophils: Will increase during the healing process

(continued)

Exam	Code	Cost	Results
			▪ Monocytes: Are the second defense mechanism against bacterial and inflammatory illnesses. Slower to respond than neutrophils but are bigger and can ingest larger organisms or foreign bodies ▪ Lymphocytes: Increase after chronic bacterial and viral infections ● RBCs: Carry O$_2$ from the lungs to the body. ● Hematocrit: A measure of the number of RBCs in a space. ● Hemoglobin: Protein substance that carries oxygen and gives RBCs their color. It is a good measure to determine the ability of the blood to carry oxygen throughout the body. ● MCV: Determines the volume of the RBCs. ● MCH: Shows the amount of hemoglobin contained in the average RBC. ● MCHC: Measures the concentration of the hemoglobin in an average RBC. ● Platelets: The platelets play an important role in blood clotting. If there are too few platelets, uncontrolled bleeding can occur. If there are too many, a blood clot can form in the artery.
CMP	80053	$49	● Glucose level: Elevated levels are seen in patients with diabetes, adrenal gland dysfunction, stress, burns, and most important, infection. ● Creatinine clearance: Decreased levels could be an indicator of renal impairment. ● Alkaline phosphatase, alanine aminotransferase, aspartate aminotransferase: These are all diagnostic tests that indicate how the liver is functioning.

CBC, complete blood count; CMP, complete metabolic panel; MCH, mean corpuscular hemoglobin; MCHC, mean corpuscular hemoglobin concentration; MCV, mean corpuscular volume; RBC, red blood cell; WBC, white blood cell.

CLINICAL DECISION MAKING

Case Study Analysis

Sudden onset of a large 3 × 3 cm nontender, hard, nonmobile lymph node localized to the anterior cervical chain. Patient complains of occasional night sweats but denies fever or chills. Rule out pharyngitis, dental caries and abscess, and lesions.

> **Diagnosis:** *Lymphadenopathy*

Since the development of the swelling the patient has not had a change in appetite, change in weight, or onset of fatigue. Because of ongoing exposure to infections from babysitting a grandchild, the patient should be evaluated for mononucleosis. Recommend a complete blood count (CBC) and complete metabolic panel (CMP) be drawn. The CBC will also provide information to determine if non-Hodgkin's lymphoma is present. Depending upon results of blood studies, further examination may be required from infectious disease or oncology.

EYE DISCHARGE

Case Presentation: A 6-year-old female presents with left eye redness and crusting for 2 days. She arrives in the company of her mother.

INTRODUCTION TO COMPLAINT

- Multiple conditions can lead to eye discharge
- Viral or bacterial conjunctivitis, also known as "pinkeye"; this is the most common type
- In newborns, ophthalmia neonatorum can, if not treated, lead to permanent scarring and blindness
- Viral conjunctivitis is often accompanied by an upper respiratory infection (URI)
- Viral herpes zoster, which, if not closely monitored and treated, can lead to blindness
- Allergic conjunctivitis: generally affects both eyes and is accompanied by other allergic symptoms, such as rhinitis
- Dacryostenosis is an obstruction of the nasolacrimal duct due to incomplete formation or cyst formation within; it can lead to tearing and matting in newborns
- Eyelid condition, such as blepharitis, ingrown lashes, hordeolum, or chalazion
- Injury: corneal abrasion or ulcer can lead to excessive tearing and mucoid discharge, with the possibility of superinfection

HISTORY OF COMPLAINT

Symptomatology

Ask about the following characteristics of each symptom using open-ended questions:

- Onset
- Location
- Duration, timing, frequency
- Character of the discharge or presence of pain
- Associated symptoms
- Aggravating factors
- Alleviating factors
- Effect on daily activities

Directed Questions to Ask

- Does the symptom involve one eye or both?
- Describe the discharge. Is it mucoid, pus-like, tearing, crusting? Is there any matting of the eyelashes?

- Is it worsening, improving, or remaining stable?
- Any recent illness or associated symptoms?
- Rate her discomfort on a pain scale. Is it persistent or intermittent?
- Does anything make it better (keeping eyes closed, darkening the room) or worse (light exposure, etc.)?
- Does she wear contacts?

Assessment: Cardinal Signs and Symptoms

General
- Fever, chills, malaise, pain

Eyes
- Visual disturbance, pain/itching/foreign body sensation, eyelid involvement

Head, Ears, Nose, Throat (HENT)
- Headache, photophobia, visual disturbance, runny nose, congestion, sneezing, facial swelling

Respiratory
- Cough, wheezing, dyspnea

Skin
- Rashes, local swelling

Lymph
- Swollen nodes

Medical History: General

- Medical history: medical conditions (treated and untreated), surgeries, allergies, current medications, and over-the-counter therapies
- Family medical history: medical conditions in close, blood-related relatives
- Social history: substance use (drugs/alcohol), leisure activities, recent travel/exposures

Medical History: Specific to Complaint

- Matted lashes
- Decreased visual acuity
- Tearing of the eyes
- Stringy discharge

PHYSICAL EXAMINATION

Vital Signs

- Heart rate (HR)
- Respiration
- Blood pressure (BP)
- Oxygen saturation (SpO_2)
- Temperature
- Pain scale

General Appearance
- Calm or distressed

Visual Acuity
- Corrected with glasses if patient has baseline diminished acuity
- Measure each eye in isolation as well as both together

HENT
- Lesions (especially surrounding eyes, ear canals, tip of nose)
- Rhinorrhea
- Boggy turbinates or hyperemia
- Allergic shiners
- Local swelling or swelling over nasolacrimal duct

Eyes
- Unilateral or bilateral
- Pupils equal, round, and reactive to light and accommodation (PERRLA)
- Extraocular movements
- Eyelid involvement
- Evert eyelids for examination
- Matting of lashes
- Conjunctival injection
- Ciliary flush
- Fluorescein uptake (extent, location, pattern)
- Peripheral vision
- Corneal opacity/cloudiness

Neck
- Lymphadenopathy

CASE STUDY
History

Directed Question	Response
Which eye is bothering her? Or is it both?	*Left eye.*
Can you describe the drainage for me?	*There is a stringy discharge during the day. It's crusty, and gets on her eyelashes at night.*
When did it begin?	*She woke up with it yesterday morning.*
Has she had any injuries or exposures?	*No.*
Is it worsening, improving, or remaining stable?	*It's worst in the mornings, and it seems to be worse today than yesterday.*
Has she had any recent illness?	*Upper respiratory infection. She's had a runny nose for a week. No fever.*
Are there any associated symptoms?	*Just the runny nose; itchy throat.*
Has she complained of eye pain?	*No, she hasn't complained at all, she just keeps rubbing and wiping it.*

Directed Question	*Response*
Does she have any medical problems that you are aware of?	*She was premature (2 weeks) and she had a hernia repair. Nothing else significant.*
Do you have any concerns for her vision?	*I don't think so.*
How does it feel? Does it hurt? Is it itchy?	*Patient: It scratches me! [rubbing eyes].*

Physical Examination Findings

- VITAL SIGNS: temperature 98.6°F (oral); RR 20; HR 90; BP 128/80; SpO$_2$ 96% room air; no pain
- GENERAL APPEARANCE: alert, very active, and friendly
- VISUAL ACUITY: oculus dexter (OD) 20/40; oculus sinister (OS) 20/40-1; oculus uterque (OU) 20/40
- HENT: no rashes or lesions; moderate mucoid rhinitis; tympanic membrane dullness bilaterally
- EYES: PERRLA 3+, extraocular movement intact (EOMI); fluorescein examination—no uptake, except for slight mucoid drainage to inner canthus; left eye—both eyelids everted for examination; mild injection in left eye, no ciliary flush; minimal crusting noted to lower lateral lashes; no lid lesions or swelling; rubbing eyes frequently throughout examination
- NECK/LYMPH: supple, no lymphadenopathy
- CARDIOVASCULAR: regular rate and rhythm (RRR), no murmurs
- LUNGS: clear to auscultation (CTA), good air entry bilaterally, no respiratory distress
- SKIN: warm and dry with good color; no rashes noted

DIFFERENTIAL DIAGNOSIS

Clinical Observations	Bacterial Conjunctivitis	Viral Conjunctivitis	Allergic Conjunctivitis	Dacryostenosis	Injury	Gonorrhea/ Chlamydia	Blepharitis
History	Possible known history of exposure, especially among children	Often associated with URI symptoms but may occur in isolation	Possible known or suspected exposure; consider environmental as well as topical (makeup, etc.) or aerosolized agents	Noted at or shortly after birth	Often recalls specific incident of foreign body to the eye or irritant exposure	Born vaginally to mother with active chlamydia/gonorrhea infection or no prenatal care; can also be self-inoculated by touching infected genitals and then eyes	May have concurrent history of seborrheic dermatitis
Age	Most common in children, can occur at any age	Most common in children, can occur at any age	Usually adult onset	Most common in newborns, usually resolves within first year of life	Any	Neonate (generally 5–14 days after delivery), or concurrent genital infection	Any
Discomfort	Irritation	Itching, gritty sensation, or burning	Itching, gritty sensation, or burning		Pain or foreign body sensation	Irritation	Irritation
Discharge	Copious purulent; may be white, yellow, or green with morning matting; accumulates in corners of the eye and on lid margins	Mucoid and crusting	Tearing and mucoid (stringy)	Chronic or intermittent tearing, often eyelash matting; tears/mucoid discharge with palpation of lacrimal duct	Tearing	Can begin as watery discharge, progresses to mucopurulent	Crusting at lid margins, or greasy flakes

(continued)

Clinical Observations	Bacterial Conjunctivitis	Viral Conjunctivitis	Allergic Conjunctivitis	Dacryostenosis	Injury	Gonorrhea/ Chlamydia	Blepharitis
Rhinitis	No	Common	Common		No	No	No
Unilateral or bilateral	Unilateral or bilateral	Often unilateral at first and proceeds to bilateral in 1 to 2 days	Bilateral (unless unilateral direct contact with irritant)	Usually unilateral	Usually unilateral	Bilateral in ophthalmia neonatorum; unilateral or bilateral in the adult	Bilateral
Eyelid involvement	No	No	Sometimes			Yes	Yes, reddened, often with dry flaking skin; waxy secretions may occur at Meibomian gland openings
Other	Tarsal conjunctivae injected	Tarsal conjunctivae injected	Tarsal conjunctivae injected	May find swelling of skin overlying nasolacrimal duct	Special attention in patients wearing contact lenses	Eye discharge may become blood-stained and pseudomembrane may form; referral is indicated	Inflammation at lid margins; tear film irregularity

URI, upper respiratory infection.

DIAGNOSTIC EXAMINATION

Exam	Code	Cost	Results	Notes
Rapid adenovirus test	87809QW	$15	Positive = viral conjunctivitis	An inconclusive test that does not help with diagnosis; acceptable sensitivity and specificity; can help prevent antibiotic misuse
Fluorescein examination	92225–92260	NA	Uptake indicates disruption in corneal surface	
Visual acuity	99172	NA	Red flag: gross loss of vision	Test corrected vision if possible
Culture	87040–87255	$35	Positive = bacterial conjunctivitis Rapid onset	Must be collected from everted eyelid, simple exudate collection insufficient because sample must include conjunctival epithelial cells

CLINICAL DECISION MAKING

Case Study Analysis

The advanced practice provider performs the assessment and physical examination on the patient and describes 36 hours' duration of unilateral pinkeye with crusting. Left eye exhibits mild but diffuse injection, including injection of the tarsal conjunctiva. The child also exhibits a copiously runny nose. Her history and examination are notable for the absence of periorbital edema or eye pain. On fluorescein examination there is no uptake of dye to suggest a corneal abrasion. Visual acuity is 20/20.

Considering the recent history of a URI, persistent nasal drainage, and ongoing wiping of the eye, allergic conjunctivitis most likely can be ruled out. The symptoms are most likely not caused by an injury or blepharitis. Other potential causes for conjunctivitis can be ruled out based upon the patient's age and symptoms.

> **Diagnosis:** *Viral conjunctivitis*

- At times, a patient will present with a confusing history regarding the nature of the discharge that does not effectively point toward a viral or bacterial cause
- Swab for adenovirus can be helpful
- Those who present with classic viral conjunctivitis require good handwashing, gentle and frequent cleansing of crusting, and the passage of time
- Excessive itching can often be improved with the use of artificial tears (or eye lubricant ointment) for comfort or, if needed, topical ophthalmic antihistamine/decongestant drops
- Antibiotics are not indicated
- Anticipatory guidance should include that it may worsen over the next few days and/or spread to the other eye, and recovery may take 2 weeks or more; a cool compress may provide comfort in the interim, along with gentle eyelid cleansing from the inner canthus outward along closed eyelids

The patient should be instructed on handwashing and the mother should be reminded to isolate the patient's face cloths and towels to prevent spreading the infection to other family members.

EYE PAIN

> **Case Presentation:** *A 74-year-old man is complaining of left eye pain, which began when he woke up from a nap. The pain worsened rapidly and he has a headache, nausea, and blurred vision in the affected eye.*

INTRODUCTION TO COMPLAINT

Primary causes of eye pain are:

- Ocular trauma
  - Corneal abrasion
- Infection
  - Bacterial conjunctivitis
- Inflammation
  - Iritis/uveitis
  - Scleritis
- Increased intraocular pressure (IOP)
  - Acute angle glaucoma

HISTORY OF COMPLAINT

Symptomatology

Ask about the following characteristics of each symptom using open-ended questions:

- Onset
- Duration, timing, frequency of pain
- Location
- Character of pain
- Associated symptoms
- Aggravating factors
- Alleviating factors
- Effect on daily activities

Directed Questions to Ask

- Can you tell me about your eye pain?
- Was the onset sudden or gradual?
- Where exactly in the eye is your pain?
- Are both eyes involved or is the pain only in your left eye?
- How would you describe your pain: is it like stabbing, throbbing, burning, sharp, aching pain, or a "something in my eye" feeling?
- Is your pain continuous or intermittent and, if it is intermittent, how long does it last?
- If 0 is no pain and 10 is the worst pain you have ever had, what number is this pain?

- Is the pain worse when you move your eyes?
- Is there anything that precipitates or aggravates your symptoms?
- Is there anything that alleviates your pain?
- Did something get into your eye?
- How is your vision? Is it blurred or do you feel blind spots that suddenly appear?
- Do you have photophobia or double vision?
- Is the eye dry or watering?
- Do you have eye itching?
- What other symptoms do you have?
- What concerns you most about the pain?
- Did you ever have this type of eye pain before? If yes, what was the treatment you received?

Assessment: Cardinal Signs and Symptoms

Head
- Headache? Unilateral or bilateral? Throbbing or aching
- On a scale of 0 to 10, if 0 is no pain and 10 is the worst pain you ever had, how bad is the pain?
- Is the pain continuous or intermittent?

Nose and Sinuses
- Facial tenderness, pain, or pressure
- Nasal/sinus congestion or stuffiness
- Nasal congestion on one or both sides
- Loss of smell

Ears
- How is your hearing?
- Any history of hearing loss
- Ear ache or pain in the ear

Other Associated Symptoms
- Fever
- Cough
- Nausea or vomiting
- Anxious or stressed

Medical History: General

- Medical conditions like diabetes, high blood pressure (BP), high cholesterol, tuberculosis (TB), or any previous herpes infections like cytomegalovirus (CMV)
- Stroke or family history of stroke or other neurologic problems
- Chronic headache or migraine
- Heart problems or history of cardiovascular disease like heart failure, heart attack, or cardiovascular occlusion
- Breathing or respiratory problems in the past
- Surgeries in the past
- Allergies to foods, medications, or plants
- Seasonal allergy
- Sinusitis
- Current use of medications, including prescription medications
- Use of over-the-counter medications
- Use of any herbal preparations or traditional therapies

Medical History: Specific to Complaint

- Frequent eye pain or infections
- Diagnosis of glaucoma, retinopathy, or retinal hemorrhage
- Trauma to eyes
- Past eye surgery
- Exposure to chemicals

PHYSICAL EXAMINATION

Vital Signs

- Temperature
- Respiration
- Heart rate
- Blood pressure

General Appearance

- Overall appearance
- Any signs of obvious distress
- Skin color, turgor, capillary refill response
- Difficulty with gait or balance

Head

- Inspect for lesions or trauma
- Inspect for involuntary movement

Eyes

- Inspect for any redness in eyes
- Any change in vision
- Photophobia

Ear

- Hearing

Nose and Sinus

- Drainage and edema
- Inspect for tenderness

Neurologic

- Mental status
- Cranial nerves
- Motor system
- Reflexes

CASE STUDY

History

Directed Question	Response
Can you tell me about your eye pain?	I can't open my eyes; it hurts so bad.
Was the onset sudden or gradual?	It was sudden and I'm scared.
Where exactly in the eye is your pain?	It seems to come from inside my eye.

Directed Question	*Response*
Are both eyes involved or is it only in your left eye?	*Only my left eye hurts.*
Is your pain radiating to anywhere else?	*Yes, to the back of my eye.*
How would you describe your pain?	*It's like a hot poker in the center of my eye.*
Is your pain continuous or intermittent?	*It is continuous.*
On a scale of 0 to 10, with 10 being the worst pain you have ever had, what number is this pain?	*13, the pain is so bad that I don't think I can take it anymore.*
Is the pain worse when you move your eyes?	*No.*
Is there anything that precipitates or aggravates your symptoms?	*Light increases the pain.*
Is there anything that alleviates your pain?	*Nothing seems to help.*
Did something get into your eye?	*No.*
How is your vision: Is it blurred or do you see blind spots?	*I think I can see well.*
Do you have double vision?	*No.*
Is the eye dry or watering?	*No.*
Does your eye itch?	*No.*
What other symptoms do you have?	*I have a constant headache. This pain affects my thinking.*
What concerns you most about the pain?	*The pain is so bad I'm afraid.*
Did you ever have this type of eye pain before?	*No.*

Physical Examination Findings

- VITAL SIGNS: temperature 98.6°F; respiratory rate 22, regular; pulse 92, regular; blood pressure 135/82
- GENERAL APPEARANCE: appears distressed and in pain; difficulty answering questions and keeping his eyes open; skin pale and sweaty
- HEAD: free of lesions or evidence of trauma; normocephalic, normal hair distribution; brows symmetrical
- EYES: clear; patient complains of blurred vision, and visual acuity test reveals the ability to detect only hand movements; patient unable to identify numbers and letters on distance charts or near cards; cornea and scleral injection and ciliary flush are present; the obviously edematous and cloudy cornea obscures funduscopic examination; extremely hard to examine left eye due to patient's complaint of pain; increased IOP (normal limit, 10–20 mmHg) and ischemia result in pain on eye movement, a mid-dilated nonreactive pupil, and a firm globe

DIFFERENTIAL DIAGNOSIS

Clinical Observations	Cerebrovascular Accident	Uveitis	Traumatic Hyphema	Acute Angle Closure Glaucoma	Migraine
Onset	Sudden	Gradual/ abrupt	Abrupt	Sudden	Sudden
Pain	Pain	Aching	Yes	Severe	Severe
Vision loss	Blurred/loss	Blurred	Yes	Blurred	Blurred
Bleeding eye	No	Yes	Yes	No	No
Light sensitivity	Photophobia	Photophobia	No	No	Photophobia
Numbness/ weakness/paralysis	Yes	No	No	No	No
Pupil	No	No	No	Nonreactive	No
Headache	Severe	Rare	No	Severe	Severe
Nausea/vomiting	Common	Rare	Common	Yes	Yes
Intraocular pressure	No	Rare	Common	High >21	No
Red eye	No	Common	No	Yes	No
Floaters	No	Common	Rare	Rare	No
Photophobia	No	No	No	No	Common

DIAGNOSTIC EXAMINATION

Exam	Code	Cost	Results
Physical examination	99397	$250	• Nonreactive pupils can also be a sign of intracranial injury.
Tonometry	89.11	Cost varies depending on age and comorbid factors	• Tonometry measures the pressure within the eyes. Most glaucoma cases are diagnosed with pressure exceeding 20 mmHg. In IOP, it will be more than 21 mmHg in most of the cases. • This examination helps to determine the angle where the iris meets the cornea • If the angle is narrow and closed, then it is closed-angle glaucoma

(continued)

Exam	Code	Cost	Results
Perimetry	92083	Cost varies depending on age and comorbid factors	• Perimetry is a visual field test that determines how much of the vision is affected • Checks peripheral vision
CT scan of the brain	70450	$1,250	• Visualizes components of the brain, size, location, and integrity

IOP, intraocular pressure.

CLINICAL DECISION MAKING

Case Study Analysis

The provider performs the physical examination on the patient and finds the following data: sudden onset of left eye pain, worsening eye pain 30 minutes after the complaint, with headache, nausea, and blurred vision. The reaction to light of the left pupil is sluggish compared to the right eye; unable to examine left eye. Even though the onset of pain was sudden, it is unlikely to be caused by a cardiovascular accident due to the absence of other physiological symptoms. Headache is localized within the eye and absence of photophobia rules out a cardiovascular accident, uveitis, and a migraine.

> **Diagnosis:** *Acute angle closure glaucoma*

Pressure inside the eye rises suddenly. Symptoms include severe eye pain, nausea and vomiting, headache, and decreased vision. These symptoms are an emergency and need immediate treatment to prevent blindness.

The patient is directed to the nearest emergency department for emergency ophthalmologic care.

EYE REDNESS

Case Presentation: *A 12-year-old female patient complains of red left eye and edematous eyelids. Her mother states the child complains of "sand in my left eye."*

INTRODUCTION TO COMPLAINT

Red eyes are caused by swollen or dilated blood vessels on the sclera. Red eyes can be accompanied by itching, pain, discharge, swelling, and visual acuity changes.

Viral Infections

- Red eyes can be caused by viral illness, such as those caused by adenovirus, picornavirus, rhinovirus, and herpes simplex virus.
- Viral conjunctivitis has a gradual onset with unilateral symptoms and no pain.
- Visual acuity is intact.
- Watery discharge is apparent.
- Blepharitis is the most common cause of inflammation of the eyelid. It is bilateral and associated with conjunctivitis.

Bacterial Infections

- A bacterial infection can also cause red eyes.
- *Staphylococcus aureus, Streptococcus pneumonia,* group A *Streptococcus, Haemophilus influenza,* and *Neisseria gonorrhoeae* are the most common causes of bacterial conjunctivitis.
- Bacterial conjunctivitis has a gradual onset, unilateral early, bilateral late; scratchy (no pain); photophobia (not generally present).
- The thick crusty discharge that is present in bacterial infections may cause "blurry" vision.
- Blepharitis can also be caused by bacterial infections.

Irritants and Injuries

- Trauma to the eye can also cause red eyes.
- Improper contact lens care can cause keratitis or fungal eye infections and lead to red eyes.
- Subconjunctival hemorrhage can cause the eye to appear red due to broken blood vessels present in the conjunctival tissues.

Allergic Conjunctivitis

- Allergic conjunctivitis is a chronic and seasonal condition that can cause the eyes to be bilaterally red and itchy. It is painless and causes a mucoid discharge.

HISTORY OF COMPLAINT

Symptomatology

Ask about the following characteristics of each symptom using open-ended questions:

- Chronology
- Current situation (improving or deteriorating)
- Location
- Radiation
- Quality
- Timing (frequency, duration)
- Severity
- Precipitating and aggravating factors
- Relieving factors
- Associated symptoms
- Effects on daily activities
- Previous diagnosis of similar episodes
- Previous treatments
- Efficacy of previous treatments

Directed Questions to Ask

- When did you first notice the redness and tearing?
- Was the onset gradual or sudden?
- Do you have any known allergies?
- Have your symptoms gotten worse since you first noticed them?
- What symptom did you notice first and how did your symptoms progress?
- Have you been around anyone who has had an eye infection?
- Do you have any pain in either eye?
- Have you had any symptoms other than redness, tearing, swelling, and "sand in eye feeling" (such as nausea, vomiting, sore throat, fever, coughs, etc.)?
- Do you have any thick discharge from or crusting of either eye?
- Have your symptoms affected your ability to see well?
- Have you injured your eye?
- Do you wear contacts?

Assessment: Cardinal Signs and Symptoms

Head, Eyes, Ears, Nose, Throat
- Sore throat recently
- Runny nose
- Sneezing
- Enlarged lymph nodes
- Itchy eyes
- Crust in eyes

Medical History: General

- Medical conditions and surgeries
- Allergies
- Medication currently used, including over-the-counter medications
- Herbal or traditional therapies

Medical History: Specific to Complaint

- Frequent eye infections
- Glasses or contacts
- Last eye examination
- Double vision, blurred vision, spots, specks, flashing lights

PHYSICAL EXAMINATION
Vital Signs

- Weight
- Temperature
- Pulse
- Respiration
- Oxygen saturation (SpO_2)
- Blood pressure (BP)

General Appearance

- Apparent state of health
- Appearance of comfort or distress
- Color
- Nutritional status
- State of hydration
- Hygiene

Eye Inspection

- Position and alignment of eyes
- Eyebrows: noticing their quantity and distribution, scaliness of underlying skin
- Eyelids: width, edema, color, lesions, condition, and direction of eyelashes, adequacy with which the eyelids close
- Lacrimal apparatus: inspect lacrimal gland and sac for swelling, excessive tearing, or dryness
- Conjunctiva and sclera
- Cornea and lens
- Iris
- Pupils

Palpation

- Tenderness, enlargement, mobility, contour, and consistency of nodes and masses
- Nodes: pre- and post-auricle, occipital, tonsillar, submandibular, submental

CASE STUDY
History

Directed Question	Response
When did you first notice the redness and tearing?	*3 days ago.*
Was the onset gradual or sudden?	*Gradual.*
Do you have any known allergies?	*None known.*
Have your symptoms gotten worse since you first noticed them?	*Yes.*

Directed Question	*Response*
What symptoms did you notice first and how did your symptoms progress?	*Redness when I first woke up this morning then pain due to gritty feeling.*
Have you been around anyone who has had an eye infection that you were aware of?	*[Mother] Yes, my little girl was exposed to another child in her class with eye infection.*
Do you have any pain in either eye?	*No, just feels like I have something in my eye.*
Have you had any symptoms other than the redness, tearing, swelling, and "sand in eye feeling" (such as nausea, vomiting, sore throat, fever, coughs, etc.)?	*No.*
Do you have any thick discharge or crusting of either eye?	*Yes, crust around my left eye, difficult to open it up this morning.*
Have your symptoms affected your ability to see well?	*Yes. With difficulty opening up my eye when the crust builds up.*
Have you injured your eye?	*No.*
Do you wear contacts?	*No.*

Physical Examination Findings

- VITAL SIGNS: temperature 98.2°F; respiratory rate (RR) 18; heart rate (HR) 78; BP 128/82; SpO$_2$ 96% room air; weight 110 lb
- GENERAL APPEARANCE: well-developed, healthy, 12 years old
- EYES: very red sclera with dried, crusty exudates; unable to open eyes in the morning— with the left being worse than the right
- EARS: no edema; no exudates
- NOSE: no edema; no exudates; no boggy turbinates
- MOUTH: no edema; no exudates
- PHARYNX: moderately large; no exudates
- NECK: no edema; no palpable nodes; neck is supple; thyroid not enlarged

DIFFERENTIAL DIAGNOSIS

Clinical Observations	Bacterial Conjunctivitis	Blepharitis	Viral Conjunctivitis	Allergic Conjunctivitis
Both eyes	Yes	Yes	No	Yes
Sclera	Red	Red	Red	Red
Itchiness	Yes	Yes	Yes	Yes
Exudate	Yes	Yes	Yes	Yes
Epiphora	Yes	Yes	Yes	Yes
Boggy turbinates	No	No	No	Yes

DIAGNOSTIC EXAMINATION

Exam	Code	Cost	Results
Vision screening	V72.0	$50 to $100	Determine visual acuity
Eye examination	V72.0	$50 to $100	Examine corneal light reflex, accommodation, strabismus, and extraocular movements
Eye culture and sensitivity	372.3	$35 to $55	Identify whether bacteria is present
Wood's lamp test	V72.0	Part of the eye examination	Assess for corneal abrasion
Transillumination of the sinus cavity	V72.0	Part of the physical examination fee, which varies between providers	Assess for consolidation of the sinuses

CLINICAL DECISION MAKING

Case Study Analysis

The advanced practice provider performs the assessment and physical examination on the patient and finds the following pertinent positives: bilateral redness of sclera, exudates, profuse tearing, and edematous eyelids. The patient complains of "sand" in left eye. The pertinent negatives are no loss of vision, history of trauma, or severe eye pain. Absence of boggy turbinates rules out allergic conjunctivitis. Since both eyes are affected, viral conjunctivitis can be ruled out. And since the sclera is reddened and not the eyelids, blepharitis can be ruled out.

> **Diagnosis:** *Bacterial conjunctivitis*

It is important to remember that eye infections are treated empirically with antibiotic eye drops. It is not necessary to culture the eye discharge. The symptoms usually resolve in 2 to 3 days. Persistent redness, vision change, or pain warrants immediate referral to an ophthalmologist.

FAINTING

Case Presentation: *A 74-year-old female presenting with a complaint of fainting spells.*

INTRODUCTION TO COMPLAINT

Syncope is a symptom in which transient loss of consciousness occurs; it is usually brief and self-limiting and spontaneously terminates after the episode of cerebral nutrient delivery deficit is corrected. It is most commonly caused by a transient fall in systemic blood pressure, below the level required to provide the brain with adequate cerebral blood flow; however, other causes exist.

Determining the cause of the fall in blood pressure is vital as it is the mechanism that requires treatment within the patient's system. Such causes can be vasovagal/Valsalva-maneuver related, arrhythmias (brady or tachy), cerebrovascular disease, orthostatic hypotension/autonomic dysfunction, drug-induced, dehydration, or hyperventilation.

HISTORY OF COMPLAINT

Symptomatology

Ask about the following characteristics of each symptom using open-ended questions:

- Onset
- Chronology
- Current situation
- Timing (frequency, duration)
- Severity
- Precipitating/aggravating factors
- Alleviating factors
- Associated symptoms
- Effects on daily activities
- Previous diagnosis of similar episodes
- Previous treatments and their effectiveness in symptom relief

Directed Questions to Ask

- Describe how you feel when it happens.
- Is it sudden or gradual when it happens?
- Which activities are you doing when it happens?
- How does it resolve itself? Does it resolve quickly or slowly?
- Do you notice any limb-specific weakness or numbness, is it on one side of your body?
- Does it occur more during the morning, during the day, or at night?

- How frequently does it happen?
- Do you have fatigue?
- Have you sustained any injuries from falling?
- What medications do you take? Do any of them make you sleepy or dizzy?
- Does anyone in your family have a history of heart attack or stroke?
- Have you ever had a heart attack or stroke?
- Do you feel out of breath before or when it happens?
- How have these episodes kept you from doing your normal routine?

Assessment: Cardinal Signs and Symptoms

General
- Fatigue
- Anxiety
- Unexplained weight loss or gain

Cardiac
- Arrhythmia
- Tachycardia
- Murmurs
- Sensation of pounding or fluttering in the chest or neck

Neurologic
- Vision changes
- Tingling or numbness
- Dizziness
- Previous loss of consciousness or head trauma

Respiratory
- Wheezing
- Shortness of breath
- Tachypnea
- Orthopnea
- Air hunger

Head, Eyes, Ears, Nose, Throat (HEENT)
- Tinnitus
- Loss of balance

Musculoskeletal
- Swelling in lower extremities
- Weakness
- Impaired gait

Medical History

- Medical conditions: osteoarthritis, diabetes mellitus type 2, stress incontinence, hyperlipidemia, seasonal allergies
- Surgery: right hip hemiarthroplasty 2009, tubal ligation 1977
- Patient denies history of heart attack, arrhythmia or stroke, father died of heart attack at age 60, mother died of heart attack at age 66
- Psychiatric: denies depression, anxiety, suicidal ideation or domestic violence
- Patient has not had a primary care visit in over 18 months

- Medications: metformin 500 mg twice a day with meals, simvastatin 20 mg HS, loratadine 10 mg daily as needed for allergies, ibuprofen 400 mg every 6 hours as needed for arthritis pain
- Allergies: no known drug allergies (NKDA)
- Patient denies illicit drugs, denies ever having smoked, drinks 1 glass of wine every Sunday at family dinner
- Diet/exercise: she states she used to walk 1 mile every day at the local YMCA but has not done so in six months as she feels she "does not have the energy" recently; she states she tries to follow diabetic diet at home but enjoys pastries and sweets "at family meals" and does not check her blood sugar regularly because "the doctor said my numbers were good last time"

PHYSICAL EXAMINATION

Vital Signs

- Temperature
- Pulse
- Respiration
- Oxygen saturation (SpO_2)

General Appearance

HEENT

- Symmetry
- Pupils equal and reactive

Neck

- Carotid bruit
- Jugular vein distention (JVD)
- Lymph node swelling
- Thyroid swelling

CV

- Heart sounds
- Murmurs
- Rate and rhythm
- Cap refill
- Cyanosis

Neurologic

- Vision changes
- Numbness/tingling
- Deficits

Respiratory

- Breath sounds
- Dyspnea
- Cough
- Orthopnea

CASE STUDY
History

Directed Question	Response
Describe how you feel when it happens	I just feel light-headed and like I can't get my balance until I have to sit down, if I don't sit down right away I'm afraid I will fall.
Is it sudden or gradual when it happens?	It usually catches me by surprise and happens suddenly.
Which activities are you doing when it happens?	Walking up the stairs or carrying groceries or laundry into the house.
How does it resolve itself? Does it resolve quickly or slowly?	As long as I sit down right away, the feeling passes in a few moments. But then I sit longer to make sure my spell is over.
Do you notice any limb-specific weakness or numbness, is it on one side of your body?	No, I haven't noticed any numbness but my fingertips sometimes tingle when it happens. It goes away when I feel better.
Does it occur more during the morning, during the day, or at night?	It usually happens during the day when I'm walking around or doing housework.
How frequently does it happen?	Maybe once or twice a week.
Do you have fatigue?	I have been feeling more tired lately, I think my allergies are just flaring up, so I can't breathe as well as I usually do.
Do you feel out of breath before or when it happens?	Almost always, but I'm always breathing a little harder these days up and down the stairs. I'm out of shape because I haven't done my walking in a few months because of my allergies.
Have you sustained any injuries from falling?	I fell on my butt in the kitchen the past week when I was carrying groceries to the sink, I couldn't get to a chair fast enough to sit down. But I think my groceries were too heavy and pulled me off balance.
What medications do you take? Do any of them make you sleepy or dizzy?	I take metformin, simvastatin, and Claritin every day. I don't like the heavy pain pills, I'm afraid I'll get addicted to them so I just take Advil when my arthritis is bothering me.
Does anyone in your family have a history of heart attack or stroke?	Mom and Dad both passed away of heart attacks in their sixties. That's why I try to stay active and watch my cholesterol.
Have you ever had a heart attack or stroke?	No, and I haven't had any chest pain ever so I think I would know if I had a heart attack.
How have these episodes kept you from doing your normal routine?	I don't walk at the Y anymore because I feel tired and out of breath, and I'm having a harder time sleeping soundly at night. I'm most comfortable sleeping in my recliner nowadays.

Physical Examination Findings

- VITAL SIGNS: temperature 98.4°F; 20 R/min; 90 bpm; 140/96; 96% on room air
- GENERAL APPEARANCE: patient is well-groomed, age-appropriate in appearance and in no apparent distress
- HEENT: face symmetrical, no ptosis or droop noted, pupils equal, round, and reactive to light and accommodation (PERRLA)
- NECK: no lymphadenopathy noted, no carotid bruit upon auscultation, JVD noted
- CARDIOVASCULAR: S3 heart tone heard, regular rhythm, no rub or murmur heard, +1 pitting edema of bilateral ankles, nonpitting edema of fingers; capillary refill longer than 2 seconds, mild cyanosis in toenail beds
- RESPIRATORY: lungs with diffuse crackles at bases, symmetrical chest wall movement, moderate dyspnea with exertion, per patient report
- NEUROLOGIC: no vision changes, denies numbness/tingling, complains of feet constantly feeling "cold"
- GASTROINTESTINAL: denies nausea, vomiting; more than 15 lb weight gain "recently my pants don't fit my belly," bowel sounds active in all four quadrants, abdomen firm and nontender, hepatomegaly noted; patient states bowel movements remain daily and regular
- MUSCULOSKELETAL: normal, active range of motion (ROM) in all extremities, nonpitting swelling of finger and knees joints, 5/5 strength in all extremities
- SKIN: bilateral lower extremities pale and slightly cool, intact, dry with no discolorations noted

DIFFERENTIAL DIAGNOSIS

Clinical Observations	Arrhythmia	Transient Ischemic Attack	Heart Failure	Carotid Stenosis
Onset	Sudden	Sudden	Gradual	Gradual
Dyspnea	Yes/No	No	Yes	No
Duration	Varies	Short	Months to years	Until treatment
Fatigue	Yes/No	Yes/No	Yes	No
Weight changes	Yes/No	No	Yes	No
Edema	Yes/No	No	Yes/No	No
Dizziness	Varies	Common	Varies	Common
Effect of respiratory effort	Yes/No	None	Yes	None
Numbness/tingling	Rare	Common	Varies	Common

DIAGNOSTIC EXAMINATION

Exam	Code	Cost	Results
EKG	93000	$41	**Normal (negative results):** Normal sinus rhythm with no electrical changes • PR interval <0.2 seconds • QRS interval <0.12 seconds • T waves: no depression or elevation >1 mm • No U waves • Intervals regular **Abnormal (positive results):** Atrial arrhythmia—absence of P waves, irregularity between matching of P to QRS waves (not coordinated, extra P waves to QRS, no relationship between the two). Ventricular arrhythmia—might indicate no P waves with QRS complexes, abnormal QRS complex (notched, wide, multifocal) indicative of heart blocks or conduction failure
Stress echocardiogram	A69.21	$547	**Normal (negative) results:** EF 50%–80% Intracardiac dimensions LV diameter systolic = 2.3–3.5 cm (in women) LV diameter diastolic = 4.0–5.2 cm No abnormal wall movements are noted, no regurgitation through the valves is noted, no thrombi within the heart are noted During stress portion, no decompensation of heart function and cardiac output is noted with increased workload on heart **Abnormal (positive) results:** EF is less than or equal to 40% Areas of akinesis or unsynchronized movement of the heart wall muscles Regurgitation of blood through the heart valves, incomplete emptying of the heart chambers Heart valve stenosis, vegetation or calcification noted on valves Intracardiac dimensions outside of normal ranges i.e., systolic/diastolic measurements larger than expected Presence of thrombi within the heart chambers Defects in heart wall integrity and shunting of blood are noted i.e., patent foramen ovale During stress portion, heart is unable to maintain cardiac output, congestion within heart chambers is noted
Chest x-ray	R91.8	$67	**Normal results:** organs pictured are size appropriate and located in correct anatomical position with no densities or opacities within the lung tissues. Both lungs are expanded without obstruction or compression. No adventitious air or fluid within the chest cavity **Abnormal results:** heart is enlarged or shifted out of its normal location. Densities are present within the lung fields, which could indicate inflammation, fluid, mass, foreign body. Fluid is present behind lungs (pleural effusion) or air/fluid is compressing the lung to prevent it from fully expanding (pneumo/hemothorax)

(*continued*)

Exam	Code	Cost	Results
CMP	R68.89	$28	**Normal results:** Glucose 70–99 mg/dL (fasting), 70–125 mg/dL (nonfasting) Sodium 136–144 mEq/L — Potassium 3.7–5.2 mEq/L Chloride 96–106 mmol/L — CO_2 20–29 mmol/L BUN 7–20 mg/dL — Creatinine 0.8–1.4 mg/dL BUN/creatinine ratio 10:1–20:1 — Calcium 8.5–10.9 mg/dL Magnesium 1.8–2.6 mEq/L — Protein 6.3–7.9 g/dL Albumin 3.9–5.0 d/dL — Globulin 2.0–3.5 g/dL Albumin/globulin ratio 1.7–2.2 — Bilirubin 0.3–1.9 mg/dL ALP 44–147 IU/L ALT 8–37 IU/L AST 10–34 IU/L Glomerular filtration rate 90–120 mL/min/1.73 m^2 Abnormal results: values outside of normal range can be indications of dehydration, kidney/liver dysfunction, malnutrition or malignant disease process
Troponin	R82.5	$26 Repeat thrice at 3, 6, and 12 hours	Troponin is a protein within the muscle fibers of the heart. When heart tissue damage occurs, such as during ischemia or chronic myopathy, these levels become elevated. Troponin becomes elevated within 3–4 hours after cardiac injury and can remain elevated for up to 2 weeks. **Normal results:** less than 0.01 ng/mL **Abnormal results:** >0.01 ng/mL An increase in serum troponin levels greater than 0.2 ng/mL should have repeat lab testing at 3, 6 and 12 hours to determine trend and whether this is an acute or chronic heart condition
BNP	L35526	$66	A hormone made within the heart and released in response to increased pressure within the heart itself. Often used to determine fluid overload status within heart failure patients **Normal:** 0–74 years = BNP <125 pg/mL 75–99 years = BNP <400 pg/mL **Abnormal:** BNP >900 pg/mL in patients 50+ years old
CBC	R68.89	$29	Measures the different blood cell components and assists in diagnosis of nutrient/oxygen delivery dysfunction, infective process, and further blood cell production Hemoglobin is responsible for delivering oxygen to cells, normal female 13.5–17.5 g/dL. A decrease in this number is indicative of anemia and can result in impaired oxygen delivery to tissues Hematocrit is the total percentage of blood composed of red blood cells, normal female 40%–55%. A decrease in this number can indicate anemia or dilution of blood with fluid WBCs attach themselves to foreign cells, infected tissues, and wounds to promote phagocytosis and removal of dangerous products. A decrease in WBCs can be a sign of bone marrow damage, dysfunctional cell production or leukemia; an elevated WBC count is a sign of an active infection process within the body Normal 5,000–10,000/mL Platelets are the cells that aid in clotting, whether it be helpful (tissue damage and cuts) or malignant (thrombi formation). Decreased platelets indicate the potential to have uncontrolled bleeding in response to an assault, while an increased count can indicate the patient is at increased risk for DVT/PE/clots. Normal 150k–400k/mL

ALP, alkaline phosphatase; ALT, alanine amino transferase; AST, aspartate amino transferase; BNP, brain natriuretic peptide; BUN, blood urea nitrogen; CBC, complete blood count; CMP, complete metabolic panel; DVT, deep vein thrombosis; EF, ejection fraction; PE, pulmonary embolism; WBC, white blood cell.

CLINICAL DECISION MAKING

Case Study Analysis

After physical assessment and detailed history of onset, the patient had an EKG performed, which indicated a left bundle branch block but no arrhythmia or acute T wave changes. Voltage parameters for left ventricle hypertrophy were met, indicating that a previous ischemic event occurred that caused a change in the electrical conduction of the heart as well as remodeling of the left ventricle as its walls grow thicker to accommodate the increased pressure within the chamber.

The patient's lab work indicated a troponin with a low-grade elevation of 0.4 ng/mL, although trended results thereafter indicate this is stable and not increasing to indicate an acute cardiac injury. Her brain natriuretic peptide (BNP) was elevated at 1,500 pg/dL, indicating her heart was stretching more to accommodate higher pressures as a result of fluid overload. Nonfasting glucose levels were elevated at 200 units, indicating poor diabetic control. Liver enzymes, aspartate amino transferase/alanine amino transferase (AST/ALT), were slightly elevated at 40 IU/L, possibly indicating a liver dysfunction. Her stress echo revealed some partial akinesis of the septal wall and impaired emptying of the left ventricle as well as left ventricular hypertrophy; ejection fraction = 40%. Her chest x-ray indicated some pulmonary edema and pulmonary vein congestion.

> **Diagnosis:** *Congestive heart failure (CHF), New York Heart Association (NYHA) class 2 with syncopal episode*

- No single test can indicate CHF, but thorough assessment of symptoms and interpretation of tests can lead to the diagnosis.
- Stress echo is positive for decreased left ventricle ejection fraction, as well as manifestations of the heart remodeling to accommodate the increased workload with decreased functionability (i.e., left ventricle hypertrophy).
- B-type natriuretic peptide >900 pg/mL is indicative of fluid overload.
- Symptoms such as dyspnea, orthopnea, fluid retention, and syncope are all indicative of a cardiac dysfunction that has impaired cardiac output and is manifesting in other systems.
- Dyspnea, weight changes, and edema are not associated with a transient ischemic attack or carotid stenosis, so these health problems can be ruled out.
- The cardiac changes, BNP level, and results of diagnostic testing do not support the diagnosis of transient ischemic attack or carotid stenosis.
- NYHA Failure Classification is important for grading the degree of disability associated with heart failure; treatment regimens will change based on the NYHA class.
- American Heart Association CHF guidelines indicate this patient should be treated with a beta-blocker, angiotensin-converting enzyme (ACE) inhibitor, and diuretic medications, which should be done under close supervision of her primary care provider with low and slow titration to decrease the likelihood of adverse medication reactions such as angioedema, bradycardia, hypotension, and kidney injury related to dehydration.
- Additional teaching appropriate for this patient includes a low-sodium diet and encouragement to resume a walking program.

FATIGUE

Case Presentation: A 64-year-old female presents with the chief complaint of fatigue for the past month.

INTRODUCTION TO COMPLAINT

- The chief complaint of fatigue is nonspecific
- It can be characterized as the inability to initiate activity (generalized weakness), reduced ability to maintain activity (easy fatigued), and mental fatigue
- Fatigue must be distinguished from dyspnea (at rest and on exertion), somnolence, and muscle weakness
- All of these signs may accompany fatigue; however, they are in fact different
- Fatigue can be additionally characterized as: acute, lasting 1 month or less: prolonged, lasting longer than 1 month but less than 6 months: and chronic, lasting longer than 6 months

HISTORY OF COMPLAINT

Symptomatology

Ask about the following characteristics of each symptom using open-ended questions:

- Onset of complaint
- Sudden or gradual
- Chronology of events
- Currently improving, stable, or deteriorating
- Timing
- Precipitating or aggravating factors
- Relieving factors
- Effects on daily activities
- Previous treatments

Directed Questions to Ask

- When did your fatigue start?
- Was it sudden or gradual?
- What events have accompanied it?
- How often does it occur?
- When do you feel the most fatigued?
- Where does it occur?
- What other symptoms do you feel during the fatigue?
- What helps your symptoms?
- How has your thought process been?
- How have you been sleeping?

- What activities does the fatigue keep you from?
- How has your appetite been?

Assessment: Cardinal Signs and Symptoms

General
- Fatigue
- Fever
- Chills
- Malaise
- Pain

Head, Eyes, Ears, Nose, Throat (HEENT)
- Swollen lymph nodes
- Goiter

Mental
- Agitated
- Anxious
- Depression

Neurologic
- Weakness
  - Generalized
  - Localized
  - Ascending
  - Descending
- Headache
- Decreased deep tendon reflexes (DTRs)
- Paresthesia

Cardiac
- Tachycardia
- Chest pain
- Palpitations
- Edema
- Murmur
- Displaced point of maximum impulse (PMI)

Pulmonary
- Dyspnea
- Tachypnea
- Accessory muscle use
- Cough
- Chest tightness

Gastrointestinal
- Ascites
- Gastroesophageal reflux disease (GERD)
- Diarrhea
- Melena

Hematological
- Active hemorrhage
- Bruising

Integumentary
- Cyanosis
- Clubbing

Medical History
- Current medications: Protonix 40 mg orally daily, Benadryl 50 mg orally nightly PRN, hydrochlorothiazide 25 mg orally daily

Past Medical History
- Allergies: penicillin
- Medical: hypertension (HTN); GERD
- Surgical: knee replacement at 55 years
- OB: two pregnancies, two live births
- Psychological: no previous history

Family History
- Unknown
- Patient states parents died of old age

Social History
- Tobacco: patient denies smoking
- Ethanol (ETOH): patient states she has a glass of wine with dinner on the weekends
- Sexual: patient not sexually active
- Illicit drug use
- Diet
- Emotional support
- Occupational
- Health maintenance
- Socioeconomics

PHYSICAL EXAMINATION
Vital Signs
- Temperature
- Pulse
- Respiration
- Oxygen saturation (SpO_2)
- Blood pressure (BP)

General Appearance
- Apparent state of health
- Appearance of comfort or distress
- Color
- Nutritional status
- State of hydration
- Hygiene
- Match between appearance and stated age
- Difficulty with gait or balance

Neurologic Assessment
- Alert, oriented, and cooperative
- Thought process coherent
- Romberg: maintains balance with eyes closed

- No pronator drift
- Gait with normal base
- Good muscle build and tone
- Strength 5/5 throughout
- Rapid alternating movements (RAMs): finger to nose. Hand flip flop and serial finger opposition intact. Cranial nerves (CNs) II through XII intact. DTR—brachioradialis, biceps, triceps, patellar, Achilles DTR 2+ bilaterally. Negative Babinski reflex

HEENT
- No thyroid enlargement. Neck supple, no tonsillar enlargement, Mallampati airway score 1, soft pallet low lying. No goiter present

Respiratory
- Chest expansion even, tachypnea. No cyanosis or pallor. Lung sounds clear throughout; no crackles, rhonchi, or rales; slight expiratory wheeze heard throughout. Cough productive with sputum, trachea midline

Cardiovascular
- Tachycardia, but regular rhythm, +3 radial pulses bilaterally. PMI dime-sized, fifth intercostal space, midclavicular line. No murmurs, rubs, or gallops. S1 and S2 clearly auscultated. No edema

Gastrointestinal
- Abdomen soft, flat, not distended; no fluid wave present; bowel sounds active

Musculoskeletal
- Full weight bearing; full range of motion (ROM) in all extremities; capillary refill <3 seconds in toes and fingers bilaterally; 3+ radial and pedal pulses bilaterally; normal gait

Integumentary
- No cyanosis, skin warm and intact

Hematological
- No ecchymosis present

CASE STUDY

History

Directed Question	Response
When did your fatigue start?	*About 1 month ago.*
Was it sudden or gradual?	*Gradual.*
What events have accompanied it?	*None that I am aware of.*
How often does it occur?	*All the time.*
When do you feel the most fatigued?	*At the end of the day or after activity.*
Where does it occur?	*Everywhere.*
What other symptoms do you feel during the fatigue?	*I feel like I can't catch my breath and my heart is racing.*
What helps your symptoms?	*Sitting or lying down.*
How has your thought process been?	*It's been tough focusing on simple tasks.*

Directed Question	Response
How have you been sleeping?	*About the same.*
What activities has the fatigue stopped you from doing?	*I can't walk to get the mail or up a flight of stairs without feeling really tired.*
How has your appetite been?	*About the same.*

Physical Examination Findings

- VITAL SIGNS: temperature 99.0°F; respiratory rate (RR) 20; heart rate (HR) 65, regular; BP 128/74; SpO2 97%
- GENERAL APPEARANCE: well developed, healthy appearing female who presents with obvious non-verbal cues of discomfort
- NECK: no thyroid enlargement or nodules/masses
- CARDIOVASCULAR: heart regular/rhythm, no murmur or gallop
- RESPIRATORY: lungs clear
- ABDOMEN: no evidence of distention, pain with palpation; no organomegaly; hyperactive bowel sounds in all four quadrants

DIFFERENTIAL DIAGNOSIS

Signs and Symptoms of Patient	Disorder			
	Multiple Sclerosis	Heart Failure	Iron Deficiency Anemia	Pernicious Anemia
Fatigue	Yes	Yes	Yes	Yes
Dyspnea on exertion	No	Yes	Yes	Yes
Palpitations	No	Yes	Yes	Yes
Tachycardia	No	Yes	Yes	Yes
Tachypnea	No	Yes	Yes	Yes

DIAGNOSTIC EXAMINATION

Exam	Code	Cost	Results	Justification
CBC with differential	D64.9	$21	Platelet count: decreased (normal 150,000–400,000) Hemoglobin: decreased (normal 12–16) Hematocrit: decreased (normal 37%–47%) Reticulocyte count: increased or decreased (normal 0.5%–1.5%) MCV: increased or decreased (normal 76–96) RBC count: decreased (normal 4.1–5.5 x 106/mm³) MCH: decreased (normal 27–32) MCHC: decreased (normal 30–35)	A CBC with differential is required to investigate for anemia.

(*continued*)

Exam	Code	Cost	Results	Justification
CMP	I10	$22	Albumin: 3.4–5.4 g/dL Alkaline phosphatase: 44–147 IU/L ALT 10–40 IU/L AST 10–34 IU/L BUN 6–20 mg/dL Calcium: 8.5–10.2 mg/dL Chloride: 96–106 mEq/L CO_2: 23–29 mEq/L Creatinine: 0.6–1.3 mg/dL Glucose: 70–100 mg/dL Potassium: 3.7–5.2 mEq/L Sodium: 135–145 mEq/L Total bilirubin: 0.3–1.9 mg/dL Total protein: 6.0–8.3 g/dL	A CMP is required to investigate for electrolyte abnormalities and kidney function. Items will affect treatment.
BNP	CPT Code: 83880	$88	0–99 pcg/mL, >100 in heart failure	A BNP is required to investigate for heart failure.
Troponin	R79.89	$26	0 in normal conditions; >0.01 if an MI has occurred	A troponin is tested to assess for MI.
Ferritin	R77.8	$36	24–336 mcg/L, low in iron deficiency anemia	Ferritin is a protein used to store iron. This level is drawn to assess for iron deficiency anemia
Reticulocyte count	R71.8	$21	RBC count: 3.9 x 106/mm3 (normal 4.1–5.5 x 106/mm^3)	Reticulocytes are young RBCs. This level is low in certain anemia.
Transferrin	D50.1	$34	Normal transferrin is 170–370 mg/dL, elevated in iron deficiency anemia.	This protein carries iron in the blood. It is drawn to assess for iron deficiency anemia.
TIBC	D50.9	$45		TIBC is a reflection of how much transferrin is available to bind to iron.

(continued)

Exam	Code	Cost	Results	Justification
Serum iron	D50.7	$17	55–160 µg/dL in men and 40–155 µg/dL in women	Low iron indicates iron deficiency.
Folic level: serum	D50.6	$39	2–20 ng/mL, decreased in pernicious anemia	Tested to assess for pernicious anemia.
Vitamin B$_{12}$ level	53.8	$38	150 and 400 ng/L, decreased in pernicious anemia	Tested to assess for pernicious anemia.
sTfR	D50.2	Not found	1.8–4.6 mg/L, increased in iron deficiency anemia	Drawn to differentiate iron deficiency anemia from anemia of inflammation or renal failure.
Blood smear	D50	$12	Megaloblasts are indicative of pernicious anemia while microblasts indicative of iron deficiency anemia.	Tested to assess for anemia.
EKG	93000	$31	Performed to assess for ongoing cardiac dysrhythmias and heart failure	Performed to assess for ongoing cardiac dysrhythmias and heart failure.
TTE	A69.20	$413	A TTE in a patient with mild heart failure could show a variety of anatomical changes	Performed to assess for heart failure and valve disorders.

ALT, alanine amino transferase; AST, aspartate amino transferase; BNP, brain natriuretic peptide; BUN, blood urea nitrogen; CBC, complete blood count; CMP, complete metabolic panel; CO_2, carbon dioxide; MCH, mean corpuscular hemoglobin; MCHC, mean corpuscular hemoglobin concentration; MCV, mean corpuscular volume; MI, myocardial infarction; RBC, red blood cell; sTfR, soluble transferrin receptor; TIBC, total iron binding capacity; TTE, transthoracic echocardiogram.

CLINICAL DECISION MAKING

Case Study Analysis

- The complaint of fatigue is nonspecific and hard to analyze because of the multitude of conditions it accompanies.

- Additionally, the symptoms must be distinguished but not forgotten in the investigation of the chief complaint.
- After investigation of the patient's history the provider finds the patient is both a vegetarian and on a *proton pump inhibitor* (PPI).
- These two findings put the patient at risk for both iron deficient anemia and pernicious anemia.
- The patient has no peripheral edema, jugular venous distention (JVD), hepatomegaly, or fluid wave.
- Diagnostic exams will differentiate the two and produce a clear diagnosis. However, until an electrocardiogram, brain natriuretic peptide (BNP), and transthoracic echocardiogram (TTE) are completed, treatment should be focused on correcting the anemia.
- Heart failure must be still be considered until ruled out with EKG, BNP, and TTE.

Diagnosis: *Possible iron deficient and pernicious anemia*

Rule Out Heart Failure

The patient appears undernourished. A complete dietary history needs to be completed to analyze the patient's sources of iron. The length of time the patient has been taking Protonix for GERD needs to be determined and alternative treatment may need to be considered. Iron supplementation needs to be prescribed along with counseling on vitamin supplements.

Scheduled to return in 2 days to have an EKG, TTE, and BNP level drawn. Further treatment will depend upon the results of these tests.

FEVER

Case Presentation: A 39-year-old African American male presents with a complaint of fever for 10 days and swelling to his left thigh and knee for 1 week causing him to have difficulty ambulating.

INTRODUCTION TO COMPLAINT

- Cellulitis
- Deep vein thrombosis (DVT)
- Gas gangrene
- Septic arthritis
- Joint effusion
- Thrombophlebitis
- Transient synovitis
- Hematoma
- Fibrosarcoma
- Eosinophilic granuloma
- Osteosarcoma
- Gout
- Osteomyelitis

HISTORY OF COMPLAINT

Symptomatology

Ask about the following characteristics of each symptom using open-ended questions:

- Onset
- Chronology
- Current situation
- Timing
- Severity
- Precipitating and aggravating factors
- Relieving factors
- Associated symptoms
- Effects on daily activities
- Previous diagnosis of similar episodes
- Previous treatments

Directed Questions to Ask

- When did the fever and leg swelling begin?
- What were you doing when it started?
- Is the fever intermittent or continuous?
- Do you have any other complaints besides the fever and swelling?
- Did you take any medication to make it better?
- Does anything make it better?
- How has your daily activity been affected by this?
- Are you on any new medications?
- Have you had a recent head cold or flu-like symptoms?
- Have you had any recent trauma?
- Have you recently traveled?
- Have you had any recent bug bites?
- Have you had any recent surgery?

Assessment: Cardinal Signs and Symptoms

General
- Fatigue
- Weakness
- Lethargy

Head, Eyes, Ears, Nose, Throat (HEENT)
- Drainage from sinus tracts

Cardiac
- Tachycardia

Respiratory
- Shortness of breath

Gastrointestinal
- Nausea

Genitourinary
- Decreased urination

Musculoskeletal
- Pain and tenderness over the affected bone
- Decreased range of motion in adjacent joints

Integumentary
- Erythema and drainage

Other Associated Symptoms
- None

Medical History

- Surgical: Right knee replacement two weeks ago
- Allergies: Penicillin

- Medication: Folic acid 1 mg daily; multivitamin 1 daily; vitamin D 400 U daily; metformin 1,000 mg twice a day; percocet 10/325 mg every 4 hours for pain as needed
- Psychosocial: Denis tobacco use; no drugs/drinks alcohol occasionally
- Health Maintenance/Immunization: Received influenza and pneumococcal vaccines

Medical History
- Diabetes
- Sickle cell
- Vitamin D deficiency

Family History
- Sickle cell
- Diabetes
- Hypertension (HTN)

PHYSICAL EXAMINATION
Vital Signs
- Temperature
- Heart rate (HR)
- Respiration
- Blood pressure (BP)
- Oxygen saturation (SpO_2)

General Appearance
- Moderate distress
- Normal physic

HEENT
- Tenderness or drainage noted
- No adenopathy

Cardiac
- Tachycardia
- No murmurs, gallops
- Right pedal pulse 1+

Respiratory
- Lung sounds are clear bilaterally

Gastrointestinal
- Soft and nontender
- Nausea

Genitourinary
- No pain with palpation

Musculoskeletal
- Edema, heat, and pain in right knee joint, right lower thigh

Integumentary
- Erythema to right knee and thigh

CASE STUDY
History

Directed Question	Response
When did the leg swelling and fever begin?	The swelling has been there since my surgery 2 weeks ago. The fever has been there a week and a half.
When did the pain begin?	The pain has been dull since surgery but it has gotten worse in the past week.
What is your pain on the scale of 0–10?	Right now 9/10.
Can you describe the pain?	It's a sharp aching pain.
Does the pain go anywhere else?	It radiated from my knee to my right hip.
Does anything make it worse or better?	The pain is less when I'm resting. Prolonged standing and walking makes it worse.
Is the fever continuous?	No, it comes and goes.
Did you take any medication to make it better?	I've taken Percocet.
Did you have other symptoms?	I have had a bad runny nose, chills, body aches, some shortness of breath, my thigh is red and painful to touch.
When did the shortness of breath begin?	Around the same time as my fever.
Have you had any chest pain?	No.
Have you had any recent travel?	No.
Is your shortness of breath at rest or with activity?	Activity.
When did the redness start in your thigh?	It started about a week and a half ago.
Has the redness spread?	Yes, at first it was just at my knee; now it's swollen and red halfway up my thigh.
Have you had any recent bug bites or bumps you may have scratched?	No.
Has your incision healed?	It has a small area that is open.
Do you have any drainage from your incision?	Yes, a little yellow drainage.
How has your daily activity been affected by this?	I can barely walk or put pressure on my leg because of the pain.
Have you started any new medications?	No.
Is there anything else you would like to tell me about?	I don't think so.

Physical Examination Findings

- VITAL SIGNS: temperature 101.9°F; RR 22; HR 112; BP 147/86; SpO$_2$ 96% on RA
- GENERAL APPEARANCE: normal male in moderate distress; restless, having severe pain
- HEENT: head symmetric, round; pupils equal, round, and reactive to light and accommodation (PERRLA) 3 mm; eye, ears, with no drainage, redness, tenderness, or trauma; drainage and redness to bilateral nares; tympanic membrane visualized, intact and opaque; mucous membrane moist, pink, and intact; no lesion or sores; nasopharynx reddened, visualized clear turbinates; neck supple, no adenopathy
- CHEST/CARDIOVASCULAR: regular rate and rhythm; no murmurs, gallops, or rubs; capillary refills <2 seconds; edema to right knee and thigh; pulses + in right lower extremity
- RESPIRATORY: lung sounds clear through all lung fields, no adventitious sounds; symmetrical; no cough
- ABDOMEN: soft, nontender without mass or organomegaly; bowel sounds in all four quadrants
- SKIN: intact with no rashes, lesions, or ulcerations; erythema to right knee and right lower thigh
- EXTREMITIES: joint pain, swelling, tenderness, and redness to right knee and lower thigh; no crepitus; swelling noted to lateral part of lower thigh, diffuse with ill-defined border; swelling soft in consistency, tender to touch, and warm; the left thigh measures 3 cm larger in circumference to the normal right side; transillumination test was negative and no bruit heard; negative Homan's sign
- MUSCULOSKELETAL: gait antalgic with persistent left knee flexion; all movements of hip were normal; unable to perform Trendelenburg's test due to pain; movement 0 to 30 degrees right knee, 0 to 130 degrees left knee

DIFFERENTIAL DIAGNOSIS

Clinical Observations	Osteomyelitis	Cellulitis	Effusion	DVT
Onset	Gradual	Sudden	Gradual	Gradual
Fever	Yes	Yes	Yes/No	No
Joint pain	Yes	No	Yes	Yes/No
Joint swelling	Yes	No	Yes/No	No
ESR	Yes	Yes	Yes/No	No
Short of breath	Yes	No	No	Yes/No
Fatigue	Yes/No	Yes/No	No	No
Lung sounds	Varies	Clear	Varies	Varies

(*continued*)

Clinical Observations	Osteomyelitis	Cellulitis	Effusion	DVT
Fever	Moderate to high	Low to moderate	Varies	Negative
Other symptoms	Red, inflamed, pain, hot to touch	Red, inflamed, pain, hot to touch	Varies, determined by what type	Homan's sign

DVT, deep vein thrombosis; ESR, erythrocyte sedimentation rate.

DIAGNOSTIC EXAMINATION

Exam	Code	Cost	Results
CBC with differential	D64.9	$25–$100	WBC: Determines infectious or inflammatory source. Elevated WBC indicative of active infection and possible source Hemoglobin: Oxygen-carrying capacity. Decreased amount may indicate anemia, blood loss or need for transfusion. Differential: Elevated neutrophil count can determine an acute bacterial infection. Decreased neutrophil count can determine severe infection. Elevated lymphocyte count can determine viral infections or chronic inflammatory disorders. Elevated monocyte count may indicate chronic or fungal infections. Decreased monocyte and lymphocyte count can indicate autoimmune or bone marrow disorders.
Anterior–posterior and lateral knee radiograph	73560	$200–$500	Radiographic films: X-rays can reveal damage to your bone. However, damage may not be visible until osteomyelitis has been present for several weeks. More detailed imaging tests may be necessary if your osteomyelitis has developed more recently.
MRI	70544	$2,700–$4,000	MRI: Using radio waves and a strong magnetic field, MRI scans can produce exceptionally detailed images of bones and the soft tissues that surround them.
Gram stain synovial fluid	87020	$75–$200	Positive results: Most common bacteria, Streptococcus. Other bacteria, e.g., *Staphylococcus aureus*, in sickle cell disease, Salmonella.
Blood culture	87076	$75–$100	The most commonly encountered organisms in osteomyelitis are *Staphylococcus aureus*, coagulase-negative streptococci, aerobic Gram-negative bacteria, and anaerobes including *Finegoldia* (formerly *Peptostreptococcus*) species.
Sedimentation rate	85652	$75–$150	The sedimentation rate measures how quickly red blood cells (erythrocytes) settle in a test tube in 1 hour. When inflammation is present in the body, certain proteins cause red blood cells to stick together and fall more quickly than normal to the bottom of the tube.
C-reactive protein	86140	$50–$100	The C-reactive protein correlates with clinical response to therapy and may be used to monitor therapy.

(continued)

Exam	Code	Cost	Results
Bone biopsy	20240	$1,200–$3,000	A bone biopsy is the gold standard for diagnosing osteomyelitis, because it can also reveal the microorganism that is the cause of the infection.

CBC, complete blood count; WBC, white blood cell.

CLINICAL DECISION MAKING
Case Study Analysis

- The patient presented with fatigue, intermittent fever for 10 days, chills, rigors, and right knee joint pain.
- Patient is 2 weeks post-op after having a right knee replacement and has diabetes and sickle cell.
- He developed worsening pain, erythema, and edema to his right knee that has gone into in his right lower thigh over the past 7 days.
- The edema is static at its current size. The fever is mostly at night but subsides with Percocet. The pain is sharp, continuous and is aggravated by prolonged standing or ambulation.
- He reports shortness of breath, but denies chest pain. After history and examination, diagnostic tests were completed. Complete blood count (CBC) revealed leukocytosis 18,000.
- Normal basic metabolic panel (BMP).
- Patient with temperature 101.9°F and concerning for cellulitis, DVT, and osteomyelitis. Blood cultures pending. Right knee aspirate culture and sensitivity (C&S), and Gram stain pending.
- Symptoms of fatigue, fever, joint edema, and erythema.
- Anterior–posterior and lateral view of femur and knee revealed there was a periosteal sclerosis and cortical thickening noticed on the shaft of right femur with osteolytic and sclerosis changes seen in the medulla to both ends of the bone.
- Soft tissue swelling noted; right knee with normal surgical hardware.
- Patient admitted to the hospital for analgesics, intravenous (IV) antibiotics, antipyretics, knee immobilization, blood glucose control, and rest.
- Beta-lactams and vancomycin are commonly used as initial empiric therapy.
- Antibiotic therapy for hematogenous osteomyelitis should be pathogen-directed, based on the results of bone biopsy or blood cultures.
- The patient will receive clindamycin 600 mg IV every 6 hours due to penicillin allergy. Antibiotic therapy may change based on culture results.
- Absence of a Homan's sign ruled out the possibility of a DVT.
- Absence of joint pain, swelling, and elevated temperature ruled out the possibility of cellulitis.
- X-ray evaluation ruled out the possibility of an effusion
- Once discharged, recovery from the hip replacement can resume to include physical therapy and progressive ambulation and continued treatment for chronic health problems.

Diagnosis: *Osteomyelitis of right femur*

FOOT PAIN

Case Presentation: A 30-year-old female reports pain in her left foot for the past 4 weeks.

INTRODUCTION TO COMPLAINT
- 64.8% of foot pain is from calluses/corns
- 29.6% of foot pain is caused by hypertrophic nails
- 21.2% is from hallux deformities (bunion)
- 15.9% is from absent arterial pulses

Forefoot Pain
- Ingrown toenails
- Metatarsalgia
- Interdigital neuromas: Morton neuroma
- Hallux rigidus
- Sesamoiditis
- Bunionette
- Callus
- Corns
- Warts
- Metatarsal stress fracture

Midfoot Pain
- Osteoarthritis
- Midfoot planter fasciitis
- Planter fibromas
- Tarsal tunnel syndrome
- Pes planus
- Pes cavus

Hindfoot Pain
- Planter fasciitis

Posterior Heel Pain
- Achilles tendinitis, Haglund's deformity
- Retrocalcaneal bursitis
- Pre-Achilles bursitis
- Achilles rupture

Planter Heel

- Planter surface planter warts

Other Causes

- Possible compartment syndrome
- Deep vein thrombosis (DVT)
- Sprain of a ligament
- Other fracture aside from stress fracture
- Ruptured tendon

HISTORY OF COMPLAINT

Symptomatology

Ask about the following characteristics of each symptom using open-ended questions:

- Chronology: onset/duration
- Current situation
- Characteristics of pain on a scale of 0 to 10
- Swelling or bruising

Directed Questions to Ask

- When did the symptoms start?
- Did the pain start suddenly or was it gradual over time?
- When does the pain occur?
- Is it worse at night when lying down or when you first stand up?
- Are there any precipitating factors?
- Are there any other associated symptoms?
- Have you had a previous diagnosis of similar episodes?
- Have you had previous treatments for foot pain?
- Past surgical history?
- What medications do you take?

Assessment: Cardinal Signs and Symptoms

In addition to the general characteristics outlined previously, additional characteristics of specific symptoms should be elicited.

Feet

- Swelling
- Achilles tendon nodules or tenderness
- Heel tenderness
- Malleolus tenderness
- Tenderness over metatarsophalangeal joints
- Range of motion (ROM)
- Pedal pulses
- Deep tendon reflexes
- Ankle alignment
- Bruising
- Sensation

Medical History: General

- Medical conditions and surgeries
- Allergies

Medical History: Specific to Complaint

- Recent trauma to foot or ankle

PHYSICAL EXAMINATION

Vital Signs

- Temperature
- Pulse
- Respiration
- Oxygen saturation (SpO_2)
- Blood pressure (BP)

General Appearance

- Apparent state of health
- Appearance of comfort or distress
- Color
- Nutritional status
- State of hydration
- Hygiene
- Match between appearance and stated age
- Difficulty with gait or balance

Ankle and Foot

- INSPECT: observe all surfaces of the ankles and feet
- PALPATE: palpate anterior aspect of each ankle joint, note any bogginess, swelling, or tenderness, feel the Achilles tendon for nodules and tenderness, palpate the heel for tenderness, palpate the medial and lateral malleolus for tenderness, and palpate the metatarsophalangeal for tenderness and compress the forefoot between the thumb and fingers
- ROM AND MANEUVERS: assess flexion and extension at the ankle joint; assess the inversion and exertion at the subtalar and transverse tarsal joints

Associated Systems for Assessment

- A complete assessment should include the nervous system (i.e., deep tendon reflexes)

CASE STUDY

History

Directed Question	Response
When did the pain begin?	*Pain began after I started walking 5 miles a day.*
What is your current situation?	*Have had to stop walking due to pain.*

Directed Question	Response
What are the characteristics of the pain on a scale of 0 to 10?	*Pain a 5 during the day but 10 when I first put my foot down in the morning.*
Is it accompanied by swelling or bruising?	*No.*
When did the symptoms start?	*When I put my foot down on the floor in the morning.*
Did the pain start suddenly or was it gradual over time?	*Started suddenly but gradually getting worse.*
When does the pain occur?	*When I am walking or standing.*
How does the pain affect your daily activities?	*I can't walk for long.*
Have you had a previous diagnosis of similar episodes?	*No.*
Have you had previous treatments for your foot pain?	*No.*
Past surgical history?	*No.*
What medications do you take?	*None.*
Have you recently taken Levaquin (r/t tendons rupture in some patients)?	*No.*
Ask the patient to point to the pain?	*Points to plantar surface anterior heel.*
Was there an acute injury or overuse from repetitive use of the body part?	*Just walking.*
Is there tenderness, warmth, or redness?	*No.*
Is there swelling, stiffness, or decreased range of motion?	*No.*
What aggravates or relieves the pain?	*Just walking.*
What are the effects of exercise, rest, and treatment?	*Rest helps.*
Are there any fever or chills?	*No.*
Do you have any history of osteoporosis or inflammatory disorders?	*No.*
Do you use alcohol or tobacco?	*No.*
Do you have any family history of fracture in a first-degree relative?	*No.*
Do you use corticosteroids?	*No.*
How much do you weigh?	*117 lb.*

Physical Examination Findings

- VITAL SIGNS: temperature 99.2°F; respiration rate 22; pulse 102; BP 117/72; SpO$_2$ 98%
- GENERAL APPEARANCE: 17-year-old female, 5'3½", 117 lb
- FEET: ankle and foot have normal color, landmarks, and alignment; both feet are warm with capillary refill less than 1 second; there is tenderness to palpation along the anterior–medial heel of the left foot; nontender along the Achilles tendon, tarsals, and metatarsals; full ROM of the ankle and foot without pain; dorsalis pedis pulse is 2+ and equal; sensation is intact to light touch, sharp, and dull

DIFFERENTIAL DIAGNOSIS

Clinical Observations	Plantar Fasciitis	Stress Fracture	Embolic Arterial Occlusion	Deep Vein Thrombosis	Compartment Syndrome
Forefoot	No	Yes	No	No	No
Midfoot	Yes	No	No	No	No
Heel	Yes	No	No	No	No
Swelling	No	Yes	No	Yes	Yes
Tenderness on palpation	Yes	Yes	No	No	No
Cold/pallor	No	No	Yes	No	No

DIAGNOSTIC EXAMINATION

Exam	Code	Cost	Results
Foot x-ray (two views)	73620	$300	These diseases or medical conditions may be diagnosed by, screened for, or associated with foot x-ray: broken foot, broken toe(s), mass or lump in the foot, ligament or cartilage tear, foreign object, infection of the foot, inflammation of the foot.
Ultrasound, leg (Doppler)	93971	$100	A Doppler ultrasound test uses reflected sound waves to see how blood flows through a blood vessel. It helps doctors evaluate blood flow through major arteries and veins, such as those of the arms, legs, and neck.
MRI, foot	73723	$1,500	MRI uses a magnetic field and pulses of radio wave energy to make pictures of organs and structures inside the body. In many cases, MRI gives different information about structures in the body that can be seen with an x-ray, ultrasound, or CT scan. MRI may also show problems that cannot be seen with other imaging methods.

(*continued*)

Exam	Code	Cost	Results
CT scan foot	73700	$1,100	CT: A diagnostic x-ray or radiological scan in which cross-sectional images of a part of the body are formed through computerized axial tomography and shown on a computer screen.
Bone scan	78300	$200	A bone scan is a test to help find the cause of your back pain. It can be done to find damage to the bones, find cancer that has spread to the bones, and watch problems, such as infection and trauma to the bones. A bone scan can often find problems days to months earlier than a regular x-ray test.

CLINICAL DECISION MAKING

Case Study Analysis

The pertinent positives are a history of sudden pain when getting out of bed. Pain is located over the anterior–medial heel, which is the area of the plantar fascia and is worse with weight bearing and relieved with rest. Pertinent negatives are the absence of trauma, swelling, or decreased pulses. The absence of swelling and the location of the pain rules out a stress fracture, DVT, and compartment syndrome. The skin color and presence of pulses rules out an arterial occlusion.

> **Diagnosis:** *Plantar fasciitis of the left foot*

The patient was counseled to limit long-distance walking at this time. Treatment is conservative to include heat/cold application, elevation, support, and over-the-counter analgesics. Suggest following up with the orthopedic clinic if symptoms do not subside within 2 weeks since splinting may need to be considered.

FREQUENCY OF URINATION

Case Presentation: A 22-year-old female reports experiencing increased frequency of urination for the past 2 days.

INTRODUCTION TO COMPLAINT

- Frequency of urination may vary from individual to individual based on bladder capacity, drinking habits, or personality traits
- Urinary frequency for the individual is defined as the need to urinate more often than one's usual/typical pattern of urination
- Urinary frequency can manifest secondary to an imbalance or disease process in the urinary tract: the kidneys, the ureters, the bladder, and the urethra
- Additionally, inflammation and infections of the vaginal tissue can result in increased frequency of urination due to extension of the inflammation/infection to the urethral tissue

HISTORY OF COMPLAINT

Symptomatology

Ask about the following characteristics of each symptom using open-ended questions:

- Onset (sudden or gradual)
- Chronology
- Current situation (improving or deteriorating)
- Location
- Radiation
- Quality
- Timing (frequency, duration)
- Severity
- Precipitating and aggravating factors
- Relieving factors
- Associated symptoms
- Effects on daily activities
- Previous diagnosis of similar episodes
- Previous treatments
- Efficacy of previous treatments

Directed Questions to Ask

- How many times a day do you typically urinate?
- How long have you been experiencing the increased urinary frequency?

- Since you have experienced increased urination, have you increased your fluid intake?
- Are you having any pain with urination?
- Have you had a fever since noting the increased frequency of urination?
- Have you had any chills since noting the increased frequency of urination?
- Have you had any nausea and/or vomiting since noting the frequency of urination?
- Have you had a sore throat recently, onset preceding the noted increased frequency of urination?
- Have you changed personal hygiene products recently?
- Had you increased your vaginal penetration sexual activities recently?
- Have you noted any changes in the color or odor of your urine?

Assessment: Cardinal Signs and Symptoms

- Urinary frequency
- Urinary urgency
- Pain with urination
- Burning with urination

Medical History: General

- Medical conditions and surgeries
- Allergies (seasonal as well as others)
- Medication currently used (prescription, birth control pill [BCP], and over the counter [OTC])
- Herbal preparations and traditional therapies

Medical History: Specific to Complaint

- Increased frequency of urination
- Symptoms associated with the increased frequency of urination
- Changes in color or odor of urine accompanying increased frequency of urination
- Recent sore throat

PHYSICAL EXAMINATION
Vital Signs

- Temperature
- Pulse
- Respiration
- Oxygen saturation (SpO_2)
- Blood pressure (BP)

General Appearance

- Apparent state of health
- Appearance of comfort or distress
- Color
- State of hydration

Mouth and Throat
- Inspect oral cavity for breath odor, color, lesions; throat and pharynx for color, exudates, tonsillar enlargement

Neck
- Inspect for symmetry, swelling, masses
- Palpate for tenderness, enlargement, lymph node chain

Abdomen
- Inspect for size and contour
- Auscultate for bowel sounds
- Palpate for pain, masses, bladder tenderness and/or distention, costovertebral angle tenderness

Pelvis
- Inspect external genitalia, condition of vaginal tissues
- Palpate for cystocele, adnexal tenderness

CASE STUDY
History

Directed Question	Response
How many times a day do you typically urinate?	*Two to three times.*
How long have you been experiencing an increase in the times you would typically urinate?	*About the past couple days . . . I have been going almost every hour or two.*
Since you have experienced increased urination, have you increased your fluid intake?	*No.*
Are you having any pain with urination?	*Not really.*
Have you had a fever since noting the increased frequency of urination?	*Not noted one.*
Have you had any chills since noting the increased frequency of urination?	*No.*
Have you had any nausea and/or vomiting since noting the frequency of urination?	*No.*
Have you had a sore throat recently, onset preceding the noted increased frequency of urination?	*No.*
Have you changed personal hygiene products recently?	*No.*
Had you increased your vaginal penetration sexual activities recently?	*Um . . . yes, I got a new vibrator and I tried it out quite a bit for a couple days.*
Have you noted any changes in the color or odor of your urine?	*No.*

Physical Examination Findings

- VITAL SIGNS: temperature 97.1°F; respiratory rate (RR) 16; heart rate (HR) 70, regular; BP 113/71; SpO_2 99%
- GENERAL APPEARANCE: well-developed, healthy-appearing female, who is a bit "fidgety"
- MOUTH: no oral lesions
- PHARYNX: no erythema; no tonsillar enlargement; no exudate
- NECK: no palpable lymph nodes
- ABDOMEN: soft, nontender without mass or organomegaly; no CVA tenderness
- PELVIS: mild edema of external genitalia, mild edema of vaginal tissues noted; no vaginal discharge noted; no cystocele or adnexal tenderness

DIFFERENTIAL DIAGNOSIS

Clinincal Observations	Lower Urinary Tract Infection	Kidney Infection	Kidney Stone	Vaginal Inflammation/ Infection
Urinary frequency	Typical	Typical	Possible	Possible
Pain with urination	Typical	Typical	Typical	Possible
Fever	Not typical	Typical	Not typical but possible	Not typical

DIAGNOSTIC EXAMINATION

Exam	Code	Cost	Results
Urine dipstick	81000	$10	For presence of infection
Complete urinalysis, includes microscopy	81015	$49	For indicators of kidney problems
Comprehensive metabolic panel	80053	$49	For glucose level and renal function
Postvoid urine residual	51798	Modest cost of bladder scan: average $30	To evaluate the amount of urine remaining in the bladder after the patient voids—normal <50 mL
Urodynamic Study— uroflowmetry	51726	Varies: average $266	Measures urine speed and volume. Measurements can be used as evaluators of strength of bladder muscles and potential blockages to urine flow

CLINICAL DECISION MAKING

Case Study Analysis

The advanced practice provider (APP) performs the assessment and physical examination on the patient and finds the following data: increased frequency of vaginal penetration/manipulation with a vibrator; urine dipstick negative for nitrites or leucocytes.

The absence of a fever ruled out the possibility of a kidney stone, kidney infection, or lower urinary tract infection. Inconsistent pain with urination also ruled out a urinary tract or kidney infection, and a kidney stone.

Since the urine dipstick was negative for cystitis, the APP recommended that the patient use RepHresh OTC (vaginal pH balancer) for a few days to see if her symptoms subside. Additionally, proper hygiene measures pertaining to vibrator use were reviewed with patient. Suggested following up in 2 weeks to 1 month if symptoms do not subside or worsen.

> **Diagnosis:** *Urinary frequency, secondary to a vaginal inflammation process*

HAND PAIN AND SWELLING

Case Presentation: A 30-year-old female reports intermittent pain, stiffness, and swelling of her hands for 2 months.

INTRODUCTION TO COMPLAINT

Joint pain in the hands that is not associated with trauma falls into three general categories:

- Degenerative arthritis: osteoarthritis (OA)
- Inflammatory arthritis: rheumatoid, psoriatic, systemic lupus, gout, undifferentiated arthritis
- Joint infection: parvovirus B19, Lyme disease, or septic joint

HISTORY OF COMPLAINT

Symptomatology

Ask about the following characteristics of each symptom using open-ended questions:

- Onset
- Location
- Duration/timing
- Character of the pain
- Intensity of the pain
- Triggering factors
- Alleviating factors
- Associated symptoms
- Effect on daily activities
- Previous similar symptoms
- Previous treatment

Directed Questions to Ask

- Is the onset abrupt or gradual?
- What specific joint or joints are affected?
- How long does pain last and is it intermittent or constant?
- Is it an ache, burn, sharp pain, or pressure?
- On a scale of 0 to 10 how severe is the pain?
- Are you stiff when you wake up in the morning? If yes, for how long?
- How many joints are involved?
  - Monoarthritis: Is it in one joint?
  - Polyarthritis: Is it in four or more joints?

- Where is the joint pain?
- Is the joint pain symmetrical?
- Do you have fever, weight loss, malaise, or fatigue?
- How long have the symptoms been present?
- Do you have any rashes?
- Are there any functional losses?
- Do you have other joints that are bothering you now or have bothered you in the past?

Assessment: Cardinal Signs and Symptoms

The following symptoms are associated with joint pain in the hand.

Symptom	Disorder
Constitutional	
Fever, weight loss, and fatigue	SLE, RA
Head, eyes, ears, neck, throat	
Hair loss	SLE, RA
Eye pain, vision loss	Uveitis, temporal arteritis
Conjunctivitis	Reiter's disease
Periorbital edema with violaceous hue	Dermatomyositis
Dry mouth	Sjogren's disease
Mouth sores	SLE, Behcet's syndrome
Respiratory	
Shortness of breath, pleuritic pain	SLE
Cardiovascular	
Chest pain, palpitation	SLE and RA
Gastrointestinal	
Abdominal pain, nausea, and vomiting; diarrhea	SLE
Gastroenteritis	Reactive arthritis
Genitourinary	
Urethral discharge, urethritis	Reiter's syndrome

(*continued*)

Symptom	Disorder
Psychiatric	
Personality change	SLE
Neurologic	
Headaches, numbness tingling, seizures	SLE
Skin	
Malar rash, photosensitive rashes	SLE
Slapped cheek	Human parvovirus B19
Annular red plague (*erythema migrans*)	Lyme disease
Violaceous papules/plaques on hand	Dermatomyositis
Psoriatic plaque, nail pitting	Psoriatic arthritis

RA, rheumatoid arthritis; SLE, systemic lupus erythematosus.

Medical History: General

- Active problem, list of past medical problems
- Past surgeries
- Current medications and drug allergies
- Family history of inflammatory arthritis, inflammatory bowel disease, thyroiditis
- Occupation, living situation, exercise, alcohol, nicotine, illicit drugs

Medical History: Specific to Complaint

- Family history of inflammatory arthritis, inflammatory bowel disease, thyroiditis
- Pain with range of motion to hand and wrist
- Inability to hold heavy objects
- Localized swelling

PHYSICAL EXAMINATION

Vital Signs

- Blood pressure (BP)
- Oxygen saturation (SpO_2)
- Temperature
- Respiration
- Pulse or heart rate (HR)
- Height
- Weight

General Appearance

Eyes
- Inspect for conjunctivitis or excessive dry eye

Mouth
- Inspect for sores or dry mouth

Heart
- Listen for murmur, rub, or abnormal rhythm

Abdomen
- Palpate for enlarged liver or spleen

Musculoskeletal
- Palpate all joints and note deformity, swelling, redness, heat, or tenderness
  - OA tends to have bony enlargement of the DIP and PIP joints
  - RA tends to have a spongy texture (synovial effusion) over the joints
  - Gout is too tender to touch
  - Psoriatic arthritis occurs in the DIP joints and may appear as a "sausage digit" with swelling of the tendon sheath of the finger; nail pitting may be observed

Skin
- Observe the skin for rashes, especially in sun-exposed areas of the face

CASE STUDY
History

Directed Question	Response
Was the onset of your joint pain sudden or gradual?	*Gradual, over days.*
Can you show me what joints are bothering you?	*[Points to all metacarpals].*
How long have you had the joint pain?	*About 2 months.*
Is it constant or intermittent?	*It started coming and going and now it is constant.*
Have you had it before?	*Yes, it was there a month ago.*
Does anything seem to trigger it?	*No, I have felt fine till this.*
Does anything make it better?	*Ibuprofen helps a bit.*
Can you describe how the pain feels?	*It is a constant ache.*
On a scale of 0 to 10 how severe is the pain?	*Probably 5 or 6.*
Do you have swelling or redness with the pain?	*Yes, especially in the morning.*
Are your hands stiff?	*Yes, all day, so stiff.*
Has it affected your daily activities?	*Yes, it is hard to button things.*
Has anyone ever had this in your family?	*Yes, my mom had rheumatoid arthritis.*

Directed Question	Response
Do you have any fevers, weight loss, or fatigue?	*No, the pain is tiring.*
Do you have any hair loss or rashes?	*Not that I've noticed.*
Do any other joints hurt you?	*Right now, just my hands.*

Physical Examination Findings

- VITAL SIGNS: temperature 98.8°F; respiratory rate 16; heart rate 64; BP 90/60; height 5′2″; weight 110 lb
- GENERAL APPEARANCE: healthy-appearing female in no acute pain
- EYES: no injection, pupils equal, round, and reactive to light and accommodation (PERRLA)
- NARES: patent, no discharge
- MOUTH: mucous membranes moist, no oral lesions or dental caries
- NECK: thyroid is not palpable, no adenopathy
- HEART: normal S2 and S2 without murmur gallop or rub
- ABDOMEN: soft, nontender without mass or organomegaly

Hands
- INSPECTION: hands reveal mild swelling of the MCP and PIP joints; faint redness
- PALPATION: notable for effusion of the joints with moderate tenderness and warmth
- RANGE OF MOTION: limited in flexion of the MCP and PIP joints; normal extension
- STRENGTH: hand grip is 4/5 bilaterally

Wrist
- INSPECTION: moderate swelling of the joints bilaterally, no redness
- PALPATION: notable for effusion of the wrists, moderate tenderness
- RANGE OF MOTION: limited flexion, normal extension
- STRENGTH: 4/5 flexion and extension, ulnar and radial deviation
- JOINT SURVEY: sternoclavicular (SC), acromioclavicular (AC) shoulder, elbow, hip, knee, ankle, feet no evidence of joint swelling, redness, tenderness, decreased range of motion or limitations in strength

Neurovascular
- PULSES: brachial, dorsalis pedis, and radial pulse 2+ and equal
- SENSATION: intact to light touch, sharp distal extremities

DIFFERENTIAL DIAGNOSIS

Disease	Risk Factors	Common Symptoms	Common Signs	Other	Diagnostic Test
Rheumatoid	female:male 3:1 Family history Common	Gradual onset of symmetric pain in small joints of hands and feet with prolonged arm stiffness	Joint effusions, tenderness, restricted motion MCP, wrists	Fatigue, fever, weight loss	Positive rheumatoid factor anti-CCP, high ESR, and CRP

(continued)

Disease	Risk Factors	Common Symptoms	Common Signs	Other	Diagnostic Test
Systemic lupus	F:M 9:1, African American three times greater, age 13 to 40, family history	Gradual onset of symmetric arthritis, morning stiffness with systemic symptoms	Joint effusion, tenderness, restricted motion MCP, wrists, malar rash, pleuritis, pericarditis	Fatigue, photosensitive skin rash, oral ulcerations, psychiatric illness, paresthesia	Positive ANA antidouble stranded DNA, anti-Smith antibody, anemia, proteinuria
Human Parvovirus	Exposed to small children	Gradual onset of symmetrical joint pain in MCP, PIP <6 weeks	Small joints of hands, wrists, and feet, restricted motion	Slapped-cheek rash	IgM antibodies to human parvovirus B19 +
Fibromyalgia	F:M 9:1, age 30 to 50, genetic, environmental	Muscle pain, aching, fatigue, stiffness, poor sleep	No joint swelling or tenderness, muscle tenderness, + trigger points	Fatigue is common but no fever or rash	Clinical diagnosis + tender points 11/18

ANA, antinuclear antibody; CCP, citrullinated peptide; CRP, C-reactive protein; ESR, erythrocyte sedimentation rate; F:M, female:male; IgM, immunoglobulin M; MCP, metacarpal; PIP, proximal interphalangeal RF, rheumatoid factor.

DIAGNOSTIC EXAMINATION

Exam	Code	Cost	Results
X-ray or plain film	73130	$250	Early in inflammatory joint disease and arthritis, radiographic findings are subtle or absent. In RA you may see erosions, deformities, and demineralization of bone. Good to get a baseline for future reference of joint changes
Rheumatoid factor	86430	$180	Positive in 85% of patients with RA, nonspecific, can be elevated in other inflammatory or infectious processes
Anticitrullinated protein antibody	86200	$275	Specific to RA; present in 50% to 80% of patients
ANA	86038	$180	Positive ANA and specific nuclear antibodies are present in RA and SLE
C-reactive protein	86140	$150	Nonspecific but elevated in most inflammatory arthritis
Erythrocyte sedimentation rate	85652	$75	Nonspecific but elevated in most inflammatory arthritis, slower to rise and lower than CRP

(*continued*)

Exam	Code	Cost	Results
Complete blood count	85025	$75	Inflammatory arthritis is associated with anemia of chronic disease; septic joint will have elevated white blood count
Basic metabolic panel	80048	$119	Systemic inflammatory arthritis is associated with nephritis or renal failure
Urinalysis	81003	$25	Establishes presence or absence of proteinuria or red cell cast + SLE
Liver enzymes and function	83516	$120	Usually negative unless autoimmune hepatitis; establish baseline for future drug treatment
Lyme titer Western blot	86618	$180	In endemic areas especially in the presence of erythema migrans
Parvovirus B19 antibodies IgM and IgG	83520	$200	If polyarthritis is less than 6-week duration, can rule out parvovirus; if positive for IgM antibody, recent infection is present

ANA, antinuclear antibodies; CRP, C-reactive protein; IgG, immunoglobulin G; IgM, immunoglobulin M; RA, rheumatoid arthritis; SLE, systemic lupus erythematosus.

The 2010 American College of Rheumatology Classification for Rheumatoid Arthritis

Who should be tested?
1. Patients with at least one joint with definite synovitis on examination
2. Patients with synovitis not explained by any other disease

Joint Involvement	Score
One joint	0
Two to 10 joints	1
One to three small joints	2
Four to 10 small joints	3
Greater than 10 joints	4
Serology	
Negative RF and CCP antibody	0
Low-positive RF or low-positive CCP antibody	2
High-positive RF or high-positive CCP antibody	3

(continued)

Joint Involvement	Score
Acute-phase reactants	
Normal CRP and normal ESR	0
Abnormal CRP or normal ESR	1
Duration of symptoms	
<6 weeks	0
>6 weeks	1

A score of 6 out of 10 indicates the patient has RA.

CCP, citrullinated peptide; CRP, C-reactive protein; ESR, erythrocyte sedimentation rate; RA, rheumatoid arthritis; RF, rheumatoid factor.

CLINICAL DECISION MAKING

Case Study Analysis

The advanced practice provider (APP) notes that the patient's test results are as follows:

- Normal CBC and complete metabolic panel
- Elevated C-reactive protein (CRP) and erythrocyte sedimentation rate (ESR)
- Negative rheumatoid factor
- Negative antinuclear antibody
- Elevated citrullinated peptide (CCP) antibody
- X-rays show joint effusions of the MCP and PIPs, but no erosions

The APP evaluated the 30-year-old woman who presented with recurrent episodes of symmetric pain and swelling in MCP joints and wrists for 2 months and noted that family history is significant as patient's mother suffers from RA. She does not have systemic symptoms of fevers, weight loss, fatigue, or rashes, which could indicate possible systemic lupus. Her symptoms have been present for over 6 weeks making the diagnosis of human parvovirus unlikely. Examination reveals symmetric joint pain and effusions of the MCP and wrists, both common findings in RA. She meets the criteria for diagnostic testing and her laboratory test confirms the presence of the CCP antibody, elevated CRP and ESR. Her x-rays do not reveal an erosive arthritis, but this is common in the early stage of the disease. Rheumatoid factor can be nonspecific even when the disease is present.

> **Diagnosis:** *Rheumatoid arthritis*

Reviewed the results of the testing with the patient and made a follow-up appointment with the rheumatology clinic in 2 weeks.

HEADACHE

Case Presentation: *A 25-year-old Hispanic female presents to the clinic with a headache.*

INTRODUCTION TO COMPLAINT

This is one of the most common and most complicated complaints that a nurse practitioner treats. Over 90% of headaches are benign, and most are either migraine or tension headaches. However, there are several quite serious etiologies that must first be ruled out.

Common Headache Without Fever

Migraines are familial and most often unilateral. Photophobia, nausea, and vomiting are common presenting symptoms. Tension headaches are often bilateral and are accompanied by muscular neck and shoulder pain. Cluster headaches are more common in men and are sharp and of short duration. They occur several times in a short time period. Often they are accompanied by unilateral rhinitis and tearing of the eye.

Other Headaches Without Fever to Consider

Sinusitis, rhinosinusitis, space-occupying lesions, cancer, hypertension (HTN), posttraumatic stress, vessel abnormalities, and bleeding within the brain need to be assessed.

Headache With Fever

If a fever is present along with the headache, then the most common reason is infectious meningitis. This is accompanied by meningeal signs of pain (nuchal ridigity) to the neck that increase when the head is flexed and the knees are bent (Brudzinski and Kernig signs). It is also possible to have a headache as a reaction to a systemic disease or a brain abscess.

Other

A few rare etiologies for headache are familial hemiplegic migraine, pituitary apoplexy, and malignancy of the central nervous system (CNS).

Triggers

Migraines have specific triggers that, when avoided, can prevent onset. These are often tension, lack of sleep, red wine, avocados, and aged cheese, but can be anything. In women, the menstrual cycle can be a trigger.

HISTORY OF COMPLAINT

Symptomatology

Ask about the following characteristics of each symptom using open-ended questions:

- Onset (sudden or gradual) of current headache and age of onset of headaches
- Location
- Duration, frequency, intensity of each episode
- Character (aching, sharp, dull, burning)
- Associated symptoms (presence or absence of aura, fever, rhinitis)
- Radiation
- Timing (morning, evening, after exercise or stress)
- Severity
- Precipitating and aggravating factors
- Relieving factors
- Effects on daily activities
- Previous diagnosis of similar episodes
- Previous treatments
- Efficacy of previous treatments
- Family history of similar episodes
- History of past workup (CT, MRI)

Directed Questions to Ask

- Was the onset sudden (thunderclap) or gradual?
- Do you have fever (intracranial, systemic, local infection)?
- Is this the first or worst headache of your life (intracranial hemorrhage, CNS abnormality)?
- Worsening pattern (mass, subdural hemorrhage [SDH], overuse)?
- Focal neurologic signs/symptoms other than typical visual or sensory aura (mass, arterial/ventricular malformation, collagen vascular diagnosis)?
- Rapid onset with strenuous activity, especially if preceded by trauma (carotid artery dissection or intracranial hemorrhage)?
- History of cancer (metastasis)?
- History of Lyme disease (meningoencephalitis)?
- HIV+ (opportunistic infection or tumor)?
- Pregnant or postpartum (cortical vein or venous sinus thrombosis, carotid dissection, pituitary apoplexy)?

Assessment: Cardinal Signs and Symptoms

In addition to the general characteristics outlined previously, additional characteristics of specific symptoms should be elicited.

Head, Eyes, Ears, Nose, Throat (HEENT)
- Eye tearing
- Vision changes
- Rhinitis, allergies, recent upper respiratory illness
- Pain over sinuses
- Ear pain

Neck
- Pain to the musculature and to shoulders
- Increased pain when flexing the head or bending the knees

Other Associated Symptoms

- Fever
- Nausea, vomiting, flashing lights, aura, or prodromal
- Change in mental status, personality, or level of consciousness
- High blood pressure (BP)

Medical History: General

- Medical conditions and surgeries
- Allergies (seasonal as well as others)
- Herbal preparations and traditional therapies

Medical History: Specific to Complaint

- Sinusitis
- Seasonal allergies
- Past headaches and effective treatments
- Recent trauma (can be as long as 3 months prior to onset of headache)
- Cancer
- Exposure to meningitis
- Meningococcal vaccine

PHYSICAL EXAMINATION

Vital Signs

- BP (would be very high with pheochromocytoma)
- Heart rate (HR)
- Temperature
- Respiration

General Appearance

- Appearance of comfort or distress
- Wearing dark glasses or in darkened room

HEENT

- SCALP/TEMPLES: palpate for areas of tenderness (trauma/temporal arteritis over temples in middle-aged women)
- EYES: clear sclera, fundoscopy looking for papilledema (increased intracranial pressure [ICP]), presence of tearing (cluster); visual field defects (lesion of the optic pathway, pituitary mass), impaired vision or seeing "holes" around a light (glaucoma, subacute angle closure glaucoma); blurred vision when bending forward that improves with sitting up (elevated ICP); blurred vision relieved with recumbency and exacerbated with upright posture (low ICP); complete sudden loss of vision unilaterally (optic neuritis)
- EARS: tympanic membranes grey with light reflex, clear canals (acute otitis media)
- NARES: edema, discharge (rhinosinusitis)
- SINUS CAVITIES: tenderness with tapping, increase in pain with forward flexion (sinusitis)
- Flex neck (Brudzinski) assessing for increased headache pain that causes flexion of the knees for relief (meningitis, subarachnoid hemorrhage [SAH], encephalitis)
- NUCHAL RIGIDITY: inability to flex neck (meningitis)
- Palpate trapezius and sternocleidomastoid (SCM) muscles and cervical vertebrae (tension)
- Carotid bruits (heard on the opposite side as the arteriovenous malformation [AVM])

Abdomen
- Assess for tenderness (if nausea/vomiting present)

Neurologic
- Pupils equal, round, and reactive to light and accommodation (PERRLA); extraocular movements (EOMs) intact and without pain to movement
- Cranial nerves
- Equal strength to head, upper extremity (UE), and lower extremity (LE)
- Sensation equal bilaterally to face, UE, and LE
- Deep tendon reflexes (DTRs) 2+, equal bilaterally (cerebellar abnormalities)
- Functional neurologic examination: get up from seated position without support, walk on tiptoes and heels, tandem gait; cerebellar: Romberg, pronator drift. Finger to nose, rapid alternating fingers

CASE STUDY

History

Directed Question	Response
Have you had this before?	Yes, it started when I was 15, with menses.
Is this headache similar to past ones?	Yes, it is just the same.
How often do you have them?	Usually once a month for about 3 days.
What helps?	Usually rest, ibuprofen, and sleep, but it is annoying to have to sleep all day.
Have you tried any medicine?	No.
Does anyone else have this?	Yes, my mom. She gives me a shot that helps.
Where does it hurt?	Right temporal.
Does your neck hurt?	No.
Have you noticed a change to vision, your mental status, or speech?	No.
Did it start gradually?	Yes, it was not that bad at first, then increased.
What is the quality and severity?	It is an 8 to 10 right now and stabbing and throbbing.
Do you have trouble with light, sound?	Yes, I have to wear dark glasses, sound is okay.
Any nausea or vomiting?	No vomiting, but I am very nauseous.
Have you been able to drink water?	Not as much as I should. I am so nauseous.
Have you had a fever? Neck pain?	No. No.
Have you had any injury to your head?	No.
Have you had vision change, dizziness?	No.

Directed Question	*Response*
Any new stressors?	*No, I go to school, but it's always stressful.*
Chronic nasal stuffiness or sinusitis?	*Seasonal allergies, but not now.*
Any pain with urination, flank pain?	*No.*
What do you think brought this one on?	*Well, it seems to be related to starting my period. Mine is due. It usually happens just before my period starts. I also notice red wine and I did drink a glass the night before it started. I read about avocados and cheese, but I don't notice anything with them.*
Do you use any drugs? Smoke?	*No.*
Have you ever been pregnant?	*No.*
What is your menstrual cycle?	*28 days, regular, with 3 days of flow.*
What other health problems do you have?	*Seasonal allergies and headaches.*
Surgery?	*No.*
What medications do you take?	*Claritin and ibuprofen as needed, Ortho Tri-Cyclen Lo.*
Allergies to medicine?	*No.*
Tell me about your family history?	*My mom has migraines and fibromyalgia; my dad has kidney stones.*
Family history of arteriovenous malformation, tumors, cancer, hypertension, myocardial infarction, cerebrovascular accident?	*No.*

Physical Examination Findings

- VITAL SIGNS: temperature 98.6°F; respiratory rate (RR) 16; HR 86, regular; BP 100/60
- GENERAL APPEARANCE: well-developed, healthy-appearing female wearing dark glasses in a dim room; she is not smiling, but is answering appropriately
- EYES: no injection, anicteric, PERRLA, EOMs intact, without pain to movement; normal vision
- NOSE: nares are patent; no edema or exudate of turbinates
- Tympanic membranes grey with light reflex, canals clear
- OROPHARYNX: no lesions, edema, exudates, or erythema; good dentition
- NECK: supple, full range of motion (FROM) without pain to palpation over the cervical vertebrae or the trapezius, SCM muscles; no increase in pain with neck flexion
- No carotid bruits
- CHEST: lungs are clear in all fields; heart S1, S2 no murmur, gallop, or rub
- ABDOMEN: soft, nontender without mass or organomegaly
- SKIN: no rashes
- EXTREMITIES: equal strength bilaterally to head, UE, and LE; no edema
- NEUROLOGIC: cranial nerves II to XII intact; sensation intact, DTRs 2+ throughout
- Functional neurologic examination is normal

DIFFERENTIAL DIAGNOSIS

Clinical Observations	Common Symptoms	Signs
Migraines	Unilateral, N/V, photophobia	Normal neurologic examination, appears uncomfortable, wearing sunglasses
Tension	Entire head or band, often with neck/shoulders, stressors	Neck pain, normal neurology
Cluster	Unilateral, male, short duration Occurs in clusters	Unilateral rhinitis, tearing
Sinusitis	Rhinitis, frontal pressure	Nare edema, sinus cavities TTP
Meningitis	Nuchal rigidity, photophobia HA	Appears ill, Kernig/Brudzinski positive
Temporal arteritis	>55, HA, fatigue, malaise, night sweats	Tender to temples
Overuse HA	Daily HA, using meds daily	Depends on type of HA
Brain tumor	New/worse HA, vision change	Neurologic changes
Posttraumatic	Pain at site of injury, head injury	Neurologic changes
Systemic reaction	Fever, associated illness symptoms	Relieves with lower temperature

HA, headache; N/V, nausea and vomiting; TTP tender to palpation.

DIAGNOSTIC EXAMINATION

Exam	Code	Cost	Results
Fundoscopy	NA	Part of examination	If you are seeing engorgement of the veins without pulsation, hemorrhages near the optic disc, blurring of the optic margins, or elevation of the optic disc, this is a sign of papilledema, which is indicative of increased intracranial pressure. You may also see "Paton's lines," which are radial retinal lines that originate at the optic disc and radiate outward
CBC	85025	$32–$75	You will see an elevated WBC count in systemic infection
LP: concern for SAH with a negative CT *or* suspected infection	62270	$190–$350	This is not done in a clinic; the patient would be sent to the emergency department or scheduled for interventional radiology if nonemergent; the CSF would not be clear and there would be bacteria, crystals, WBCs in the fluid; this can be further tested for bacteria or viruses

(*continued*)

Exam	Code	Cost	Results
CT: trauma with loss of consciousness or vomiting *or* nonacute HA with abnormal neurologic examination *or* for reassurance of the patient (particularly if family history of tumor)	70450	$1,290–$3,000	You could see a large mass or a hematoma signifying an area of bleeding within the brain structure; the type of bleed is determined by the location: SAH versus SDH
MRI/MRA: to see masses not seen on CT or for vessel damage (family history of AVM)	70553 or 70544	$4,097 $2,585	You could see an AVM or a mass not seen on CT or an aneurysm

AVM, arteriovenous malformation; CBC, complete blood count; CSF, cerebral spinal fluid; HA, headache; LP, lumbar puncture; MRA, magnetic resonance arteriogram; SAH, subarachnoid hemorrhage; SDH, subdural hemorrhage; WBC, white blood cell.

CLINICAL DECISION MAKING

Case Study Analysis

It is important to rule out all the danger signs first. Often this can be done with a thorough history. A neurologic examination is essential. If this is abnormal, the patient needs to be referred for imaging and to a neurologist, which is best handled in the emergency department. If there are no danger signs and no neurologic changes on the examination, you can be reassured that this is a benign headache.

The advanced practice provider performs the assessment and physical examination on the patient and finds the following: 25-year-old woman with a headache of 3 days that is similar to her history of headaches. She endorses photophobia and nausea. It is an 8 to 10 on a pain scale with throbbing and stabbing pain. There is a correlation with her menses, which is due and with red wine. Denies red flags of trauma, fever, vomiting, vision changes, and neurologic changes.

She fits the International Headache Society criteria for diagnosis of migraine: at least five attacks lasting 4 to 72 hours, unilateral, pulsating, moderate to severe intensity, causing avoidance of routine activity, associated with nausea and photophobia.

Headache from tension is ruled out because of pain location and lack of neck and shoulder involvement. A cluster headache was ruled out because of the length of time it is present and because of gender. Sinusitis was ruled out because of pain location and lack of other symptoms. Meningitis was ruled out because of the absence of nuchal rigidity. Temporal arteritis was ruled out because of the patient's age and lack of other related symptoms. A brain tumor and traumatic cause were ruled out because of lack of symptoms and lack of injury. Systemic reaction was ruled out due to lack of other related symptoms.

> **Diagnosis:** *Migraine headache*

Since the patient has trended the occurrence and precipitating factors, she was counseled to avoid red wine prior to beginning her menses. Recommend prescribing medication specific for migraine headaches. Activity should be limited during the duration and other symptoms treated conservatively. If headaches worsen over time, recommend following up at the neurology clinic.

HEARTBURN

Case Presentation: A 40-year-old Mexican American male presents stating "my stomach hurts after I eat."

INTRODUCTION TO COMPLAINT

Heartburn (pyrosis) is a common complaint in primary care practice. It is described as a burning sensation in the central chest, typically after eating:

- The majority of heartburn cases are benign and related to one of three types of problems:
  - Mucosal irritation
    - Gastroesophageal reflux disease (GERD)
    - Peptic ulcer disease (PUD)
    - Intermittent reflux due to obesity, large meals, fatty foods, caffeine, or alcohol
  - *Helicobacter pylori* infection
  - Nonulcer dyspepsia
- Other causes of heartburn-like symptoms are:
  - Mechanical: pregnancy, hiatal hernia, esophageal strictures
  - Iatrogenic: large pill volume, medication-induced, radiation-induced
  - Motility: lower esophageal hypotension, esophageal dysmotility
  - Inflammatory: eosinophilic esophagitis, scleroderma, sarcoidosis
  - Vascular: angina, intestinal ischemia
  - Cancerous: esophageal, gastric or duodenal cancers, gastrinoma
- The VBAD mnemonic (very bad) reminds you of the most alarming features to look for:
  - Vomiting
  - Bleeding: anemia
  - Abdominal mass
  - Dysphagia (pain when swallowing—especially with solids or if worsening)
- Other alarming features by body system include:
  - General: evolving—progressive symptoms, weight loss, age older than 45 years
  - Abdominal: jaundice, rigid abdomen, pulsatile abdomen
  - Stool—emesis: hematochezia, melena, hematemesis, coffee-ground emesis
  - Pain: acute onset, severe quantity, ripping, tearing quality

HISTORY OF COMPLAINT

Symptomatology

Ask about the following characteristics of each symptom using open-ended questions:

- Provocative and palliative factors
- Quantity and quality of pain or symptoms

- Region and radiation of pain or symptoms
- Symptoms associated with the chief complaint
- Time course and therapies tried
- Patient's understanding of the symptom's cause and its impact on his or her life

Directed Questions to Ask

- When did your pain begin? *or* When did you *first* have this pain?
- What makes your pain worse? *and* What makes it better?
- What words describe how your pain feels?
- If 0 is no pain and 10 is the worst pain you can imagine, what number is your pain?
- Where is your pain located; can you point to it?
- Do you also feel pain in other places at the same time—like your belly, back, or chest?
- Have you noticed any other new symptoms since your belly pain began?
- When the pain comes, how long does it last—minutes, hours, or days?
- After you eat, how long does it take before the pain starts?
- Have you tried anything to help the pain (suggest things like herbs, over-the-counter [OTC] drugs, prescriptions)?
- What do you think is causing the pain? How has it affected your day-to-day life?

Assessment: Cardinal Signs and Symptoms

General

- Nausea
- Vomiting
- Diarrhea
- Weight loss
- Difficulty swallowing

Pulmonary

- Shortness of breath, coughing, chest pain

Abdominal (involved)

- Abdominal changes (rigid or pulsatile)
- Stool changes (bright red blood or thick-black-tarry stools)
- Vomiting (hematemesis or coffee emesis)

GU

- Urine changes (dark color, bloody, painful)

Medical History: General

- Good health with no significant history
- Surgical: abdominal injury or surgery
- Medications: use of calcium channel blockers (CCBs), inhalers, tricyclics, iron, potassium, tetracycline
- Nutrition: large-volume meals
  - High-fat foods (including fast foods, oils, butter, red meats)
  - Acidic liquids (soda, citrus juices)
  - Acidic foods: liquids (citrus, tomato)

- Other foods (spices, chocolates, peppermint, garlic)
- Substances: alcohol, tobacco, recreational drugs (cocaine, heroin, marijuana)

Medical History: Specific to Complaint

- Stomach disorders (like reflux, ulcers, or cancer)
- Intestinal disorders (like irritable bowel syndrome [IBS], inflammatory bowel disease [IBD], or colitis)
- Liver–gallbladder disorders (like hepatitis, cirrhosis, or gallstones)
- Pancreatic disorders (like pancreatitis or diabetes)
- Lung disorders (like emphysema, asthma, or tuberculosis [TB])
- Renal and genital disorders (like renal failure, kidney stones)
- Unusual food or drink intake

PHYSICAL EXAMINATION

Vital Signs

- Respiration
- Blood pressure (BP)
- Pulse
- Temperature

General Appearance

- Anthropometry: body mass index (BMI), height, weight, abdominal girth

Abdominal

- Contour
- Bowel sounds: four quadrants
- Tenderness to palpation and location of tenderness
- Spleen–liver size by palpation and percussion
- Abdominal masses
- Fluid shift
- Tests and signs: McBurney's, Blumberg, Murphy, Markle, Cullen, Grey Turner

Pulmonary–Chest

- Auscultation of anterior–posterior–lateral fields
- Egophony

Cardiovascular

- Auscultation of S1, S2 for rate, rhythm, murmurs, rubs, gallops
- Abdominal bruits or pulsations
- EKG for unexplained chest pain only

Musculoskeletal

- Sternum–rib joint stability and tenderness
- Lumbar–thoracic range of motion, joint stability, and deformities

HEENT (Optional and Mostly for Detecting Atypical Reflux Sequelae)

- Dentition: presence–absence, coloration, caries, erosions, repairs
- Oral mucosal: coloration, lesions
- Oropharynx: tonsillar size, erythema, edema

CASE STUDY

History

Directed Question	Response
What brings you in today?	I have pain in my stomach—it is frustrating!
Tell me about your pain.	It hurts badly after I eat.
When did your pain begin?	Oh, I don't know. Maybe 6 months ago.
What makes your pain worse?	It happens mostly after lunch and dinner. Breakfast doesn't seem to bother it.
Does any food or drink make it worse?	It is really mostly when I have more than eight tortillas at once or carne asada (grilled beef).
What makes your pain better?	I don't really know.
What word describes your pain?	It is like a fire in my chest and a deep ache in my belly after I eat.
What number would you give your pain?	3.
Show me where your pain is.	[Places hand on epigastrium and sternum].
When you have pain in your belly, do you feel pain anywhere else—like your abdomen, back, chest, or throat?	Yes—in the center of my chest.
Are there any other symptoms you have noticed since your belly pain began?	No.
How long does the pain last?	Well, I guess it usually stays for about 2 hours or so after I eat.
Have you tried anything like vitamins, herbs, prescriptions, or over-the-counter medicines to help the pain?	Yes; Maalox seems to help it some and ibuprofen seems to make it better for a bit.
What do you think is causing the pain?	I don't know. That is why I came to see you.

Physical Examination Findings

- VITAL SIGNS: temperature 98.7°F; respiratory rate (RR) 16; heart rate (HR) 86, regular; BP 130/74; height 74″; weight 334 lb; BMI 42.9
- GENERAL APPEARANCE: no acute distress, elevated BMI
- PULMONARY: clear to auscultation anteriorly, posteriorly, and laterally without wheezes, rhonchi, or rales; no egophony; no retractions
- CARDIOVASCULAR: S1 and S2 within normal limits; no murmurs, rubs, or gallops; no S3 or S4; no abdominal bruits or palpable abdominal pulsations
- ABDOMINAL: bowel sounds present in all four quadrants, protuberant abdomen with striae; mild tenderness to palpation in epigastrium and along medial costal margins bilaterally no hepatosplenomegaly appreciated by palpation or percussion but examination limited by abdominal girth of 154 cm (at umbilicus); negative Blumberg, Murphy's, McBurney's, Markle, Grey Turner, and Cullen signs; no fluid shift
- MUSCULOSKELETAL: sternum–rib joints stable and no tenderness to palpation

DIFFERENTIAL DIAGNOSIS

Clinical Observations	GERD	PUD	Nonulcer Dyspepsia	Intermittent Reflux
30- to 60-minute postprandial onset	Common	If gastric	Common	Common
Steady discomfort for 30 to 120 minutes	Common	Common	Possible	Common
Food intake triggers pain	Common	If gastric	Common	Common
Retrosternal burning quality	Common	Uncommon	Uncommon	Common
Reflux (stomach contents in mouth or throat)	Common	No	No	Possible
Specific food triggers (fatty, spicy, acidic)	Common	Common	No	Common
Liquid triggers (sodas, alcohol, caffeine)	Common	Common	No	Common
NSAIDs trigger	Common	Common	No	Common
Epigastric pain	Common	Common	Common	Uncommon
Supine position triggers	Common	No	No	Common
Bitter taste in mouth	Common	No	No	Common
Epigastric burning	Uncommon	Common	Common	Common
Nocturnal pain awakens from sleep	Uncommon	If duodenal	No	No
Nausea: mild and intermittent	Uncommon	Uncommon	Common	No
Belching, postprandial	Uncommon	Common	Common	No
Bloating	Uncommon	Common	Common	No
Chronic cough	Uncommon	No	No	No

(*continued*)

Clinical Observations	GERD	PUD	Nonulcer Dyspepsia	Intermittent Reflux
Laryngitis (hoarseness)	Uncommon	No	No	Uncommon
Halitosis (bad breath)	Uncommon	No	No	No
Throat clearing	Uncommon	No	No	No
Hypersalivation (water brash)	Rare	No	No	No
Globus (throat fullness despite swallow)	Rare	No	No	No
Dental erosions	Rare	No	No	No
Epigastric "fullness" (postprandial)	Rare	Uncommon	Common	Uncommon
Vomiting: mild and intermittent	Rare	Uncommon	No	No
"Gnawing," "hunger-like," or "achy" quality	No	Common	No	Uncommon
2- to 5-hour postprandial onset	No	If duodenal	No	Uncommon
Food relieves pain	No	If duodenal	No	No
Early satiety	No	Common	Common	Uncommon
Psychiatric comorbidity	No	Rare	Common	No
Relapse–remitting pain pattern	No	No	Common	Common

GERD, gastroesophageal reflux disease; NSAID, nonsteroidal anti-inflammatory drug; PUD, peptic ulcer disease.

DIAGNOSTIC EXAMINATION

- Initiate lifestyle modification for heartburn trigger reduction and/or
- Conduct a "PPI test"; this is an empiric GERD therapy with a high-dose proton pump inhibitor (PPI) at least 30 to 60 minutes before meals (AC) twice daily (BID)
  - A "PPI test" is positive and suggests GERD if symptoms resolve within 4 weeks
  - Common agents are: omeprazole 20 mg or lansoprazole 30 mg
  - Diagnostic testing for heartburn is typically reserved for patients with:

- Failed PPI test
- Recurrence of symptoms within 3 months after successful suppression using a PPI
- History clearly suggestive of a non-GERD pathology (e.g., *H. pylori* or hiatal hernia)

Exam	Code	Cost	Results
Stool antigen, *H. pylori* or *H. pylori* urea breath test	87338	$25	A positive result would indicate active infection A negative result would indicate no active infection
RBC count and indices (Hgb, Hct, and MCV are part of a complete blood count)	85027	$20	Anemia is present if the total number of RBCs, Hgb, and/or Hct is below the normal range for the patient's age and sex. The MCV cutoffs for RBC size in adults are: <80: microcytic (small cells) 80–100: normocytic (normal sized cells) >100: macrocytic (large cells) However, a normocytic or microcytic anemia, if present, could suggest an active gastrointestinal bleed
Endoscopy	43200	$1,000	Referral to gastroenterology for refractory symptoms

Hct, hematocrit; Hgb, hemoglobin; H. pylori, Helicobacter pylori; MCV, mean corpuscular volume; RBC, red blood cell.

CLINICAL DECISION MAKING

Case Study Analysis

The clinician's examination does not identify a focal cause of the patient's heartburn or any alarming features (such as hypotension, tachycardia, or abdominal masses). However, the patient's positive *H. pylori* stool antigen indicates an active infection that likely caused PUD. His postprandial, gnawing epigastric pain is consistent with PUD.

> **Diagnosis:** *Peptic ulcer disease secondary to* H. pylori *infection*

- Additional PUD risks include heavy alcohol use, nonsteroidal anti-inflammatory drug (NSAID) use, and central adiposity
- The patient's normal red blood cell (RBC) indices suggest the ulcer is not causing significant blood loss
- Causes of heartburn are not mutually exclusive and can often overlap; however, key symptoms inhibit prostaglandins that protect the mucosal wall from stomach acidity
- Alcohol intake can damage the mucosa directly due to acidity
- Central adiposity may compress the esophageal sphincter and promote reflux

The patient was counseled on the cause for the discomfort and treatment to include antibiotics and PPI medication. Additional teaching focused on weight management, food choices, and portion control. It was explained how NSAIDs may precipitate/worsen the discomfort and enteric coated analgesics were suggested going forward for pain control. Recommend beginning prescribed medication and following up in 1 month. If symptoms persist after antibiotics are completed, recommend further testing through the gastroenterology department.

HEAVY MENSTRUAL FLOW

Case Presentation: A 16-year-old female described a prolonged heavy menstrual flow with increased cramping over the past 8 days. This was unlike her normal menses, which were normal in the past.

INTRODUCTION TO COMPLAINT

Heavy menstrual bleeding can be caused by:

- Hormonal imbalance
- Uterine fibroid tumors
- Cervical polyps
- Endometrial polyps
- Infection
- Cervical cancer
- Endometrial cancer
- Intrauterine devices (IUDs)

HISTORY OF COMPLAINT

Symptomatology

Ask about the following characteristics of each symptom using open-ended questions:

- Onset (sudden or gradual)
- Chronology
- Improving or deteriorating
- Quality and quantity
- Timing (frequency, duration)
- Severity
- Precipitating and aggravating factors
- Relieving factors
- Associated symptoms
- Effects on daily activities
- Previous diagnosis of similar episodes
- Previous treatments
- Efficacy of previous treatments

Directed Questions to Ask

- How long have you had menstrual irregularities?
- Age of menarche (when you had your first menstrual period)?
- Duration of the menstrual period?

- Is the menstrual interval regular?
- What is the interval of your menstrual cycle?
- How old are you now?
- How saturated are the pads you use? Do you get clots, if yes, how big were the clots?
- Dysmenorrhea?
- Intermenstrual bleeding, that is, spotting between your menstrual periods?
- Bleeding after intercourse?
- Have you experienced painful intercourse?
- Do you have excessive vaginal discharge? If so, describe the discharge.

Assessment: Cardinal Signs and Symptoms

- Dysmenorrhea
- Polymenorrhea
- Oligomenorrhea
- Menorrhagia
- Metrorrhagia
- Postcoital bleeding
- Premenstrual syndrome

Medical History: General

- Allergies to medications
- Smoking or drinking alcohol
- Previous medical history or surgeries
- Medications
- Sexually active
- Last sexual encounter
- Birth control or barrier devices
- Last gynecological exam
- Family members with problems of heavy bleeding

Medical History: Specific to Complaint

- Start of menses
- Regularity of periods
- Color of flow
- Length of flow
- Number of pads used per day
- Bleeding between cycles
- Cramping, then and now
- Pregnancies
- Miscarriages or abortions
- Consistency of the bleeding now

PHYSICAL EXAMINATION

Vital Signs

- Temperature
- Pulse
- Respiration
- Blood pressure (BP)
- Oxygen saturation (SpO_2)

General Appearance

- Apparent state of health
- Hygiene, age-appropriate dress and demeanor

Skin

- Observe color and torgur

Abdomen

- Inspect for distress, cramping, low back pain

Nutrition

- Observe appropriate weight and body mass index

Musculoskeletal

- Observe difficulty with gait or balance

CASE STUDY

History

Directed Question	Response
Do you have allergies to medications?	No.
Do you smoke cigarettes or drink alcohol?	No.
Do you have a previous medical history or surgeries?	No.
Do you use any medications?	No.
How long have you had menstrual irregularities?	Since my first period.
Age of menarche (when you first got menstrual period)?	11.
Duration of the menstrual period?	5 to 7 days.
Is the menstrual interval regular?	Yes.
What is the interval of your menstrual cycle?	26 days.
How old are you now?	16.
With heavy menstrual bleeding, how many pads or tampons do you use per day?	I change my tampons every hour and always wear a pad for extra protection.
With the heavy bleeding do you experience large clots?	Yes, there have been large clots for the past year, the size of a half dollar.
Dysmenorrhea?	Yes, bad cramps.
Intermenstrual bleeding (i.e., spotting between your menstrual periods)?	No.
When was your last gynecological exam?	When I was 15 and the exam was normal.

Directed Question	*Response*
Do any family members have problems with heavy bleeding?	*When my mom was my age she had heavy menstrual flow.*
Are you sexually active?	*No. [advanced practice provider had doubts about this response].*
When was your last sexual encounter?	*A month ago. I had a boyfriend but we broke up.*
Do you use any type of birth control or barrier devices?	*No.*
Bleeding after intercourse?	*No.*
Do you experience painful intercourse? If so, is the discomfort within the vagina or deep within the abdomen?	*Deep.*
Have you experienced vaginal discharge between periods?	*No discharge.*
Was the onset of the bleeding gradual or sudden?	*Sudden.*
What is the consistency of the bleeding now?	*Very heavy, with big clots of dark blood.*
Have you had any fever?	*No.*
Have you had any cramping?	*Yes.*
Do you normally have cramps with your period?	*No.*
On a scale of 0 to 10, rate your pain.	*3 or 4.*
Have you ever been pregnant?	*No.*
Do you have fatigue?	*Yes, very tired, sleeping a lot, don't feel like doing anything.*
Have you had any nausea or vomiting?	*I feel queasy.*
Any breast tenderness?	*No.*
Is your abdomen tender?	*Yes, very.*
Are you bleeding at this time?	*Yes.*
How many days have you had the heavy bleeding?	*8 days.*

Physical Examination Findings

- VITAL SIGNS: temperature 98.2°F; respiratory rate 20; pulse 92; BP 110/70; SpO$_2$ 98%
- GENERAL APPEARANCE: patient is a 16-year-old, well-developed, overweight, Caucasian female; skin is cold and clammy to touch; her height is 5'6" and weight is 162 lb; her BMI is 26.1

- HEAD, EYES, EARS, NOSE, THROAT (HEENT): head and neck are within normal limits; pupils equal, round, and reactive to light and accommodation (PERRLA); extraocular movements are intact; nonicteric sclerae; nares are patent; no edema or exudate of the turbinates is noted; all teeth present with no apparent gum hyperplasia; tonsils are normal; no redness or exudate is noted; neck range of motion is within normal limits; there is no lymph node enlargement on palpation; thyroid is not enlarged
- CHEST: lungs are clear
- HEART: S1 and S2 are normal; no murmur, gallop, or rub noted
- ABDOMEN: excess fat in abdomen; tender to deep palpation, pain is worse in the right and left lower quadrants of abdomen; no distention is noted; suprapubic tenderness present upon examination
- BACK: pain and tenderness located in the lower back on palpation
- PELVIC: no discharge is noted; heavy bleeding and blood clots noted; cervix is normal in color and round; extreme tenderness and pain are noted on cervical motion; the cervical os is closed; the uterus is enlarged and tenderness is noted in the posterior aspect of the abdomen; fundal height is noted at 4 cm; the hymen is not intact; palpation of the ovaries does elicit some tenderness bilaterally; the ovaries are noted to be 2 to 4 cm in size
- EXTREMITIES: within normal limits; no edema is noted

Specific to OB/GYN

- GENERAL: the patient is a 16-year-old female who is complaining of abdominal cramping with heavy menstrual flow for the past 8 days; the patient has a history of heavy menstrual periods; however, this is different from her normal menstrual periods; she is quite pale and her skin is cold and clammy; she is 5′6″ in height and weighs approximately 162 lb; her BMI is 26.1; she states she does not exercise and is not active in sports; she is an overachiever scholastically as evidenced by taking prerequisite classes in high school for entry into law school; she is disciplined in this endeavor and involved in her journal club
- BREASTS: states she has no tenderness or soreness and none is elicited on exam
- ABDOMEN: has excess fat on her abdomen; she is very tender to deep palpation, stating the pain is worse in the right and left lower quadrants of her abdomen; she raises her legs due to the pain elicited on deep palpation; there is no evidence of bloating or distention; when questioned about nausea or vomiting, the patient states "I have some queasiness"; there is suprapubic tenderness also
- BACK: has pain in her lower back; she states this is a constant ache; she states that she had really bad lower back pain when abdomen palpated; she states the pain in her lower back, on a scale of 0 to 10, is a 3 or 4; the pain is made worse on palpation of the lower back
- PELVIC: on general inspection, there is no discharge from the vagina; large blood clots and heavy bleeding are noted; a pediatric speculum was used and the hymen is noted to be not intact; the cervix is normal in color and round; there is extreme tenderness noted in the cervical area on movement, and the patient complains of pain; the cervical os is closed; no discharge is noted from the cervical os; vaginal mucosa appears normal; on bimanual exam the uterus is noted to be enlarged and tender in the posterior aspect; fundal height is noted at 4 cm; palpation of the ovaries reveals no masses; however, there is slight tenderness bilaterally; the ovaries are 2 to 4 cm in size

DIFFERENTIAL DIAGNOSIS

Clinical Observations	PID	Spontaneous Abortion (Miscarriage)	Threatened Abortion	Ectopic Pregnancy	Fibroids/ Polyps
Dysmenorrhea	Rare	Yes	Yes	Common	Common
Abdominal pain/ cramping	Common	Yes	Yes	Common	Not a common complaint, unlikely
Uterus enlarged on examination	Rare	Yes	Yes	Yes/No	Common
Painful uterus on examination	Rare	Yes	Yes	Yes/No	Yes/No
Painful cervix on examination	Yes	Rare	Yes	Yes	No
Fever	Yes	Rare	Rare	No	No
Acute bleeding in a normally regular menstrual cycle	Rare	Yes	Yes	Rare	Common
Nausea/vomiting	Yes	Common	Yes	Rare	Rare
Dizziness/fainting	Rare	Rare	Yes	Yes	Rare

PID, pelvic inflammatory disease.

DIAGNOSTIC EXAMINATION

Exam	Code	Cost	Results
CBC	85025	$75	CBC: typically has several parameters: • WBC count: when an infection is present, the WBCs elevate in number • WBC differential: ▪ Neutrophils: the most abundant of the white blood cells; respond more rapidly to areas of tissue injury and infection ▪ Eosinophils: allergic or parasitic illnesses ▪ Basophils: will increase during the healing process ▪ Monocytes: second defense mechanism against bacterial and inflammatory illnesses; slower to respond than neutrophils but are bigger and can ingest larger organisms ▪ Lymphocytes: increased after chronic bacterial and viral infections • RBCs: carry oxygen from the lungs to the body • Hematocrit: this is the amount of space the RBCs take up in the blood

(continued)

Exam	Code	Cost	Results
			• Hemoglobin: carries oxygen and gives the RBCs their color; determines the ability of blood to carry oxygen throughout the body • Mean corpuscular volume: shows the size of RBCs • MCH: shows the amount of hemoglobin contained in the average RBC • MCHC: measures the concentration of the hemoglobin in an average RBC • Platelets: The platelets play an important role in blood clotting. When bleeding occurs, the platelets swell, clump together, and form a stick plug that helps stop bleeding. If there are too few platelets, uncontrolled bleeding can occur. If there are too many, a blood clot can form in the artery.
Qualitative urine hCG test	81025	$64	A urine pregnancy test is one of the easiest and less expensive laboratory and diagnostic studies to confirm or exclude a pregnancy. If a more sensitive test is needed, the serum hCG can be used.
Pelvic examination	89.26	$155	A pelvic examination can assist with determining a diagnosis by assessing and palpating the uterus, uterus size, cervix, and cervical size, whether or not the cervical os is open or closed
Ultrasound transvaginal Ultrasound pelvic	76830 76856	$130	Can detect complications of pregnancy, such as ectopic pregnancy or a threatened abortion or absence of conception; cysts or polyps can be identified as well

CBC, complete blood count; hCG, human chorionic gonadotropin; MCH, mean corpuscular hemoglobin; MCHC, mean corpuscular hemoglobin concentration; RBC, red blood cell; WBC, white blood cell.

CLINICAL DECISION MAKING

Case Study Analysis

The assessment on the patient is completed and data analysis is as follows: A 16-year-old female with an 8-day history of prolonged heavy menstrual flow and increased cramping that presents with a hematocrit level of 20. The patient had extreme tenderness on pelvic examination to include an enlarged uterus with the posterior part of uterus positive for tenderness. When the cervix was palpated, the patient was noted to have discomfort. Fundal height of the uterus is measured at 4 cm. An enlarged uterus and cervical discomfort are not associated with pelvic inflammatory disease (PID). Abdominal pain and cramping are not associated with uterine fibroids. A urine pregnancy test done on the patient is positive. The diagnosis is threatened abortion. A referral to OB/GYN is made as well as counseling the patient on birth control methods for the future. A transvaginal ultrasound will most likely be completed during the OB/GYN appointment to confirm the diagnosis.

Diagnosis: *Threatened abortion*

HIP PAIN

Case Presentation: *A 66-year-old African American woman reports a complaint of hip pain from a fall she had 3 weeks ago.*

INTRODUCTION TO COMPLAINT

Hip pain can occur from a fall and subsequent damage to the hip joint. Damage can also occur from a number of causes including sports-related injury, exercises, old age, overuse, and falls. Also, certain diseases lead to hip pain, including osteoarthritis, rheumatoid arthritis, avascular arthritis, and bone cancer.

Injuries That Cause Hip Pain

Hip Dislocation
- An injury to a joint in which the ends of the bones are forced from their normal positions
- This injury immobilizes the hip joint and results in sudden and severe pain

Hip Fracture
- Usually occurs in the joint area where the head of the femur is fractured. This results in extreme pain and immobility
- Multiple medications

Hip Labral Tear
- Tear involves the labrum that follows the outside rim of the socket of the hip joint
- The labrum acts like a socket to hold the ball at the top of the femur in place

Compartment Syndrome
- Results from bleeding or swelling after an injury into a compartment space
- High pressure in compartment syndrome impedes the flow of blood to and from the affected tissues

Osteoporosis
- Causes bones to become weak and brittle so that a fall or even mild stresses, like bending over or coughing, can cause a fracture
- Physical findings include palpable tenderness over the area of compression fracture
- Osteoporosis-related fractures most commonly occur in the hip, wrist, or spine, especially in older people

Bursitis
- Affects the bursae
- Occurs when bursae become inflamed and patient experiences pain

Tendinitis
- Inflammation or irritation of a tendon
- Causes focal pain and tenderness just outside a joint due to trauma-related activities
- One of the most common sites is hip

Diseases That Cause Hip Pain

Osteoarthritis
- Most common form of arthritis
- Often called wear-and-tear arthritis
- Occurs when the protective cartilage on the ends of the bones wears down over time

Rheumatoid Arthritis
- Affects the synovial membranes, causing edema
- Results in bone erosion and damage to ligaments and tendons
- An autoimmune disorder

Paget's Disease
- Disrupts body's normal bone recycling process
- Old bone tissue is gradually replaced with new bone tissue
- Over time, the affected bones become fragile and can cause pain and tenderness

HISTORY OF COMPLAINT

Symptomatology

Ask about the following characteristics of each symptom using open-ended questions:

- Quality and severity of the pain
- Location
- Range of motion
- Relieving factors
- Radiation
- Ability to walk
- Gait and balance affected
- Able to complete activities of daily living
- Is the pain continuous or intermittent?
- What makes the pain worse: walking, bending, or extending the knee?
- Relief from pain with rest
- Medications or treatments tried
- Burning, cramping, or aching pain

Directed Questions to Ask

- How is your balance?
- Are you able to walk straight?
- Are you able to bear weight on both legs? Which leg hurts more when you walk?
- Are you able to raise your left hip? Right hip?
- Did you notice the shortening of any one leg?
- Did you notice any external rotation of your leg/hip?
- Do you have any redness or swelling?
- Did you notice any bulge in your inguinal area?
- Did you notice any lymph nodes in your groin area?
- Do you feel any pain in your groin area?
- Did you have any pain in your ischiogluteal area? Sciatica?
- Are you able to flex your hip (bend your knee)?
- Are you able to extend your hip (lie face down, then bend your knee and lift it up)?
- Are you able to abduct your leg (lying flat, moving your leg away from the midline)?

- Are you able to adduct your legs (lying flat, bend your knee and move your lower leg toward the midline)?
- Are you able to rotate the leg internally (lying flat, bend your knee and turn your lower leg and foot away from the midline)?

Assessment: Cardinal Signs and Symptoms

- Extreme localized pain in the affected area
- Inability to abduct or adduct the affected limb
- Paresthesia
- Swelling or edema

Other Associated Symptoms

- Chills or fever
- Malaise
- Nausea or vomiting
- Pain or swelling or any joint pain
- Restricted or limited movement of any other joints

Medical History: General

- Weight/diet
- Hypertension
- Diabetes
- Falls
- Coronary artery disease

Medical History: Specific to Complaint

- Swelling
- Pain
- Numbness
- Tingling
- Medications

PHYSICAL EXAMINATION

Vital Signs

- Blood pressure (BP)
- Pulse
- Respiration
- Temperature

General Appearance

- Body mass index (BMI)
- Height, weight
- Abdominal girth

Musculoskeletal

- Hip adduction
- Hip abduction
- Range of motion
- Pain

CASE STUDY
History

Directed Question	Response
How is your general state of health?	I am obese. I don't brush my teeth enough and have several cavities. My skin is warm and dry.
Do you have any history of medical conditions like diabetes, high blood pressure, high cholesterol, or cancer?	Yes, I have high blood pressure.
Did you have any heart problems or a history of cardiovascular disease?	No.
Did you have any breathing or respiratory problems?	No.
Did you have any stomach or gastric problems in the past?	Yes, I have GERD.
Did you have any surgeries in the past? Any hospitalization?	No.
Are you allergic to any medication, food, or plants? Any seasonal allergies?	No.
Do you have any history of lupus, psoriasis, Lyme disease, gonococcal infection, rubella, or rheumatic fever?	No.
Are your immunizations up to date?	I don't know.
Do you currently use any medications that include any prescription medications?	Yes, I take Prilosec for GERD and a calcium channel blocker and hydrochlorothiazide for hypertension.
Do you use any over-the-counter medications?	No.
Did you use any herbal preparations or traditional therapies?	I use Biofreeze for my hip pain.
Do you have any weakness in any of your extremities?	No.
Any changes in your activities?	I am not able to wear my high-heel shoes now. I feel wobbly.
Do you have any trauma, injury, or fracture of your hip before?	No.
Do you have arthritis?	I believe I have arthritis in my right knee. But no doctors told me that.

Directed Question	Response
Do you have any unsteady gait? Do you use any assistive devices?	No.
Do you drink or smoke?	No.
Do you have trouble falling asleep at night?	No.
Are you sleeping more than usual, such as taking naps throughout the day?	No.
Do you feel like your appetite has increased or decreased?	No, I am obese.
Where do you live, and who lives with you (spouse, son, daughter)?	With my daughter and grandkids.
How well do you get along with your household members?	Good.

GERD, gastroesophageal reflux disease.

Physical Examination Findings

- VITAL SIGNS: temperature 98.6°F (oral); respiratory rate 24 beats/min; pulse 72 beats/min; BP 142/92 mmHg (supine), 138/90 mmHg (sitting), 138/92 mmHg (standing)
- GENERAL APPEARANCE: older adult, obese, African American female, who was admitted due to syncope with a complaint of hip pain from a fall; she is in a fair state of health and concerned about the episode of her fainting spell; she is 5'4" tall and weighs 213 lb; appears neat and clean, however, with poor dentition; her appearance matches with her age; her mood looks worried and anxious; skin looks normal; nutritional status is fair, drinks eight glasses of water per day; she has difficulty with gait or balance; states feeling wobbly when walking due to her obesity and right knee pain
- ACCU-CHEK: random blood glucose 82 mg/dL
- SKIN: skin is warm and dry with no open lesions; quarter-sized, yellowish green old bruise on right hip
- CARDIAC: EKG reveals normal sinus rhythm; echocardiogram was normal
- PULMONARY: oxygen saturation 96%; respirations regular and even; lungs clear
- GASTRIC: abdomen obese, soft, nontender; bowel sounds normoactive
- HIP/MUSCULOSKELETAL:
  - Bilateral hips no swelling or deformity
  - Right hip has quarter size, yellowish green old bruise
  - Mild irritation and tenderness on internal rotation of the right hip
  - Hands with degenerative changes and stiffness
  - Right knee with moderate effusion and tenderness
  - Both feet have bunions
  - All other joints with good range of motion; no other deformity or swelling

DIFFERENTIAL DIAGNOSIS

Clinical Observations	Muscle Injury/Strain	Compartment Syndrome	Hip Fracture	Labral Tear	Tendon Injury
Location of the pain	Hip muscle pain	Persistent deep ache in the hip and right knee	Pain in the hip, lower groin	Groin pain, buttocks and thigh pain	Pain in the affected area where the injured tendon is located or may radiate out from the joint area
Quality of the pain	Muscle tightness, weakness	Pain that seems greater than expected for the severity of the injury, bruising	Severe pain and swelling	Sharp deep pain	Tenderness, redness, warmth/swelling near the injured tendon
Course of the pain	Inability to fully stretch the injured muscle	Persistent everyday pain, hurts when pressure is applied to the area	Inability to walk or move hips, abnormal appearance and shortening of the affected leg	Worse with extension, episodes of deep clicking, feeling of hip giving away	Pain and stiffness may be worse during night or when getting up in the morning; pain may increase with activity
Involvement of trauma	Yes	Yes	Yes	Yes/No	Yes

DIAGNOSTIC EXAMINATION

Exam	Code	Cost	Results
Plain x-ray	M25.559	$350	An x-ray can reveal deterioration of the structure of the hip, an excess of bone on the femoral head or neck and the acetabular rim.
CT scan	M12.559	$1,500	CT scan provides digital images of the body using a thin x-ray beam to produce a more detailed, cross-sectional image of the body.
Compartment pressure measurement	20950	$150	Insert a needle into the area of suspected compartment syndrome while an attached pressure monitor records the pressure. A plastic catheter can also be inserted to monitor the compartment pressure continuously. Compartment measurement within 20 mmHg of diastolic pressure is an indication of fasciotomy.

CLINICAL DECISION MAKING
Case Study Analysis

The provider performs the assessment and physical examination on a 66-year-old female and reports the following data: the diagnosis of hip pain evidenced by bruise due to fall; physical examination revealed limited internal rotation of the right hip, with tenderness. Since weight bearing has no effect on the pain, a hip fracture can be ruled out. The lack of deep groin pain that worsens with extension rules out a labral tear. Since it is possible the patient may have a muscle injury, compartment syndrome, or tendon injury, laboratory diagnostic tests of complete blood count and blood chemistry, compartment pressure measurement, and pelvic x-ray must be done. Scheduled these tests to be performed within 2 days.

> **Diagnosis:** *Hip pain due to trauma and fall*

Until the results are provided the patient was counseled to wear low-heeled shoes, use over-the-counter analgesics for pain control, and apply heat/ice to the area to manage symptoms. Follow-up appointment made for 1 week in the orthopedic clinic where the test results will be reviewed and further treatment provided.

IMPOTENCE

Case Presentation: A 57-year-old male reports to the clinic with a complaint about his erectile quality.

INTRODUCTION TO COMPLAINT

The inability to achieve an erection firm enough for vaginal penetration or the inability to sustain an erection for completion of intercourse is defined as organic impotence. Psychogenic impotence can result from conflict around sexual issues, anxiety, depression, or feelings of guilt.

Erectile dysfunction is the term most often used to refer to impotence. Reported erectile dysfunction is the most common sexual problem that men report to their health care provider.

Risk Factors for Erectile Dysfunction

- Hormonal disorders
- Cardiovascular disease (atherosclerosis, hypertension, stroke, hypercholesterolemia)
- Diabetes mellitus
- Sedentary lifestyle/obesity
- Aging
- Tobacco/nicotine product use
- Recreational drug use
- Neurologic disorders (dementia, multiple sclerosis, Parkinson's, para/quadriplegia)
- Radical prostatectomy/history of pelvic surgery or irradiation
- Medications (some antihypertensives, antihistamines, antidepressants)
- Peyronie's disease
- Psychological issues

HISTORY OF COMPLAINT

Symptomatology

Ask about the following characteristics of each symptom using open-ended questions:

- Onset (sudden or gradual)
- Chronology
- Current situation (improving or deteriorating)
- Location
- Radiation
- Quality
- Timing (frequency, duration)

- Severity
- Precipitating and aggravating factors
- Relieving factors
- Associated symptoms
- Effects on daily activities
- Previous diagnosis of similar episodes
- Previous treatments
- Efficacy of previous treatments

Directed Questions to Ask

- How long have you had the erectile problems?
- Can you achieve an erection? If yes, is the quality satisfactory for the duration of sexual activity?
- Have you noted a decreased libido prior to or coinciding with the onset of the erectile dysfunction?
- Have there been any changes in your orgasmic capacity?
- Do you have any medical conditions/diagnoses?
- Have you had any prostate or pelvic surgeries or irradiation?
- Are you on any prescription medications?
- Do you smoke or use tobacco/nicotine products?
- Do you use recreational drugs?
- Are you experiencing any major psychological or emotional stress?

Assessment: Cardinal Signs and Symptoms

- Unsatisfactory erectile quality
- Inability to maintain an erection during intercourse activity
- Inability to achieve an erection

Medical History: General

- Medical conditions and surgeries
- Allergies (seasonal as well as others)
- Medication currently used (prescription and over the counter [OTC])
- Herbal preparations and traditional therapies

Medical History: Specific to Complaint

- Onset
- Medical risk factors
- Prescription medications
- Lifestyle choices
- Psychological issues

PHYSICAL EXAMINATION

Vital Signs

- Temperature
- Pulse
- Respiration
- Oxygen saturation (SpO_2)
- Blood pressure (BP)

General Appearance

- Apparent state of health
- Appearance of comfort or distress
- Color
- State of hydration

Neck
- Inspect for symmetry
- Palpate for masses/lumps, shape/size of thyroid

Cardiac
- Auscultate for heart sounds, check for murmurs, gallops, rubs
- Palpate peripheral pulses

Respiratory
- Auscultate lungs for crackles, and wheezing

Abdomen
- Inspect for size and contour
- Auscultate for bowel sounds
- Palpate for pain, masses

Genitourinary
- Inspect penis, scrotum
- Palpate testicles, penile shaft, prostate gland size and consistency

Neurologic
- Test for pupil reflexes and response to light; cranial nerves (CNs) II to XII, sensory capacity perineal region

CASE STUDY
History

Directed Question	Response
How long have you had the erectile problems?	*I have had a little bit of a problem here and there for a few years but now it's getting to be almost all the time.*
Can you achieve an erection? If yes, is the quality satisfactory for the duration of sexual activity?	*Most of the time. More often than not now . . . am not able to keep it for as long as she or I would like it to be there.*
Have you noted a decreased libido prior to or coinciding with the onset of the erectile dysfunction?	*Not really.*
Have there been any changes in your orgasmic capacity?	*No.*
Do you have any medical conditions/ diagnoses?	*No.*
Have you had any prostate or pelvic surgeries or irradiation?	*No.*

Directed Question	Response
Are you on any prescription medications?	No, I take some ibuprofen on occasion for minor aches and pains.
Do you smoke or use tobacco/nicotine products?	No.
Do you use recreational drugs?	No.
Are you experiencing any major psychological or emotional stress?	Not really.

Physical Examination Findings

- VITAL SIGNS: temperature 97.6°F; respiratory rate (RR) 16; heart rate (HR) 88, regular; BP 132/82; SpO_2 99%
- GENERAL APPEARANCE: well-developed, healthy-appearing male in no acute distress
- NECK: nontender, no thyroid enlargement or masses/nodules noted
- CARDIOVASCULAR: heart regular rate/rhythm, no murmur or gallop
- RESPIRATORY: lungs clear
- ABDOMEN: round, nontender without mass or organomegaly
- GENITOURINARY: no abnormalities of penis noted, no testicular abnormalities noted
- NEUROLOGIC: pupil reflexes/responses intact, CNs II to XII intact, perineal sensory capacity intact

DIFFERENTIAL DIAGNOSIS

Risk Factors/Etiologies	Imaging/Visualization Studies of Value	Lab Tests of Value
Hormonal disorders	Not typically	TSH, free T3, free and total testoterone, prolactin level
Cardiovascular disease	Not typically	Fasting lipid panel
Diabetes	Not typically	Comprehensive metabolic panel, Hgb A1C, fasting lipid panel
Sedentary lifestyle, obesity	Not typically	Insulin level
Recreational drug use	Not typically	Drug screen panel – urine and/or serum
Neurologic disorders	Possibly CT of the head	Not typically
Peyronie's disease	Ultrasound of the penis	Not typically
Psychological issues	Not typically	TSH, free T3, free and total testosterone, prolactin level

DIAGNOSTIC EXAMINATION

Exam	Code	Cost	Results
Total testosterone level	84403	$79	To evaluate for hypogonadism
TSH	84443	$49	To evaluate for hormonal contributors to the erectile dysfunction problem
Comprehensive metabolic panel	80053	$49	Fasting for evaluation of serum glucose level
Lipid panel	80061	$49	Fasting for evaluation of hypercholesterolemia

TSH, thyroid-stimulating hormone.

CLINICAL DECISION MAKING

Case Study Analysis

The advanced practice provider performs the assessment and physical examination on the patient and finds the following data: history and physical examination findings are negative for the primary risk factors for erectile dysfunction with the exception of "aging." Blood specimens sent for testosterone, thyroid-stimulating hormone (TSH), complete metabolic panel (CMP), and lipid panel. Testosterone level normal for the patient's age. TSH was within normal limits. CMP findings all within normal limits. Lipid panel was within normal limits.

Based on the laboratory data, the diagnosis of age-related erectile dysfunction is made. The patient is provided with a sample trial of Cialis. The patient is also reminded that alcohol, tobacco, and other substances can adversely affect achievement of an erection.

A follow-up appointment is suggested in 2 weeks to evaluate the effectiveness of prescribed medication and to plan further intervention if required.

> **Diagnosis:** *Erectile dysfunction, age related*

INCONTINENCE

Case Presentation: *A 44-year-old female reports to the clinic with a complaint of "peeing" herself anytime she exercises, coughs, or sneezes.*

INTRODUCTION TO COMPLAINT

The prevalence of urinary incontinence is as high as 30% for women 30 to 60 years of age. The two most common types are "stress incontinence" and "urge incontinence."

While men, particularly older men or men with enlarged prostate glands, can experience urinary incontinence the discussion herein will be devoted to the female patient who reports with incontinence symptoms.

A detailed history is key in making the diagnosis.

HISTORY OF COMPLAINT

Symptomatology

Ask about the following characteristics of each symptom using open-ended questions:

- Onset (sudden or gradual)
- Chronology
- Current situation (improving or deteriorating)
- Location
- Radiation
- Quality
- Timing (frequency, duration)
- Severity
- Precipitating and aggravating factors
- Relieving factors
- Associated symptoms
- Effects on daily activities
- Previous diagnosis of similar episodes
- Previous treatments
- Efficacy of previous treatments

Directed Questions to Ask

- How long have you been having the urine leakage problem?
- How severe would you say the urine leakage is?
- Have you noticed anything that makes the urine leakage better or worse?
- How many times throughout the day do you urinate?
- Do you wake up at night to urinate?
- When you urinate, do you feel like you are able to completely empty your bladder?

- Do you smoke?
- Do you drink caffeinated beverages? If yes, how often?
- Do you drink alcohol? If yes, how often?
- How often do you eat spicy, acidic, or sugary foods?
- Are you on any prescription medications?

Assessment: Cardinal Signs and Symptoms

- Leakage of urine with any stress (e.g., cough, sneeze, exercise, laughing, lifting, etc.)
- Intense sensation to have to urinate associated with an uncontrolled loss of urine
- Constant dribbling of urine due to the perception of not being able to fully empty bladder

Medical History: General

- Medical conditions and surgeries
- Allergies (seasonal, as well as others)
- Medication currently used (prescription, birth control pill [BCP] and over the counter [OTC])
- Herbal preparations and traditional therapies

Medical History: Specific to Complaint

- Urine leakage with stress
- Intense urge to urinate followed by uncontrolled loss of urine
- Nearly constant loss of small amounts of urine such that a "pad" is worn daily
- Medications that are known to increase the volume of urine production
- Medical or surgical condition known to cause weakening of genitourinary structures

PHYSICAL EXAMINATION

Vital Signs

- Temperature
- Pulse
- Respiration
- Oxygen saturation (SpO$_2$)
- Blood pressure (BP)

General Appearance

- Apparent state of health
- Appearance of comfort or distress
- Color
- State of hydration

Abdomen

- Inspect for size and contour
- Auscultate for bowel sounds
- Palpate for pain, masses, bladder tenderness and/or distention, costovertebral angle (CVA) tenderness

Pelvis

- Inspect for external genitalia, suppleness and redundancy of vaginal tissues
- Palpate for cystocele, adnexal tenderness

CASE STUDY

History

Directed Question	Response
How long have you been having the urine leakage problem?	*The past year or so.*
How severe would you say the urine leakage is?	*Sometimes so bad that I need to change my clothes . . . so I always have a spare set of clothes with me.*
Have you noticed anything that makes the urine leakage better or worse?	*Seems like on days that I limit my coffee to only one cup a day, I have less of a problem.*
How many times throughout the day do you urinate?	*About a half dozen or so.*
When you urinate, do you feel like you are able to completely empty your bladder?	*Yes, for the most part.*
Do you smoke?	*No.*
Do you drink caffeinated beverages? If yes, how often?	*A couple cups of coffee most mornings and a couple large, unsweetened iced teas a day.*
Do you drink alcohol? If yes, how often?	*No.*
How often do you eat spicy, acidic, or sugary foods?	*I have a pretty "clean" diet . . . so I really don't do sugar, don't really like spicy, don't think I overdo acidic either.*
Are you on any prescription medications?	*Vivelle estrogen patches since my hysterectomy.*

Physical Examination Findings

- VITAL SIGNS: temperature 97.4°F; respiratory rate (RR) 16; heart rate (HR) 82, regular; BP 100/58; SpO$_2$ 99%
- GENERAL APPEARANCE: well-developed, healthy-appearing female, in no acute distress
- ABDOMEN: nondistended, nontender, active bowel sounds, no bladder distention, no CVA angle tenderness
- PELVIS: external genitalia normal in appearance, mild dryness of the vaginal tissue noted, no cystocele or adnexal tenderness

DIFFERENTIAL DIAGNOSIS

Clinical Observations	Stress Incontinence	Urge Incontinence	Overflow Incontinence	Functional Incontinence
Unexpected urine leakage	Yes	Yes	Yes	Yes/No

(continued)

Clinical Observations	Stress Incontinence	Urge Incontinence	Overflow Incontinence	Functional Incontinence
Nocturnal urine leakage	Yes/No; if experiences the stressor	Yes/No	Yes	Yes/No
Bladder distention	Yes/No; not typical	Yes/No; not typical	Yes	Yes/No; not typical

DIAGNOSTIC EXAMINATION

Exam	Code	Cost	Results
Urine dipstick	81000	$10	For presence of infection
Complete urinalysis, includes microscopy	81015	$49	For indicators of kidney problems
Comprehensive metabolic panel	80053	$49	For glucose level and renal function
Postvoid urine residual	51798	Modest cost of bladder scan: average $30	To evaluate the amount of urine remaining in the bladder after the patient voids—normal <50 mL
Urodynamic Study— Uroflowmetry	51726	Varies: average $266	Measures urine speed and volume. Measurements can be used as evaluators of strength of bladder muscles and potential blockages to urine flow

CLINICAL DECISION MAKING

Case Study Analysis

The advanced practice provider performs the assessment and physical examination on the patient and finds the following data: history of urine leakage with "stress," mild loss of vaginal tissue suppleness. Presenting symptoms do not support urge, overflow, or functional incontinence. Urine dipstick was negative for leukocytes. Urinalysis results within normal limits. Complete metabolic panel levels within normal limits. Postvoid bladder scan <10 mL. Uroflowmetry deferred at this time.

Given that the patient has identified that reducing her "coffee" intake does decrease the problem, recommend that she eliminates coffee from her diet. Recommend the patient consult with prescribing provider for her Vivelle-Dot patches about a possible dosage adjustment or the addition of vaginal estrogen application to see if improved vaginal suppleness can ease the urine leakage. Instructed on the use of Kegel exercises and encouraged to perform repetitively throughout the day. Recommended voiding every 2 hours and practice stopping the stream while voiding.

Scheduled for a follow-up appointment in 2 months, sooner if condition worsens. Should symptoms persist or worsen a urology clinic appointment may be necessary for further diagnostic testing and evaluation.

Diagnosis: *Stress incontinence*

ITCHINESS IN SKIN

Case Presentation: A 79-year-old female reports to the clinic with a complaint of itching skin.

INTRODUCTION TO COMPLAINT

Itching, also known as pruritus, refers to a sensation of the skin that leads the individual to want to "scratch"

- Pruritus can be a normal body response to external agents or parasites
- Pruritus can be due to a wide range of skin and internal diseases
- Pruritus can be caused by medications
- Pruritus can be either localized or generalized
- Pruritus without an identifiable cause is more common in older people

HISTORY OF COMPLAINT

Symptomatology

Ask about the following characteristics of each symptom using open-ended questions:

- Onset (sudden or gradual)
- Chronology
- Current situation (improving or deteriorating)
- Location
- Radiation
- Quality
- Timing (frequency, duration)
- Severity
- Precipitating and aggravating factors
- Relieving factors
- Associated symptoms
- Effects on daily activities
- Previous diagnosis of similar episodes
- Previous treatments
- Efficacy of previous treatments

Directed Questions to Ask

- How long have you been having this itching?
- Where are you experiencing this itching?
- Do you have a rash?

- Have you been bitten by an insect?
- Are you on any medications?

Assessment: Cardinal Signs and Symptoms

- Report of itching skin

Medical History: General

- Medical conditions and surgeries
- Allergies (seasonal, as well as others)
- Medication currently used (prescription, birth control pill [BCP] and over the counter [OTC])
- Herbal preparations and traditional therapies

Medical History: Specific to Complaint

- Onset of itching
- Location of the itching
- Known external offending agents/insect bites
- Medications

PHYSICAL EXAMINATION

Vital Signs

- Temperature
- Pulse
- Respiration
- Oxygen saturation (SpO_2)
- Blood pressure (BP)

General Appearance

- Apparent state of health
- Appearance of comfort or distress
- Color
- State of hydration

Skin

- Inspect for color changes, evidence of rash, evidence of insect bites
- Palpate for tenderness
- Temperature of skin

Neck

- Inspect for symmetry, swelling, masses, scars
- Palpate for tenderness, thyroid enlargement, and presence of nodules/cysts

Cardiovascular

- Inspect for capillary refill time
- Auscultate for heart sounds, check for murmurs, gallops, rubs
- Palpate for peripheral pulses

Respiratory

- Auscultate lungs for crackles, and wheezing

Abdomen
- Inspect for contour
- Auscultate for bowel sounds
- Palpate for pain, hepatomegaly, or splenomegaly

CASE STUDY
History

Directed Question	Response
How long have you been having this "itching?"	For months and it's driving me crazy.
Where are you experiencing this itching?	Mostly right in the middle of my back where I can't reach it without a back scratcher. And across the front of my belly too!
Do you have a rash?	No, I haven't noticed a rash.
Have you been bitten by an insect?	No.
Are you on any medications?	Yes, I take Cozaar for high blood pressure, Spironolactone for my high blood pressure, Axid for my GERD, gabapentin for my neuropathy, Synthroid and an aspirin a day.

GERD, gastroesophageal reflux disease.

Physical Examination Findings
- VITAL SIGNS: temperature 96.9°F; respiratory rate (RR) 18; heart rate (HR) 60, regular; BP 134/82; SpO_2 96%
- GENERAL APPEARANCE: slightly obese, elderly female in no acute distress
- SKIN: warm to touch, nontender, overall dry with mild flaking; no rashes or insect bites noted
- NECK: scar from subtotal thyroidectomy noted, no asymmetry noted, no palpable masses/nodules
- CARDIOVASCULAR: regular rate/rhythm without murmur or gallop
- RESPIRATORY: lungs clear
- ABDOMEN: soft, nontender without masses or organomegaly

DIFFERENTIAL DIAGNOSIS

Clinical Observations	External Agents	Skin Diseases	Internal Diseases	Medication Induced
Itching	Yes	Yes	Yes	Yes
Localized/generalized	Localized	Generalized	Generalized	Generalized
Age related	Yes/No	Yes/No	Yes/No	Yes/No

DIAGNOSTIC EXAMINATION

Exam	Code	Cost	Results
TSH	84443	$49	Measure TSH levels and helps to evaluate appropriateness of current Synthroid dose—dry skin can be a sign of suboptimum thyroid replacement therapy
Comprehensive metabolic panel	80053	$49	For evaluation of kidney function and hydration status—dehydration can be a causative factor of dry skin; declining renal function can be an internal cause of pruritus

TSH, thyroid-stimulating hormone.

CLINICAL DECISION MAKING

Case Study Analysis

The advanced practice provider performs the assessment and physical examination on the patient and finds the following data: overall dry skin, history of subtotal thyroidectomy at 19 years of age; itching experienced predominantly in middle of back and over abdomen. Laboratory testing for thyroid-stimulating hormone (TSH) and complete metabolic panel (CMP) was all within normal limits.

Given the positive finding of dry skin, the APP recommends a daily routine of use of a hydrating moisturizer like a shea butter product. A prescription is given for Allegra 180 mg to be taken daily to see if the patient can get relief from the "itching." Patient is instructed to use soap products without perfumes or dyes. Laundry detergent should be mild. Clothing should be cotton based and loose fitting.

The patient is encouraged to return in 2 weeks for a follow-up evaluation or sooner if symptoms persist or worsen. An appointment with the dermatology clinic may be required for further diagnostic testing.

> ***Diagnosis:*** *Pruritus, etiology unknown*

JAUNDICE

Case Presentation: A 67-year-old Mexican American man presents with jaundice.

INTRODUCTION TO COMPLAINT

- Jaundice is a yellow discoloration of the skin and eyes, which occurs when there is too much bilirubin in the blood
- Hyperbilirubinemia is from one of two categories: either an elevation of unconjugated bilirubin or elevation of both unconjugated and conjugated bilirubin
- Elevation of unconjugated bilirubin can be from:
  - Hemolysis, extravasation of blood into tissues, stress situations leading to increased bilirubin production, impaired hepatic bilirubin uptake, and impaired bilirubin conjugation
- Elevation of unconjugated and conjugated bilirubin can be from:
  - Biliary obstruction, viral hepatitis, alcoholic hepatitis, nonalcoholic steatohepatitis (NASH), biliary cholangitis, drugs and toxins, ischemic hepatopathy, liver infiltration, postsurgery, end-stage liver disease, and organ transplant
- The most common causes are pancreatic or biliary carcinoma, gallstones, and alcoholic cirrhosis
- Some people can have multiple factors that lead to jaundice, such as sickle cell anemia, organ transplant, total parental nutrition, and AIDS
- Jaundice can be emergent if it is from a massive hemolysis, such as in sepsis or malaria, ascending cholangitis, or fulminant hepatic failure. These can be life-threatening

HISTORY OF COMPLAINT

Symptomatology

Ask about the following characteristics of each symptom using open-ended questions:

- Onset
- Associated symptoms/pain
- Recent travel
- Medication use
- Use of alcohol and/or drugs
- History of abdominal surgery
- History of liver disease
- HIV status
- Exposure to toxic substances

Directed Questions to Ask

- When did you first notice this yellowing of your skin?
- Have you had any other symptoms with this change?
- Have you noticed any change to your urine or stool?
- Are you having any pain? Where? How bad on a scale of 1 to 10?
- Have you traveled outside the country recently?
- How much alcohol do you normally drink in a day? Did you drink more than that in the past couple of days?
- Do you use any illegal drugs, especially intravenous (IV) drugs?
- Have you had any abdominal surgeries?
- Do you have a history of liver disease?
- Do you practice safe sex?
- Do you know if you're HIV positive?
- Have you been taking a lot of Tylenol/acetaminophen recently?

Assessment: Cardinal Signs and Symptoms

General
- Ill-appearing
- Moderate to severe distress

Head, Eyes, Ears, Nose, Throat (HEENT)
- Yellowing of eyes
- Mucus membranes

Cardiovascular
- Tachycardia

Respiratory
- Possible shallow respirations

Gastrointestinal
- Distention
- Decreased bowel sounds
- Tenderness to palpation
- Pain
- Nausea
- Vomiting
- Anorexia
- Hepatomegaly
- Splenomegaly
- Changes in stool (oily or clay-colored)

Genitourinary
- Possibly dark urine
- Oliguria

Psychological
- Confusion

Skin
- Pruritus
- Yellow skin

Medical History

- Medical conditions
- Surgeries
- Allergies
- Medication use, including illicit drugs OTC, or herbal
- Family history
- Travel history
- Sexual history
- Exercise and diet

PHYSICAL EXAMINATION

Vital Signs

- Temperature
- Pulse
- Blood pressure (BP)
- Oxygen saturation (SpO_2)
- Respiration

General Appearance

- Coloring
- Nutritional status
- Orientation

HEENT
- Scleral coloring
- Mucus membranes

Respiratory
- Lung sounds
- Effort
- Depth of respirations

Cardiovascular
- Heart rate and rhythm
- Murmurs
- Gallops, or rubs
- Cap refill
- Distal pulses

Gastrointestinal
- Distention
- Bowel sounds
- Tenderness/pain
- Nausea
- Vomiting
- Appetite
- Organomegaly

Genitourinary
- Changes in frequency
- Hydration status
- Urine color

Skin
- Color
- Turgor

CASE STUDY
History

Directed Question	Response
When did you first notice this yellowing of your skin?	*I just noticed it today. But it freaked me out so I came to get it checked.*
Have you had any other symptoms with this change?	*Yeah. I thought I had the flu for the past few days. I had chills and felt awful. I didn't want to eat. But that's started to get a bit better.*
Have you noticed any change to your urine or stool?	*My urine looks normal. I haven't really looked at my stool.*
Are you having any pain? Where? How bad on a scale of 1 to 10?	*My stomach hurts. I'm kind of achy all over. It's maybe a 6 out of 10.*
Have you traveled outside the country recently?	*I went to Haiti in early September.*
How much alcohol do you normally drink in a day? Did you drink more than that in the past couple of days?	*I have maybe one beer or scotch a day. Sometimes I don't drink at all. I haven't had anything in the past couple of days because I felt so bad.*
Do you use any illegal drugs, especially IV drugs?	*I've never used any kind of drugs.*
Have you had any abdominal surgeries?	*No surgeries. I had my colonoscopy a couple of years ago.*
Do you have a history of liver disease?	*No.*
Do you practice safe sex?	*I'm married.*
Do you know if you're HIV positive?	*I'm not.*
Have you been taking a lot of Tylenol recently?	*No.*

IV, intravenous.

Physical Examination Findings
- VITAL SIGNS: temperature 100.4°F; RR 22; pulse 94; BP 111/72; SpO_2 96% on RA
- GENERAL APPEARANCE: patient is ill-appearing, anxious, alert, oriented times 4.
- HEENT: pupils equal, round, and reactive to light and accommodation (PERRLA), pupils 2 mm, sclera jaundiced

- RESPIRATORY: lungs clear bilaterally to auscultation, symmetric chest expansion, shallow respirations
- CARDIOVASCULAR: regular rate and rhythm, no murmurs, gallops, or rubs; capillary refill <2 seconds, peripheral pulses 2+ bilaterally
- GASTROINTESTINAL: bowel sounds present in all four quadrants; right upper quadrant (RUQ) painful to palpation, surrounding abdomen tender to palpation; murphy's sign; hepatomegaly noted, smooth liver borders; no splenomegaly
- SKIN: jaundice, turgor normal

DIFFERENTIAL DIAGNOSIS

Clinical Observations	Pancreatitis	Viral Hepatitis	Cholecystitis
Onset	Abrupt	Rapid	Abrupt
Pain	LUQ	Myalgia, RUQ	RUQ or epigastric, may radiate to right shoulder
Fever	Yes	Low grade	Maybe low grade, usually no fever
Malaise	Yes	Yes	Yes
Nausea/vomiting	Yes	Yes	Yes
Stool changes	Steatorrhea	Diarrhea, acholic stool	Acholic stool
Laboratory test changes	Amylase and lipase elevated	Large elevations of AST and ALT, elevated alkaline phosphatase	Elevated alkaline phosphatase
Ultrasound findings	May find gallstones, thrombosis, necrosis	Hepatomegaly, gallbladder wall thickening, periportal edema, bright portal vein walls	Thickened gallbladder wall, gallstones, pericholecystic fluid, dilated bile duct
Possible symptoms	Feeling of fullness, abdominal distention	Ascites, hepatomegaly, splenomegaly, anorexia	Positive Courvoisier sign, + Murphy's sign

ALT, alanine amino transferase; AST, aspartate amino transferase; LUQ, left upper quadrant; RUQ, right upper quadrant.

DIAGNOSTIC EXAMINATION

Exam	Code	Cost	Results
CBC with differential	D64.9	$21	This allows you to look at the white blood cell count and band thickness to determine if there is an infectious process; the differential helps determine the type of infection. The hemoglobin and hematocrit determine if anemia is present. Platelet counts can help to determine if there are clotting deficiencies, which could indicate liver dysfunction.

(continued)

Exam	Code	Cost	Results
LFT	R94.5	$22	The two main components of the LFT are AST and ALT. These are markers that indicate liver disease or damage based on the ratio and degree of elevation. The liver clears bilirubin from the body, so dysfunction of the liver causes a buildup of bilirubin, which can lead to jaundice. An elevated ALT and AST can also indicate pancreatitis.
Amylase	R10.9	$17	Often four to six times higher than the upper limit in an acute pancreatitis attack.
Lipase	R74.8	$18	Will be elevated with an acute pancreatitis. Can also indicate gallbladder inflammation if elevated.
Alkaline phosphatase	R74.7	$14	Alkaline phosphatase is an enzyme made in the liver cells and bile duct. This is elevated when there is a blockage of flow in the biliary tract or there is a buildup of pressure on the liver from a gallstone or scarring. This can help differentiate between liver disease and gallbladder disease.
Abdominal x-ray	74010	$57	An abdominal x-ray can show the general size and shape of organs, presence of gallstones, fluid buildup, masses, and intestinal blockages. Due to the low radiation exposure of the x-ray it is often used as a first-line imaging tool to guide treatment with the aim to avoid more radiating imaging such as CTs.
Ultrasound	76700	$365	If labs are not definitive, ultrasound may be necessary to look at the abdominal structures to assess for strictures, stones, or free fluid. It can also show enlargement of the organs, which can aid in diagnosing. Ultimately a CT scan may be needed to assess the severity of any problems found, but often laboratory tests and ultrasound can be enough for a broad diagnosis.

ALT, alanine amino transferase; AST, aspartate amino transferase; CBC, complete blood count; LFT, liver function panel.

CLINICAL DECISION MAKING

Case Study Analysis

Based on the history and physical examination findings, an abdominal x-ray was taken, and laboratory tests were ordered.

The abdominal x-ray demonstrated an enlarged liver. Abnormal laboratory testing included:

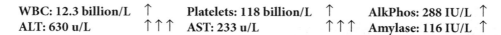

WBC: 12.3 billion/L ↑   **Platelets: 118 billion/L** ↑   **AlkPhos: 288 IU/L** ↑
ALT: 630 u/L ↑↑↑   **AST: 233 u/L** ↑↑↑   **Amylase: 116 IU/L** ↑

The liver was enlarged on x-ray; hepatomegaly present on palpation, generalized abdominal pain with myalgia, and very elevated alanine amino transferase (ALT) and aspartate amino transferase (AST) levels all indicated a disease of the liver. As the patient denies alcohol use and previous liver dysfunction, this appears to be an acute hepatitis. The recent travel, denial of IV drug use, and lack of risky sexual behavior suggests hepatitis A. The only way to differentiate between types of hepatitis is by using an acute viral hepatitis panel that is based on specific antibodies; the patient's blood was drawn and sent for this kind of analysis. The patient's symptoms are not consistent with pancreatitis or cholecystitis.

Diagnosis: *Hepatitis A*

Hepatitis A can be contracted from oral–fecal contamination. This can be from unwashed hands after using the restroom or changing a diaper, drinking contaminated water, or eating foods not properly handled, all of which could have occurred when traveling to Haiti. Many people who contract hepatitis A, especially children, do not have symptoms, but those that do often mimic any viral illness and subsequently develop jaundice as the symptoms subside. There is no treatment besides fluids and rest and a full recovery provides lifelong immunity. This patient will need to be monitored for improvement of liver enzymes to ensure there is no long-term damage.

Explained the need to rest and increase fluids. A follow-up appointment is scheduled for 1 week at which time the hepatitis panel results will be reviewed with the patient. Depending upon the results, further treatment may be required. The patient was encouraged to seek medical attention sooner if symptoms worsen. Long-term management may be required for ongoing evaluation of liver function.

JOINT PAIN

Case Presentation: *A 55-year-old presents with complaints of joint pain.*

INTRODUCTION TO COMPLAINT

- Osteoarthritis
- Bursitis
- Gout
- Sprains and strains
- Rheumatoid arthritis
- Trauma
- Inflammatory arthritis
- Ankylosing spondylitis
- Dislocation
- Hypothyroidism
- Lupus
- Juvenile rheumatoid arthritis
- Lyme disease
- Pseudogout
- Psoriatic arthritis
- Septic arthritis
- Tendinitis
- Temporomandibular joint (TMJ)

HISTORY OF COMPLAINT

Symptomatology

Ask about the following characteristics of each symptom using open-ended questions:

- Onset
- Chronology
- Current situation
- Timing
- Severity
- Precipitating and aggravating factors
- Relieving factors
- Associated symptoms
- Effects on daily activities
- Previous diagnosis of similar episodes
- Previous treatments

DIRECTED QUESTIONS TO ASK

- When did the joint pain start?
- Where is the pain?
- Can you describe the pain?
- Can you rate the pain from 0 to 10?
- Does the pain extend anywhere else?
- Do you have any other symptoms associated with the pain?
- What makes it worse/better?
- Did you take any medication to make it better?
- Did you do anything to make it better?
- How has this affected your daily activity?
- Do you perform any activity repeatedly?
- Are you on any new medication?
- Have you had a fever?
- Have you been sick or treated for illness recently?
- Have you traveled out of the country?
- Have you been bitten by ticks within the past 30 days?

Assessment: Cardinal Signs and Symptoms

General

- Fatigue
- Malaise

Head, Eyes, Ears, Nose, Throat (HEENT)

- Rash (tick bite, lupus, rheumatoid arthritis)
- Jaw stiffness/pain
- Trouble chewing
- Swelling

Respiratory

- Difficult to breathe

Musculoskeletal

- Pain
- Swelling
- Stiffness
- Warm to touch
- Deformity
- Limited range of motion (ROM)
- Unsteady gait
- Imbalance
- Muscle aches

Integumentary

- Rash

Medical History

- Surgical: Hernia repair
- Allergies: Penicillin: hives; bee stings: anaphylaxis

- Medication: Lisinopril 20 mg daily; furosemide 80 mg daily; atorvastatin 20 mg daily; metformin 500 mg BID
- Psychosocial: One six pack of beer weekly; no drugs/smoker; married; sedentary
- Health Maintenance/Immunization: Childhood vaccinations up to date; yearly flu vaccine up to date; pneumococcal vaccine up to date

Medical History
- Hypertension (HTN)
- Hyperlipidemia
- Diabetes mellitus (DM) type 2
- Cholelithiasis

Family History
- Father: gout, DM, coronary artery disease (CAD)
- Mother: DM, HTN
- Sister: breast cancer

PHYSICAL EXAMINATION
Vital Signs
- Temperature
- Heart rate (HR)
- Respiration
- Blood pressure (BP)
- Oxygen saturation (SpO_2)

General Appearance
- No signs of distress, obese

HEENT
- No trauma or stiffness

Cardiac
- Regular rate and rhythm (RRR)
- Absence of murmur, gallops, or rubs
- Capillary refill <2 seconds in all extremities
- Right knee 1+ edema

Respiratory
- Clear to auscultation bilaterally

Musculoskeletal
- Right knee with pain, swelling, redness, heat
- Difficult to walk on right leg
- All other extremities without pain, swelling, redness, heat

Integumentary
- No rash
- No trauma
- Right knee warm and red

CASE STUDY

History

Directed Question	Response
When did the joint pain start?	Suddenly last night.
Where is the pain?	Right knee.
Can you describe the pain?	It aches and throbs.
Can you rate the pain from 0 to 10?	5.
Does the pain extend to other parts of your body?	No.
What makes the pain worse?	Moving around.
What makes the pain better?	Resting.
Have you done anything to improve the pain? Did it help?	Prop on pillows. A little.
What other symptoms do you have?	My knee is hot and swelling.
When did the swelling begin?	Last night and has become worse throughout the day.
Did you have a fever?	No.
Have you been recently ill?	No.
Have you recently had any injuries?	No.
Have you experienced this before?	No.
What does your diet consist of?	I love meat and seafood.
How long have you been drinking?	For as long as I can remember.

Physical Examination Findings

- VITAL SIGNS: temperature 98.5°F; RR 18; HR 80; BP 140/85; SpO_2 99% on RA
- GENERAL APPEARANCE: no distress
- HEENT: no limitations on neck ROM; no trauma
- CHEST/CARDIOVASCULAR: RRR; no murmurs, gallops, or rubs; capillary refills <2 seconds; 1+ edema in knee; pulses 2+ in all extremities
- RESPIRATORY: CTA BBSH symmetrical
- MUSCULOSKELETAL: limited ROM of right knee, strength 3/5; all other extremities with full ROM, strength 5/5; gait unsteady
- SKIN: red and warm right knee

DIFFERENTIAL DIAGNOSIS

Clinical Observations	Gout	Sprain	Septic Arthritis	Bursitis
Onset	Sudden	Sudden	Gradual	Gradual
Pain	Yes	Yes	Yes	Yes
Swelling	Yes	Yes/No	Yes	Yes
Redness	Yes	Yes/No	Yes	Yes
Warm to touch	Yes	Yes	Yes	Yes
Bruising	No	No	No	Yes
Rash	No	No	No	Yes
Fever	No	No	Yes/No	Yes/No
Rigors	No	No	Yes/No	No

DIAGNOSTIC EXAMINATION

Exam	Code	Cost	Results
CBC with differential	R68.89	$25–$100	WBC count: Determines infectious or inflammatory source. Elevated WBC count indicative of active infectious source. Differential: Elevated neutrophil count can determine an acute bacterial infection. Decreased neutrophil count can determine severe infection, sepsis. Elevated lymphocyte count can determine viral infections or chronic inflammatory disorders. Elevated monocyte count may indicate chronic or fungal infections. Decreased monocyte and lymphocyte count can indicate autoimmune or bone marrow disorders.
Serum uric acid level	E79.0	$15–$40	Measures breakdown of purines in the body Hyperuricemia: acidosis, alcoholism, DM, medications, excessive exercise, hypoparathyroidism, lead poisoning, leukemia, kidney disease, diet, polycythemia vera Hypouricemia: Fanconi syndrome, diet, SIADH, Wilson disease
X-ray	R92.0	$260–$460	Tophi may be seen in chronic gout Rule out trauma
Synovial fluid aspiration	R65.9	$130–$660	Gram stain to reveal possible infectious source

(*continued*)

Exam	Code	Cost	Results
Urine uric acid level	R82.99	$15–$40	High levels: diet, obesity, liver or kidney disease, bone marrow disorders, metastatic cancer Low levels: lead poisoning, alcoholism, diet

CBC, complete blood count; DM, diabetes mellitus; SIADH, syndrome of inappropriate antidiuretic hormone secretion; WBC, white blood cell.

CLINICAL DECISION MAKING

Case Study Analysis

History and examination were conducted for a patient with sudden onset of right knee pain. The patient developed swelling, erythema, and pain overnight, which worsened throughout the day. Patient afebrile, no malaise-like symptoms. Elevated serum uric acid level and urine uric acid level, uric acid crystals in joint fluid with no bacterial growth, x-ray negative, and white blood cell (WBC) with differential negative. Sudden onset of symptoms rules out septic arthritis and bursitis. No history of an injury rules out a sprain.

> **Diagnosis:** *Gout*

Based on the laboratory data and symptoms, the patient is diagnosed with gout. The patient's risk is high due to gender, alcohol use, overweight, diet high in purines and diuretics. Patient denies recent trauma, injury, illness, recurrent symptoms, and is afebrile.

Patient provided with a prescription for colchicine. Instructed on a low-purine diet emphasizing the importance of avoiding alcohol. A follow-up appointment is scheduled for 1 month and the patient is encouraged to seek treatment sooner if symptoms do not subside or worsen within 2 weeks.

KNEE PAIN

Case Presentation: *A 56-year-old teacher presents to the clinic with a complaint of right knee pain for 2 weeks after playing soccer.*

INTRODUCTION TO COMPLAINT

Knee pain is a common complaint in primary care. The most common cause is osteoarthritis (OA).

Acute Knee Pain

- The knee is a joint that is frequently injured in weight-bearing sports:
  - Medial/lateral meniscus injury
    - Medial more common than lateral
  - Medial collateral ligament/lateral collateral ligament (MCL/LCL) injury
    - Medial more common than lateral
  - Anterior cruciate ligament/posterior cruciate ligament (ACL/PCL) injury
    - Anterior more common than posterior
- Gout
- Fracture

Chronic Knee Pain

- Common site of OA in population older than 50 years

Uncommon But Not to Be Missed Etiology

- Septic arthritis
- Rheumatoid arthritis (RA)
- Malignancy

Consider Mixed Etiology

- Acute injury with OA
- Systemic condition with OA or acute injury

Consider Age of Patients

- Pediatric population:
  - Osgood–Schlatter disease
  - Patellar tendinitis (jumper's knee)
  - Osteochondritis dissecans
  - Patellar subluxation

- Young adult:
  - Patellofemoral syndrome (PFS)
    - Collection of symptoms
    - More common in women than in men
    - Can be due to overuse (repetitive microtrauma)
    - Can be due to misalignment: Q angle, quadriceps weakness, patella cartilage damage
  - Chondromalacia patellae
    - Soft cartilage behind the knee
    - Requires biopsy of cartilage for definitive diagnosis
  - Patellar tendinitis (jumper's knee)
  - Reiter's syndrome
  - RA
    - Morning stiffness longer than 30 minutes
  - Bursitis (pes anserine)
  - Septic knee
  - Systemic disease (i.e., lupus)
- Older adult:
  - OA
    - Morning stiffness improves with activity
  - Gout/pseudogout
  - Baker's cyst
  - Septic knee
  - Systemic disease

Consider Location of Pain

Have the patient point to where pain is with one finger.

- Anterior knee pain:
  - Osgood–Schlatter disease
  - Patellar tendinitis (jumper's knee)
  - Patellar subluxation
  - Prepatellar bursitis
  - PFS
  - Chondromalacia patellae
  - OA
- Posterior knee pain:
  - PCL tear
  - Baker's cyst
- Medial knee pain:
  - MCL injury
  - Medial meniscus injury
  - Bursitis (pes anserine)
- Lateral knee pain:
  - LCL injury
  - Lateral meniscus injury
  - Iliotibial band syndrome

Consider Referred Pain

- Hip
- Ankle
- Neuropathy
- Malignance

HISTORY OF COMPLAINT

Symptomatology

Ask about the following characteristics of each symptom using open-ended questions:

- Previous knee pain/injury
- Systemic disease (rheumatoid conditions, diabetes mellitus [DM])
- Knee surgical history
- Allergies (medication and seasonal)
- Medications currently used daily and as needed:
  - Prescription
  - Over the counter, including herbal and traditional therapies
  - What is the effect of the medication used on the current pain?

Directed Questions to Ask

- Was the onset of pain sudden or gradual?
- If chronic knee pain—is this pain worse than your usual pain?
- What were you doing when the pain started?
- What did the pain feel like at onset?
- Was there immediate swelling and difficulty with ambulation?
- Were you able to keep doing activity or did you have to stop due to pain?
- What type of activity you were doing and on what surface?
- Was there direct contact?
- Was there an injury? If so, what was the mechanism of injury?
- Were you able to keep playing after injury?
- What is your level of pain on a 0 to 10 scale now?
  - What makes the pain worse?
  - Does the pain keep you awake at night/awaken you from sleep?
- Where is the pain? With one finger point to where the pain is.
- Describe the pain.
  - Popping, clicking, catching, buckling
- Do you have pain with range of motion (ROM)?
  - Is ROM limited?
- Is there associated weakness?
- Does pain radiate?
- Do you have numbness, tingling in feet?
- Have you had a previous diagnosis of knee pain?
  - When?
  - Are episodes increasing?
- Previous treatments:
  - Efficacy of previous treatments
- Was imaging done?
  - Findings

Assessment: Cardinal Signs and Symptoms

Hip

- Pain
- Injury
- Decreased ROM
- Past history of hip problems

Ankle
- Pain
- Recent injury
- Decreased ROM

Calf
- Pain
- Recent injury
- Lesions/discoloration

Associated Symptoms for Assessment
- Fever
- Systemic symptoms
- Paresthesias distal foot

Medical History
- Medical conditions and surgeries
- Allergies (seasonal as well as others)
- Medication currently used (prescription, birth control pill [BCP] and over the counter [OTC])
- Herbal preparations and traditional therapies

PHYSICAL EXAMINATION

Vital Signs
- Temperature
- Pulse
- Respiration
- Blood pressure (BP)

General Appearance
- Apparent state of health
- Appearance of comfort or distress
- Color and temperature of skin
- Nutritional status
- State of hydration
- Hygiene
- Match between appearance and stated age
- Difficulty with gait or balance

Knee
- Inspect (compare to unaffected knee):
  - Position in which patient is holding knee
  - Presence of effusion
  - Presence of erythema or lesions
- Palpate:
  - Presence of warmth
  - Bony tenderness: knee
    - Patella
    - Tibial plateau
  - Tenderness along MCL, LCL, popliteal, medial, or lateral joint lines
  - Tenderness or atrophy of distal quadriceps

- Evaluate ROM of knee:
  Observe for evidence of pain with ROM and if symmetrical right to left
  - Flexion 140 plus or minus
  - Extension 0 (not uncommon to hyperextend to minus 5 to 6)
- Perform tests:
  - Ballottement and/or bulge sign to determine whether effusion is present
  - McMurray test to detect meniscus injury
  - Lachman test to determine integrity of ACL (most sensitive test for ACL injury)
  - Drawer test to determine whether there is instability of ACL or PCL
  - Varus stress test to determine stability of LCL
    - Push calf laterally (abduction)
  - Valgus stress test to determine stability of MCL
    - Push calf medially (adduction)
- Evaluate ROM of hips: Does patient have pain with ROM of hips?
- Evaluate distal neurologic status if complaints of paresthesias

CASE STUDY

History

- History: positive for controlled hypertension (HTN); OA diagnosed 3 years earlier; negative for systemic illness, cardiac disease, DM
- Negative surgical history
- Medications: lisinopril 10 mg daily; currently using over-the-counter ibuprofen 400 mg two to three times per day without relief
- No known drug allergies

Directed Question	Response
Was the onset sudden or gradual?	*Sudden onset.*
If chronic knee pain—is this pain worse than your usual pain?	*Yes, since my soccer injury.*
What brought you in today?	*The pain has not improved after 2 weeks.*
What were you doing when it started?	*Playing soccer.*
What was the mechanism of injury?	*Another player ran into my lateral right knee.*
Were you able to keep playing after injury?	*Yes, but it hurt a bit.*
What is your level of pain on a 0 to 10 scale?	*Initially, 3 to 4 out of 10, today 5 to 6 out of 10.*
What makes pain worse?	*Walking.*
Describe the pain. Is there popping, clicking, catching, or buckling in the knee?	*Medial knee pain with most activities. Yes, occasionally will give way [baseline].*
Does the pain keep you awake at night/ awaken you from sleep?	*Not really.*
Do you have pain with ROM?	*Yes, especially with flexion.*
Is ROM limited?	*Yes.*

Directed Question	*Response*
Is there associated weakness?	*Not that I know of.*
Do you have numbness, tingling in your feet?	*No, that seems okay.*
Does pain radiate?	*Sometimes to back of knee with walking.*
Do you have fever or sign of infection?	*I feel okay other than my knee.*
Have you had a previous diagnosis of knee pain?	*Yes, I was told I had arthritis.*
When?	*Three years ago when first started hurting and "giving way."*
Are episodes increasing?	*Do not have episodes, have mild pain most of the time.*
Have you had previous treatments?	*Tylenol and NSAIDs usually help but not now.*
Was imaging done?	*They did an x-ray and told me that I had arthritis in my knee.*

NSAID, nonsteroidal anti-inflammatory drug; ROM, range of motion.

Physical Examination Findings

- VITAL SIGNS: temperature 98.6°F; respiratory rate (RR) 16; heart rate (HR) 82, regular; BP 138/784
- GENERAL APPEARANCE: well-developed, appropriate for age; gait favors right leg
- KNEE: no effusion, erythema, or lesions; tender to palpation along MCL; no tenderness at patellar tendon, popliteal, LCL, or joint lines; no bony tenderness of patella or tibial plateau; decreased and painful flexion at 90%; instability with valgus stress test; negative McMurray, Lachman, and Drawer tests
- HIP EXAMINATION UNREMARKABLE: symmetrical bilaterally; full ROM without pain; negative Patrick test
- CALF AND ANKLE EXAMINATION UNREMARKABLE: no erythema, effusion, warmth, tenderness, lesions; full ROM without pain; extremities' sensation intact distal foot

DIFFERENTIAL DIAGNOSIS

Clinical Observations	MCL/LCL Sprain	ACL/PCL	Meniscus Injury	Fracture	OA	Gout	Bursitis	Septic Joint
History of trauma	Yes	Yes	Yes	Yes	No	No	No	No
Onset	Sudden	Sudden	Sudden or gradual	Sudden	Gradual	Gradual	Gradual	Gradual
Knee pain	Yes	Yes	Yes	Yes	Yes	Yes	Yes	Yes

(continued)

Clinical Observations	MCL/LCL Sprain	ACL/PCL	Meniscus Injury	Fracture	OA	Gout	Bursitis	Septic Joint
Unable to bear weight	No	Yes/No	No	Yes	No	No	No	Yes/No
Decreased and painful ROM	Yes	Yes	Yes/No	Yes	Yes/No	Yes/No	Yes/No	Yes
Bony tenderness	No	No	No	Yes	No	No	No	No
Medial or lateral pain	Yes	No	Yes	Yes	Yes/No	Yes/No	Yes/No	Yes
Anterior or posterior pain	No	Yes	Yes/No	Yes	Yes/No	Yes/No	Yes/No	Yes
Locking, catching sensation	No	No	Yes	No	Yes/No	No	No	Yes/No
Knee giving way	No	Yes	Yes/No	Yes/No	Yes/No	No	No	Yes/No
Effusion	Yes/No	Yes/No	No	Yes	No	Yes/No	Yes/No	Yes
Erythema and warmth	No	No	No	No	No	Yes/No	Yes/No	Yes
Fever	No	No	No	No	No	No	No	Yes

ACL, anterior cruciate ligament; LCL, lateral collateral ligament; MCL, medial collateral ligament; OA, osteoarthritis; PCL, posterior cruciate ligament; ROM, range of motion.

DIAGNOSTIC EXAMINATION

EXAM	Procedure Code	Cost	Results
Knee x-ray	715.16	$150	Unable to visualize meniscus integrity with plain A & P films
MRI	B030Y0Z	$1,567	Osteoarthritis

- Few laboratory examinations were indicated because there was no evidence of infection.
- Imaging was indicated per Pittsburgh and Ottawa rules due to history of:
  - Age older than 55
  - Direct trauma
  - Inability to flex to 90%
- Radiograph showed osteophytes indicative of OA with possible loose body at medial aspect otherwise negative.

CLINICAL DECISION MAKING

Case Study Analysis

The advanced practice provider performs history and physical examination on the patient and finds the following pertinent positives and negatives to rule out the differential.

The pertinent positive history findings are:

- Age older than 55
- Previous diagnosis of OA of the right knee with positive radiograph x-ray findings
- Knee occasionally "giving way"
- Recent direct blow to lateral right knee
- Pain at time but able to keep playing soccer
- Describes pain along MCL with occasional clicking and locking

The pertinent negative history findings are:

- Was able to keep playing after injury (although it was painful)
- Denies fever or systemic symptoms
- Denies anterior, posterior knee pain
- Denies clicking, popping
- Denies hip pain
- Denies radiating pain or paresthesias

The pertinent positive physical examination findings are:

- Compensated gait favoring right knee
- Mild tenderness to palpation along MCL
- Decreased and painful flexion of right knee
- Instability with valgus stress test

The pertinent negative physical examination findings are:

- Normal vital signs, no fever
- No bony tenderness of patella or tibial plateau
- No tenderness along patellar tendon, popliteal, LCL, or joint lines
- No warmth, erythema
- Negative ballottement; bulge; and negative Lachman, Drawer, and McMurray tests
- No instability with varus stress test

Findings indicate no evidence of ACL/PCL, meniscus injury, fracture, gout, bursitis, or a septic joint.

> **Diagnosis:** *Right knee MCL sprain in the setting of OA*

Discussed findings with the patient and suggested splinting and minimal weight bearing until acute pain subsides. Encouraged the use of over-the-counter analgesics for pain management and application of ice for 20-minute increments several times a day. A follow-up appointment with the orthopedic clinic was scheduled for 2 weeks for further evaluation of the possible loose body at the medial aspect of the joint.

LEG PAIN

Case Presentation: A 55-year-old presents with complaints of leg pain.

INTRODUCTION TO COMPLAINT

Leg pain is a common complaint seen by providers today. Workup requires careful review and assessment of the patient's history and a physical exam.

- Osteoarthritis
- Bursitis
- Gout
- Sprains and strains
- Rheumatoid arthritis
- Trauma
- Inflammatory arthritis
- Ankylosing spondylitis
- Dislocation
- Hypothyroidism
- Lupus
- Juvenile rheumatoid arthritis
- Lyme disease
- Pseudogout
- Psoriatic arthritis
- Septic arthritis
- Tendinitis
- Temporomandibular joint (TMJ)

HISTORY OF COMPLAINT

Symptomatology

Ask about the following characteristics of each symptom using open-ended questions:

- Onset
- Chronology
- Current situation
- Timing
- Severity
- Precipitating and aggravating factors
- Relieving factors
- Associated symptoms
- Effects on daily activities

- Previous diagnosis of similar episodes
- Previous treatments

Directed Questions to Ask

- When did the joint pain start?
- Where is the pain?
- Can you describe the pain?
- Can you rate the pain from 0 to 10?
- Does the pain extend anywhere else?
- Do you have any other symptoms associated with the pain?
- What makes it worse/better?
- Did you take any medication to make it better?
- Did you do anything to make it better?
- How has this affected your daily activity?
- Do you perform any activity repeatedly?
- Are you on any new medication?
- Have you had a fever?
- Have you been sick or treated for illness recently?
- Have you traveled out of the country?
- Have you been bitten by ticks within the past 30 days?

Assessment: Cardinal Signs and Symptoms

General
- Fatigue
- Malaise

Head, Eyes, Ears, Nose, Throat (HEENT)
- Rash (tick bite, lupus, rheumatoid arthritis)
- Jaw stiffness/pain (TMJ)
- Trouble chewing
- Swelling (TMJ)

Respiratory
- Difficult to breathe

Musculoskeletal
- Pain
- Swelling
- Stiffness
- Warm to touch
- Deformity
- Limited range of motion (ROM)
- Unsteady gait
- Imbalance
- Muscle aches

Integumentary
- Rash

Medical History

General
- Hypertension (HTN)
- Hyperlipidemia

- Diabetes mellitus (DM) type 2
- Cholelithiasis

Surgical
- Hernia repair

Allergies
- Penicillin: hives
- Bee stings: anaphylaxis

Medication
- Furosemide
- Atorvastatin
- Metformin

Family History
- Father: gout, DM, coronary artery disease (CAD)
- Mother: DM, HTN
- Sister: breast cancer

Psychosocial
- One six pack of beer weekly
- No drugs, smoker
- Married
- Sedentary

Health Maintenance/Immunization
- Childhood vaccinations up to date
- Yearly flu vaccine up to date
- Pneumococcal vaccine up to date

PHYSICAL EXAMINATION
Vital Signs
- Temperature
- Heart rate (HR)
- Respiration
- Blood pressure (BP)
- Oxygen saturation (SpO_2)

General Appearance
- No signs of distress, obese

HEENT
- No trauma or stiffness

Cardiac
- Regular rate and rhythm (RRR)
- Absence of murmur, gallops, or rubs
- Capillary refill <2 seconds in all extremities
- Right knee 1+ edema

Respiratory
- Clear to ascultation

Musculoskeletal
- Right knee with pain, swelling, redness, heat
- Difficult to walk on right leg
- All other extremities without pain, swelling, redness, heat

Integumentary
- No rash
- No trauma
- Right knee warm and red

CASE STUDY
History

Directed Question	Response
When did the joint pain start?	Suddenly last night.
Where is the pain?	In my right knee.
Can you describe the pain?	It aches and throbs.
Can you rate the pain from 0 to 10?	5.
Does the pain extend to other parts of your body?	No.
What makes the pain worse?	Moving around.
What makes the pain better?	Resting.
Have you done anything to improve the pain? Did it help?	I've propped it on pillows. A little.
What other symptoms do you have?	My knee is hot and swelling.
When did the swelling begin?	Last night, and it has become worse throughout the day.
Did you have a fever?	No.
Have you been recently ill?	No.
Have you recently had any injuries?	No.
Have you experienced this before?	No.
What does your diet consist of?	I love meat and seafood.
How long have you been drinking?	For as long as I can remember.

Physical Examination Findings
- VITAL SIGNS: temperature 98.5°F; RR 18; HR 80; BP 140/85; SpO$_2$ 99% on RA
- GENERAL APPEARANCE: no distress
- HEENT: no limitations on neck ROM; no trauma
- CARDIOVASCULAR: regular rate and rhythm; no murmurs, gallops, or rubs; capillary refills <2 seconds; 1+ edema in knee; pulses 2+ in all extremities
- RESPIRATORY: CTA BBSH symmetrical

- MUSCULOSKELETAL: limited ROM of right knee, strength 3/5; all other extremities with full ROM, strength 5/5; gait unsteady
- SKIN: red and warm right knee

DIFFERENTIAL DIAGNOSIS

Clinical Observations	Gout	Sprain	Septic Arthritis	Bursitis
Onset	Sudden	Sudden	Gradual	Gradual
Pain	Yes	Yes	Yes	Yes
Swelling	Yes	Yes/No	Yes	Yes
Redness	Yes	Yes/No	Yes	Yes
Warm to touch	Yes	Yes	Yes	Yes
Bruising	No	No	No	Yes
Rash	No	No	No	Yes
Fever	No	No	Yes/No	Yes/No
Rigors	No	No	Yes/No	No

DIAGNOSTIC EXAMINATION

Exam	Code	Cost	Results
CBC with differential	D64.9	$25–$100	WBC count: Determines infectious or inflammatory source. Elevated WBC count indicative of active infectious source Differential: Elevated neutrophil count can determine an acute bacterial infection. Decreased neutrophil count can determine severe infection, sepsis. Elevated lymphocyte count can determine viral infections or chronic inflammatory disorders. Elevated monocyte count may indicate chronic or fungal infections. Decreased monocyte and lymphocyte count can indicate autoimmune or bone marrow disorders
Serum uric acid level	E79.0	$15–$40	Measures breakdown of purines in the body Hyperuricemia: acidosis, alcoholism, DM, medications, excessive exercise, hypoparathyroidism, lead poisoning, leukemia, kidney disease, diet, polycythemia vera Hypouricemia: Fanconi syndrome, diet, SIADH, Wilson disease
X-ray	73630	$260–$460	Tophi may be seen in chronic gout Rule out trauma

(continued)

Exam	Code	Cost	Results
Synovial fluid aspiration	89051	$130–$660	Gram stain to reveal possible infectious source
Urine uric acid level	84550	$15–$40	High levels: diet, obesity, liver or kidney disease, bone marrow disorders, metastatic cancer Low levels: lead poisoning, alcoholism, diet

CBC, complete blood count; DM, diabetes mellitus; SIADH, syndrome of inappropriate antidiuretic hormone secretion; WBC, white blood cell.

CLINICAL DECISION MAKING

Case Study Analysis

History and examination were conducted for a patient with sudden onset of right knee pain. The patient developed swelling, erythema, and pain overnight, which worsened throughout the day. Patient afebrile, no malaise-like symptoms. Elevated serum uric acid level and urine uric acid level, uric acid crystals in joint fluid with no bacterial growth, x-ray negative, and white blood cell (WBC) with differential negative. Symptoms occurred spontaneously without evidence of trauma. Since the symptoms occurred suddenly, septic arthritis and bursitis are ruled out.

> **Diagnosis:** Gout

Based on the laboratory data and symptoms, the patient is diagnosed with gout. The patient's risk is high due to gender, alcohol use, overweight, diet high in purines and diuretics. Patient denies recent trauma, injury, illness, recurrent symptoms, and is afebrile.

Patient provided with a prescription for colchicine. Instructed on a low-purine diet emphasizing the importance of avoiding alcohol. A follow-up appointment is scheduled for 1 month and the patient is encouraged to seek treatment sooner if symptoms do not subside or worsen within 2 weeks.

LOW BACK PAIN

Case Presentation: A 35-year-old male painter presents to the clinic with the complaint of low back pain. He recalls lifting a 5-gallon paint can and felt an immediate pull in the lower right side of his back. This happened 2 days ago and he had the weekend to rest, but after taking Motrin and using heat, he has not seen any improvement. He is having some right leg pain but no bowel or bladder changes. His pain is sharp, stabbing, and he scored it as a 9 on a scale of 0 to 10. He had a similar incident approximately 5 years ago but made a complete recovery.

INTRODUCTION TO COMPLAINT

Acute low back pain is a common problem seen in primary care practices. Most low back pain can affect approximately 80% of the population between the ages of 25 and 45 years. Fortunately, 90% of back injuries are benign and account for the fifth most common visit in primary care. Some of the important characteristics of low back pain that are critical to making the correct diagnosis are:

- Localized pain that is worse with moving due to muscle pain
- Trauma may cause a fracture and requires an x-ray
- Radiating pain into the leg along a dermatome indicates a ruptured disc
- Loss of bowel or bladder function indicates an emergency
- Back pain that is continuous and associated with a history of cancer requires diagnostic testing to rule out malignancy

HISTORY OF COMPLAINT

Symptomatology

Ask about the following characteristics of each symptom using open-ended questions:

- Chronology/onset/mechanism of injury
- Current situation (improving or deteriorating)
- Location
- Radiation
- Quality
- Timing (frequency, duration)
- Severity
- Precipitating and aggravating factors
- Relieving factors
- Associated factors
- Effects on daily living
- Previous low back injury or pain
- Previous treatments

- Efficacy of treatments
- Social history and lifestyle habits

Directed Questions to Ask

- What was the onset of your symptoms?
- What was the mechanism of injury (without trauma may suggest serious disease)?
- How did this occur?
- Where is your pain specifically? Point with one finger.
- Specifically ask about duration of pain; pain is considered chronic if it persists for more than 6 to 9 weeks.
- Are you having any numbness or tingling?
- Are you having any radiating pain?
- On a scale from 0 to 10 with 10 being the worst, could you rate your pain?
- Are you having any bowel or bladder issues? Difficulty with urination or producing a bowel movement?
- Any difficulty with sleep?
- Any problems with sitting?
- Any problems with walking?
- Have you ever suffered a similar back problem like this before today? If so, when? What kind of treatments have you had in the past and were they effective?
- Are you taking any medication for this problem? If so, what?
- Have you tried any other home self-care remedies? If so, what?
- Are you allergic to any medications?

Assessment: Cardinal Signs and Symptoms

Any history of radiculopathy, foot drop, or bowel/bladder changes needs immediate attention and possibly an MRI and referral to a neurosurgeon.

Abdomen
- Pain
- Rectal bleeding
- Bowel linkage

Urinary
- Urinary linkage or incontinence
- Painful urination

Neurologic
- Radiculopathy
- Foot drop
- Motor weakness of lower extremities (LEs)

Other Associated Symptoms
- Fever
- Rash over one side of back (shingles)
- Malaise
- Enlarged lymph nodes in groin
- Pelvic pain or discharge (females)

Medical History: General

- Age
- Allergies

- Medications currently used (prescription and over-the-counter vitamins or medications)
- Herbal and home therapies
- Supplements
- Level of daily activity
- Physical exercise
- Lifestyle questions (smoking, alcohol, and recreational drugs)
- Other medical conditions
- Previous hospitalizations or surgeries

Medical History: Specific to Complaint

- Previous back injury, including motor vehicle accident (MVA) or work-related injury
- Previous back surgeries
- History of scoliosis or lordosis
- Increased pain with sitting, standing, or sleeping
- Occupation
- Hobbies or sport activities
- Second job

PHYSICAL EXAMINATION

Vital Signs

- Temperature; fever is an ominous sign
- Pulse
- Blood pressure (BP)
- Oxygen saturation (SpO_2)
- Respiration

General Appearance

- Apparent state of health
- Observe general gait for signs of limping
- Guarding or coordination problems while walking are important to note and suggest a possible neurological problem
- Appearance of comfort versus distress
- Overall muscle tone, alignment, and abnormalities

Lumbar Spine

Inspect

- Symmetrical checking for scoliosis, kyphosis, or lordosis
- Swelling
- Masses
- Discoloration
- Signs of infection
- Bruising of the skin

Palpate

- Tenderness, noting specific location and muscle spasms

Range of Motion (ROM)

- Check forward flex
- Side to side bending

- Twisting and extension of the back
- Carefully watch the patient as he or she moves on and off the examination table

Strength
Check LE strength by asking the patient to push or lift knee up against the examiner's hand:

- Watch for weakness or limitations with the ROM activities
- Have patient perform a push-up lying prone on the table and arch back leaving stomach on the table to see how flexible the lower lumbar region is
- While patient is still on stomach, bring heel to buttocks
- On back, perform a knee-to-chest activity
- Watch the abdominal muscles when the patient sits up
- Check the gait by asking the patient to walk normally
- Walk on toes
- Walk on heel

Neurologic
- Check LE deep tendon reflexes (DTRs)
- Check sensory neurological tests by checking dermatomes

Special Test
- Straight leg raises (SLRs): Elevate each leg while the patient is lying down; if pain is indicated between 30 degrees and 60 degrees, this indicates a positive SLR and could be diagnostic of a herniated disc.

Vascular
- Pedal pulses and leg swelling

Rectal Examination
- Indicated if patient presents with a history of falling on tailbone, rectal bleeding, or you suspect a malignancy.

Pelvic Examination
- Indicated if you suspect a gynecological problem, such as pelvic inflammatory disease

CASE STUDY
History

Directed Question	Response
What was the onset of your symptoms?	Abrupt.
What was the mechanism of injury?	Lifting a heavy object (5 gallons of paint).
How did this occur?	Lifting a heavy object (5 gallons of paint).
Where is your pain specifically?	Right lower back.
Specifically how long have you had this pain?	2 days.
Are you having any numbness or tingling?	No.
Are you having any radiating pain?	Yes, down the right leg.
On a scale from 0 to 10 with 10 being the worse, could you rate your pain?	9.

Directed Question	Response
Are you having difficulty with urination or any bowel changes?	*No.*
Any difficulty with sleeping?	*Some, when I turn over in bed.*
Any problems with sitting?	*Not so much.*
Any problems with walking?	*I am walking with a slight limp.*
Have you ever suffered a similar back problem?	*Yes, about 5 years ago.*
If so, when? What kind of treatments have you had in the past?	*It just resolved on its own.*
What is your occupation? Full time or part time?	*Full-time painter.*
Do you have any hobbies or sport activities?	*I coach my son's fifth-grade baseball team.*
Do you have a second job?	*No.*
Are you taking any medication for this problem?	*Motrin.*
Have you tried any other home remedies? If so, what?	*Yes, I used a heating pad on it.*
Are you allergic to any medications?	*No.*

Physical Examination Findings

- VITAL SIGNS: temperature 98.4°F; respiratory rate (RR) 16; heart rate (HR) 82; BP 120/64; SpO$_2$ 98%
- GENERAL APPEARANCE: well-developed, healthy 35-year-old male; no gross deformities
- CHEST: lungs are clear in all fields; heart S1, S2 no murmur, gallop, or rub
- MUSCULOSKELETAL: no obvious deformities, masses, or discoloration; palpable pain noted at the right lower lumbar region; no palpable spasms; ROM limited to forward bending 10 inches from floor; able to bend side to side but had difficulty twisting and going into extension; SLRs were negative
- NEUROLOGIC: DTRs 2+ LE, SLR negative; sensory neurology intact to light touch and patient able to toe and heel walk; gait was stable and no limping noted

DIFFERENTIAL DIAGNOSIS

Clinical Observations	Lumbar Strain	Herniated Disc	Sacroiliac	Osteoarthritis	Malignancies
Onset	Abrupt	Either	Abrupt	Gradual	Gradual
Duration	<2 weeks	Varies	Acute symptoms	Many years	Many years

(continued)

Clinical Observations	Lumbar Strain	Herniated Disc	Sacroiliac	Osteoarthritis	Malignancies
Location	Lumbar region	Lumbar or thoracic region	Buttocks region	Lumbar region	Varies depending on location of malignancy
Pain	Can radiate	Can radiate	Can radiate	Can vary	Can vary
Numbness and tingling	Sometimes	Often	Sometimes	Not often	Varies
Bowel or bladder changes	No changes	Possible changes	No changes	No changes	Possible changes
DTR	Normal	Possible asymmetrical	Normal	Normal	Possible asymmetrical
Toe and heel walking	Normal	Difficulty depending on the location of the herniation	Difficulty	Normal	Normal
SLR	Normal	Abnormal or positive	Normal	Normal	Normal

DTR, deep tendon reflex; SLR, straight leg raise.

DIAGNOSTIC EXAMINATION

Exam	Code	Cost	Results
CBC, determination of erythrocyte sedimentation rate	85025	$15–$25	Used to confirm the diagnosis of infection or malignancy
Plain-film radiographs, oblique views of the spine	72010	$150–$175	Inexpensive and easily obtained. It provides two-dimensional view of motion and evidence of trauma
MRI	75571	$1,600–$1,700	Superior contrast resolution with disadvantages being: it is a costly diagnostic test; it interacts with metals in the body
CT scanning	72192	$300–$700	Detects abnormal tissue; it is a useful technique for planning areas for radiotherapy and biopsies Can also provide valuable data on the patient's vascular condition, bone diseases, bone density, and the state of the patient's spine

CBC, complete blood count.

CLINICAL DECISION MAKING
Case Study Analysis

A lumbar strain is based on history and clinical findings. A complete history may suggest the cause of the acute low back pain based on the mechanism of injury. If there is no obvious history of trauma or physical activities, it is important to consider other diagnostic tests to rule out pathology.

Because the patient's symptoms had a sudden onset, osteoarthritis and a malignancy are ruled out. Since the pain is located in the lumbar region, sacroiliac involvement is ruled out. The absence of numbness and tingling rules out a herniated disk. No x-rays are indicated for minor low back pain, but if symptoms persist, x-rays, CT scan, and MRI are often considered.

The patient was prescribed a mild muscle relaxant and encouraged to continue with over-the-counter analgesics for pain control. It was suggested to continue using heat for 20 minutes several times a day. Ice was also recommended. The patient was counseled to avoid heavy lifting until the injury resolves. Discussed the importance of maintaining normal activity to include walking and avoiding bed rest and excessive sitting.

A follow-up appointment is made for 2 weeks. If the symptoms persist or worsen, additional diagnostic testing to include spinal x-rays and possibly CT scan or MRI will be considered. Long-term management may need to be coordinated through the orthopedic or neurology clinic.

Diagnosis: Lumbar strain

LOWER EXTREMITY EDEMA

Case Presentation: *A healthy-appearing 52-year-old gentleman presents with 2 weeks of increasing bilateral lower leg edema.*

INTRODUCTION TO COMPLAINT

The most common causes of lower extremity edema are:

- Venous stasis
- Congestive heart failure
- Renal failure
- Liver failure
- Obstruction of lymphatics due to ascites from tumor
- Fluid overload from excessive intravenous (IV) rehydration

HISTORY OF COMPLAINT
Symptomatology

Ask about the following characteristics of each symptom using open-ended questions:

- Onset (sudden or gradual)
- Chronology
- Current situation (improving or deteriorating)
- Location
- Severity
- Precipitating and aggravating factors
- Relieving factors
- Associated symptoms
- Effects on daily activities
- Previous diagnosis of similar episodes
- Previous treatments
- Efficacy of previous treatments

Directed Questions to Ask

- Was the onset sudden or gradual?
- Do you have a fever?
- Do you have any pain?
- Is it hard to walk?
- Do you have any dyspnea?
- Do you have a cough?
- Have you started any new medications?

- What surgeries have you had?
- Do you have a history of any liver disease?
- Cardiac disease?
- Renal disease?
- Any history of malignancies?
- Any swollen lymph nodes?
- Previous lymph node dissection?
- Any recent prolonged travel?
- Recent insect bites/infections?
- Any history of intravenous drug abuse (IVDA), if so, how recent and where?
- Prolonged sitting?
- Recent cast/splints?
- Any recent surgeries?
- Any history of coagulopathies/family history?
- Previous pregnancy or premenstrual edema?
- Diet and/or history of malnutrition?
- Do you have a rash?

Assessment: Cardinal Signs and Symptoms

In addition to the general characteristics outlined previously, additional characteristics of specific symptoms should be elicited.

Chest
- Jugular vein distention
- Lung sounds/evidence of pulmonary congestion
- Chest wall lesions, spider angiomata
- Heart murmurs, diastolic gallop (S3)

Abdomen
- Pain
- Shifting dullness or fluid wave
- Distention or ascites

Lower Extremity
- Stasis dermatitis
- Pattern of edema pitting or nonpitting, bilateral, or unilateral
- Nausea or vomiting
- Pedal pulses
- Evidence of isolated warmth redness or pain

Other Associated Symptoms
- Fever
- Malaise
- Nausea or vomiting
- Periorbital edema
- Skin exam with spider angiomata

Medical History: General

- Medical conditions and surgeries
- Allergies (seasonal, as well as others)
- Medication currently used (prescription and over-the-counter [OTC] medicine)
- Herbal preparations and traditional therapies

Medical History: Specific to Complaint

- Frequent episodes related to activity or nonactivity
- Congestive heart failure
- Renal disease
- Hypertension
- Trauma to the lower extremities
- History of vascular surgeries
- History of methicillin-resistant *Staphylococcus aureus* (MRSA)

PHYSICAL EXAMINATION

Vital Signs

- Temperature
- Pulse
- Respiration
- Oxygen saturation (SpO_2)
- Blood pressure (BP)

General Appearance

- Apparent state of health
- Appearance of comfort or distress with gait and respirations
- Color of skin
- Nutritional status
- State of hydration
- Hygiene
- Match between appearance and stated age

Lower Extremity Examination: Inspection

- Groin, assess for inguinal adenopathy
- Assess pulses and bruits of femoral artery
- Describe as firm or soft, fixed, or mobile
- Assess for femoral hernia
- Assess in males for scrotal edema
- Inspect thigh looking for warmth, tenderness, and asymmetrical girth
- Assess popliteal fossa for popliteal pulse pulsatile or enlarged/aneurysmal
- Color of lower extremity
- Assess color of legs in dependent or raised position
- Is there asymmetric leg swelling, and if so, to what level?
- Dilated or varicose superficial veins
- Hair pattern or lack of
- Observe for ulceration of skin
- Assess for dorsalis pedis artery
- Assess for posterior tibial artery
- Nail growth

Lower Extremity Examination: Associated Systems for Assessment

- A complete assessment should include the respiratory system and abdomen

CASE STUDY

History

Directed Question	Response
Was the onset sudden or gradual?	*It was gradual.*
Do you have any pain?	*No, but my legs ache.*
If 10 is the worst pain you have ever had, what number is this pain?	*2/10.*
Do you have any shortness of breath?	*A little, only with steep long stairs.*
Do you have a cough?	*No.*
Do you have any chest discomfort or pain?	*No.*
Do you have a rash?	*No.*
Do you have fatigue?	*Yes, but I always feel that way.*
Do you have fevers?	*No.*
Do you have a sense of one leg being more uncomfortable?	*No.*
Do you have any nausea or vomiting?	*No.*
Have you had any changes in your medication?	*Sort of.*

Physical Examination Findings

- VITAL SIGNS: temperature 98.9°F; respiratory rate (RR) 18; heart rate (HR) 88, regular; BP 156/102; SpO$_2$ 97%
- GENERAL APPEARANCE: well-developed, heavy but healthy-appearing gentleman with normal voice in no acute distress
- CARDIOVASCULAR: no jugular vein distention, faint S3 appreciable; +3 femoral pulses equal, no bruits, dorsalis pedis pulse +2 equal right/left, posterior tibial pulse difficult to palpate due to edema
- CHEST: breath sounds equal, faint crackles in right and left bases, equal excursion, no fremitus, no egophony, no retractions, rate even and unlabored
- ABDOMEN: large, obese, no rashes or skin changes, no tenderness, rebound, or guarding; no appreciable fluid shift
- LOWER EXTREMITIES: no appreciable inguinal adenopathy, no hernia, no scrotal edema, skin without rashes, lesions, or excoriations; without unilateral pain, swelling, or warmth; has symmetrical edema up to about 6 cm below the knee, increasing distally

DIFFERENTIAL DIAGNOSIS

Clinical Observations	Deep Vein Thrombosis	Venous Insufficiency	Cellulitis	Lymphedema	Heart Failure
Onset	Either	Gradual	Abrupt	Gradual	Gradual

(continued)

Clinical Observations	Deep Vein Thrombosis	Venous Insufficiency	Cellulitis	Lymphedema	Heart Failure
Fever	No	No	Possible	No	No
Skin changes	Yes	Yes	Yes	No	No
Skin erythema/ warmth	Yes	No	Yes	No	No
Edema	Unilateral	Bilateral	Unilateral	Either	Bilateral
Dyspnea	No	No	No	No	Possible
Chest discomfort	No	No	No	No	Possible
Jugular vein distention	No	No	No	No	Possible
Abdominal distention	No	No	No	No	Rare
Fatigue	No	Possible	No	No	Possible
Cough	No	No	No	No	Common
Lymphadenopathy	No	No	Possible	Yes	No

DIAGNOSTIC EXAMINATION

Exam	Code	Cost	Results
Transthoracic stress echocardiogram, complete with contrast EKG	93351	$1,400–$2,500	• Evaluates all four chambers of the heart • Determines strength of the heart, the condition of the heart valves, the lining of the heart (the endocardium), and the aorta • Detects a heart attack, enlargement, or hypertrophy of the heart, infiltration of the heart with an abnormal substance • Detects weakness of the heart; cardiac tumors; measures diastolic function, fluid status, and ventricular dyssynchrony • Identifies vegetations of valves • Visualizes structures at the back of the heart, such as the left atrial appendage
Chest radiography (x-ray)	71020	$300	• Shows heart, lungs, airway, blood vessels, and lymph nodes • Shows bones of your spine and chest, including breastbone, ribs, collarbone, and the upper part of spine • Chest x-ray is the most common imaging test or x-ray used to find pathology Negative chest x-ray: normal results Positive chest x-ray: infection, consolidation, fluid

(continued)

Exam	Code	Cost	Results
EKG	93000	$500–$1,200	• Quick and noninvasive procedure • Records the electrical impulse produced by every heartbeat to gain information about a patient's heart, such as duration of heart contraction, the direction of the impulse, and the strength of the contraction
Doppler ultrasound	93970–93971	Average is $230	• Noninvasive test that can be used to measure vessel blood flow and blood pressure through high-frequency sound waves • Can estimate how fast blood flows by measuring the rate of change in its pitch (frequency) • This test may be done as an alternative to more invasive procedures, such as arteriography and venography, which involve injecting dye into the blood vessels so that they show up clearly on x-ray images • A Doppler ultrasound test may also help check for trauma/injury to veins and arteries
CBC	85025	$75	The CBC typically has several parameters that are created usually from an automated cell counter: WBC count • Indicates is the number of WBCs • High WBC can be a sign of infection, and in association with unilateral leg edema, warmth and fever might be associated with a local cellulitis • WBC count is increased in certain types of leukemia • Low WBC count can be a sign of bone marrow diseases or an enlarged spleen • Low WBC count is also found in HIV infection in some cases (*Editor's note*: The vast majority of low WBCs in our population are not HIV-related) Hgb and Hct • Hgb is the amount of oxygen-carrying protein contained within the RBCs • Hct is the percentage of the blood volume occupied by RBCs • In most laboratories, Hgb is actually measured, whereas Hct is computed using the RBC measurement and the MCV measurement • Purists prefer to use the Hgb measurement as it is more reliable; low Hgb or Hct suggests anemia • Anemia can be due to nutritional deficiencies, blood loss, destruction of blood cells internally, or failure to produce blood in the bone marrow • High Hgb can occur due to lung disease, living at high altitudes, or excessive bone marrow production of blood cells MCV • This helps diagnose a cause of an anemia. Low values suggest iron deficiency; high values suggest deficiencies of either vitamin B_{12} or folate, ineffective production in the bone marrow, or recent blood loss with replacement by newer (and larger) cells from the bone marrow PLT • This is the number of cells that plug up holes in your blood vessels and prevent bleeding

(*continued*)

Exam	Code	Cost	Results
			• High values can occur with bleeding, cigarette smoking, or excess production by the bone marrow • Low values can occur from premature destruction states, such as immune thrombocytopenia, acute blood loss, drug effects (such as heparin), infections with sepsis, entrapment of platelets in an enlarged spleen, or bone marrow failure from diseases such as myelofibrosis or leukemia • Low platelets also can occur from clumping of the platelets in a lavender-colored tube • You may need to repeat the test with a green-top tube in that case
CMP	Z13.228	$91.59	• A comprehensive metabolic panel is a blood test that measures glucose level, electrolyte and fluid balance, kidney, function, and liver function.
BNP	R79.89	$175	• A normal level rules out acute heart failure in the emergency setting. • An elevated level should never be used to "rule in" acute or chronic heart failure due to lack of specificity • Can also be used for screening and prognosis of heart failure • Typically increased in patients with left ventricular dysfunction

BNP, brain natriuretic peptide; CBC, complete blood count; CMP, comprehensive metabolic panel; Hct, hematocrit; Hgb, hemoglobin; MCV, mean corpuscular volume; PLT, platelet count; RBC, red blood cell; WBC, white blood cell.

CLINICAL DECISION MAKING

Case Study Analysis

The advanced practice provider performs the assessment and physical examination on the patient and finds the following data: Vital signs 156/102, 88 beats per minute HR, oxygen concentration 96% room air. Without jugular venous pressure (JVP) distention at 30 degrees, heart sounds reveal distant S3 gallop, breath sounds equal with faint crackles bilaterally in bases, rate 18 to 20 and unlabored at rest. Abdomen exam is soft without rebound, guarding, no distention of fluid shift, and skin is without spider angioma. Patient with notable bilateral pitting edema to below the knee with somewhat obscured ankle landmarks. Without warmth/tenderness or drainage to suggest cellulitis. Without unilateral edema, calf, or thigh discomfort. No history of coagulopathies and no previous history of pulmonary embolism or deep vein thrombosis. Without known renal disease or cancers. Complete blood count (CBC) shows normal white blood count, which is reassuring. No anemia, no thrombocytopenia, renal profile shows no electrolyte disturbance or significant acidosis. Comprehensive metabolic panel shows blood glucose normal, normal protein/normal liver function tests, and normal electrolytes. Brain natriuretic peptide (BNP) returns 242 suggestive of early heart failure; troponin 0.0; urinalysis without signs of infection, co-casts, and no hematuria. EKG in a normal sinus rhythm of 88, without ST segment elevation or depression. There is poor precordial R wave progression, and low limb lead voltage. Also notable is high precordial QRS voltage. Chest x-ray shows slight bilateral blunting of costophrenic angles, suggestive of fluid. No appreciable consolidation or effusion.

The patient is prescribed a diuretic and asked to call the clinic to provide a complete list of prescribed medications. Reviewed activities to help reduce lower extremity edema to include low-sodium diet and elevation. The patient is instructed on performing daily exercises with weights and recording his progress in anticipation for the next appointment. Antiembolism stockings/compression stockings discussed if edema worsens or causes an increase in discomfort. A follow-up appointment is scheduled for 2 weeks with the cardiology clinic. The patient is encouraged to seek medical attention if swelling becomes more severe or problematic prior to the scheduled appointment.

Diagnosis: *Early congestive heart failure*

MEMORY LOSS

> **Case Presentation:** *A 70-year-old African American female presents to the acute care clinic with complaints of "memory loss." She is accompanied by her son.*

INTRODUCTION TO COMPLAINT

- Side effect or reaction to medicines (antidepressants, antihistamines, antianxiety medications, muscle relaxants, tranquilizers, sleeping pills, or pain medications)
- Metabolic disorders or thyroid issues
- Nutritional deficiencies (B_1 or B_{12})
- Emotional/psychiatric problems/stress
- Infections (meningitis, urinary tract infection [UTI], or encephalitis)
- Dementia or Alzheimer's disease
- Illicit drug use or alcohol use
- Stroke
- Sleep deprivation
- Head injury

HISTORY OF COMPLAINT

Symptomatology

Ask about the following characteristics of each symptom using open-ended questions:

- Onset
- Situation
- Duration
- Associated symptoms
- Alleviating factors
- Timing
- Previous diagnosis of similar episodes
- Effects on daily activities

Directed Questions to Ask

- When did you notice the memory loss start?
- Was it gradual or sudden?
- How long has this been happening?
- What are your current medications? Have you recently started any new medications?
- Have you or anyone in your family ever been told you have a thyroid issue?
- Have you noticed a change in your skin or hair?
- Have you had a change in your strength or energy?
- Have you been more sensitive to heat or cold?

- Have you been running a temperature?
- Have you been around anyone sick lately?
- Do you use illicit drugs or alcohol products? How frequently?
- Have you ever had a head injury?
- How have you been sleeping lately? Is it different than normal?
- Can you tell me your name, date, time, and year?
- Have you ever noticed this happening before?
- Has this affected your daily activities?
- Has anything made this worse that you are aware of?
- Has anything happened lately in your life that has caused you stress?
- Have you had a change in diet recently?
- Has anything made this better? For example, rest?

Assessment: Cardinal Signs and Symptoms

General
- Assess for fatigue
- Weight loss
- Fever
- Night sweats, or chills

Eyes
- Vision changes

Head
- Headache
- Head trauma
- Fainting

Neck
- Thyroid enlargement

Musculoskeletal
- Decrease in strength

Neurologic
- Weakness
- Paralysis
- Trouble walking
- Memory/speech problems

Psychological
- Mood changes

Endocrine
- Heat/cold intolerances
- Unusual fatigue
- Hair loss

Medical History

- Hypertension, hyperlipidemia, cholecystectomy in 2000, and hysterectomy in 1990
- Allergies: penicillin: rash

- Current medications: hydrochlorothiazide (HCTZ) 50 mg daily, amlodipine 5 mg daily, simvastatin 40 mg daily, and multivitamin daily
- Psychiatric: never been hospitalized for psychiatric issues
- OB/GYN: gravida 2, para 2
- Diet: not on any specific diet, enjoys home cooked meals
- Occupation: retired school teacher
- Health maintenance: no longer sees an OB/GYN
- Mammogram: had in 2015
- Colonoscopy: had in 2013; she sees her primary MD every year
- Vaccinations: flu shot this year. PS23 given at age 65; Tdap in 2008
- Exercise: used to walk around the mall once a day, but has not been out since her husband died

Family History
- Mother: hypertension, type 2 diabetes
- Father: seizures, transient ischemic attack (TIA), elevated cholesterol
- Sister: alive and well, hypertension
- Brother: died in 1960 from motor vehicle accident
- Recently widowed, moved in with her son

Social History
- Current smoker; smoked ½ pack a day for 50 years
- Never used alcohol
- Not currently sexually active
- Illicit drug use, denies
- Attends weekly bridge meetings
- Attends church every Sunday
- Has not traveled to any foreign countries

PHYSICAL EXAMINATION
Vital Signs
- Temperature
- Blood pressure (BP)
- Respiration
- Heart rate (HR)
- Height
- Weight

General Appearance
- State of health
- Appearance of comfort or distress
- Hygiene

HEN
- JVD
- Pupils
- Nodes

CV
- Heart sounds
- Breath sounds

MS
- Edema
- Pulses

Neurologic
- Level of consciousness

Psychiatric
- Confusion
- Delirium
- Hallucinations

CASE STUDY

History

Son has to answer as the patient is unable to give clear answers.

Directed Question	Response
When did you notice the memory loss start?	*This morning when she got up.*
Was it gradual or sudden?	*It seemed sudden.*
How long has this been happening?	*Just this morning.*
What are your current medications? Have you recently started anything new?	*[Review medication list] No new medications.*
Have you or anyone in your family ever been told you have a thyroid issue?	*No, not that I am aware of.*
Have you noticed a change in your skin or hair?	*No.*
Have you noticed a change in your strength or energy?	*This morning she seemed very weak, hard to get out of bed.*
Have you become more sensitive to heat or cold?	*She is always cold, nothing different that I have noticed.*
Have you been running a temperature?	*We have not taken her temperature.*
Have you been around anyone sick lately?	*No.*
Do you use illicit drugs or alcohol? How frequently?	*No.*
Have you ever had a head injury?	*No.*
How have you been sleeping lately? Is it different than normal?	*She seems to be sleeping fine.*
Can you tell me your name, date, time, and year?	*She can state her name, but is disoriented to the other questions.*
Have you ever noticed this happening before?	*No.*

Directed Question	Response
Has this affected your daily activities?	*It was difficult to get her here, I had to help her in the car and then into the office. We used a wheelchair and she never has done that before.*
Has anything made this worse that you are aware of?	*Not that I can think of.*
Has anything happened lately in your life that has caused you stress?	*Her husband died a few months ago. She was scared to stay in the house by herself, so she moved in with me.*
Have you had a change in diet recently?	*My wife cooks dinner every night, home cooked meals. Mom used to cook as well, but has not since my father died.*
Has anything made this better? Like rest?	*She felt bad when she woke up this morning and had some memory loss. I was concerned but she went to lie back down and rest. When she woke up she did not seem better, so no nothing has made it better.*

Physical Examination Findings

- VITAL SIGNS: temperature 98.7°F; HR 88 regular rhythm; BP 198/100; weight 170 lb; height 5′4″; body mass index (BMI) 29.2
- GENERAL APPEARANCE: well-groomed, well-nourished Black female appearing her stated age
- HEAD/EYES/NECK: normocephalic head, pupils equal, round, and reactive to light and accommodation (PERRLA), extra ocular movement abnormal, patient unable to follow. Thyroid midline
- CHEST/CARDIOVASCULAR: lung sounds clear, HR regular rate and rhythm. No murmurs, rubs, or gallops
- MUSCULOSKELETAL: range of motion (ROM) intact
- NEUROLOGIC: alert to self, unable to answer other questions; speech is slurred; recognizes her son, but unable to recall past events; facial asymmetry noted; strength 2/5 on right, 5/5 on left; unable to complete finger to nose on right side, left intact; unable to complete heel to shin on right, left intact; unable to stand without assistance; gait unassessed due to safety

DIFFERENTIAL DIAGNOSIS

Clinical Observations	Stroke/TIA	Infection	Psych Issue	Metabolic Issue
Onset	Sudden	Gradual	Sudden/gradual	Sudden
Fever	No	Yes	No	No
Disorientation	Yes	Yes	Yes	Yes

Clinical Observations	Stroke/TIA	Infection	Psych Issue	Metabolic Issue
Vision changes	Yes	No	No	No
Neuro changes	Yes	No	Yes	No
Slurred speech	Yes	Yes/No	Yes/No	No

TIA, transient ischemic attack.

DIAGNOSTIC EXAMINATION

Exam	Code	Cost	Results
CBC with differential	D64.9	$12	Assess for infection
CMP	I10	$12	Assess electrolytes
Urinalysis	R82.90	$25	Assess for infection
Homocysteine level	83090	$64	Assess for elevated levels: possible clot or atherosclerosis
Blood glucose	R73.01	$29	Assess for low blood sugar
Lipid panel	80061	$29	Assess for abnormal cholesterol
PT/INR	R79.1	$28	Assess for blood clotting disorder
Head CT	R93.90	$1,200	Assess for hemorrhage
EKG	R94.31	$50	Assess for cardiac abnormalities
Carotid ultrasound	76870	$200–$400	Assess for blockages

CBC, complete blood count; CMP, complete metabolic panel; PT/INR, prothrombin time/international normalized ratio.

CLINICAL DECISION MAKING

Case Study Analysis

Memory loss that started this morning upon awakening. The memory loss includes disorientation. She is also weak on the right side and unable to stand/ambulate. She tried rest to relieve the symptoms with no change in symptoms. She has a history of hypertension, hyperlipidemia, and smoking. She has vision changes, asymmetry to the face, and an abnormal neurologic exam. CBC is negative for infection. Urinalysis is negative for infection. Blood sugar is 89 mg/dL. Lipid panel reveals: low density lipoprotein (LDL) 130 mg/dL; total cholesterol 201; high density lipoprotein (HDL) 35 mg/dL; triglycerides 180 mg/dL. Prothrombin time/international normalized ratio (PT/INR) is 11/0.9 units. Head CT is negative for acute changes, no hemorrhage. EKG shows normal sinus rhythm. Carotid ultrasound shows a blockage in the carotid arteries. Patient is afebrile, infection ruled out. Although she experienced the recent death of her husband, a stress incident is less likely. She is currently hypertensive. She is slightly overweight. Stable blood glucose and other laboratory findings rule out a metabolic event.

Diagnosis: *Cerebral infarction*

- She has passed the window for tissue plasminogen activator (tPA). Admit to the hospital to monitor patient
- Continuous cardiac monitoring for 24 to 48 hours
- Consult to neurology
- Monitor BP
- Physical therapy, occupational therapy, and speech therapy
- Have nursing assess gag reflex; refer to speech therapy for swallowing studies as necessary
- Monitor neurologic status every 2 hours

MOUTH LESIONS

Case Presentation: A 16-year-old Caucasian female has multiple mouth lesions. According to the patient, she had been experiencing these painful mouth lesions over the past several weeks with increasing severity.

INTRODUCTION TO COMPLAINT

- Ulcer that occurs on the mucous membrane of the oral cavity
- Usually an open lesion in the mouth
- Very common occurrence due to association with many diseases and imbalances
- Often causes pain and discomfort
- May alter patient's nutritional state

Different conditions can cause mouth sores, including:

- **Aphthous ulcer (canker sores)** appears white or yellow in the middle, and red around the edges and are caused by certain foods, infections, and biting the tongue or inside of the cheek.
- **Oral thrush** is caused by *Candida albicans*. Presents as whitish plaques in the mouth and can vary from painless to mild soreness.
- **Mouth cancer** appears on the lips or tongue. Mouth cancer can also cause the inside of the mouth, lips, or tongue to turn pale or dark in color. Symptoms are not painful and thus are discovered only after a routine medical or dental exam.
- **Leukoplakia** is white or gray patches inside the mouth or on the tongue. Patches can be thick and usually develop over time due to irritations inside of the mouth. Smoking and chewing tobacco are examples of these irritants.
- **Herpetic mucositis** is caused by the herpes simplex virus (HSV) type 1. It is ulcerative and usually presents in multiple spots in the mouth.
- **Acute necrotizing stomatitis** is caused by bacterial infections in the immune-deficient patient. Presenting symptoms include pain, fever, and necrotic or bloody ulcers.
- **Cheilitis** lips appear "chapped" and get red and scaly. Causes include windburn, licking the lips a lot, and certain medicines and foods. Two types exist: *actinic cheilitis* is caused by too much sun and can later turn into lip cancer; *angular cheilitis* is caused by a bacterial infection, and usually occurs in older people whose dentures do not fit well. Cheilitis causes redness and cracking in the corners of the mouth.
- **Mucositis** is inflammation of the mucosal surfaces throughout the body and typically involves redness and ulcerative sores in the soft tissues of the mucosa. Oral mucositis manifests as erythema, inflammation, ulceration, and hemorrhage in the mouth and throat.

HISTORY OF COMPLAINT

Symptomatology

Ask about the following characteristics of each symptom using open-ended questions:

- Onset (sudden or gradual)
- Chronology
- Current situation (improving or deteriorating)
- Location
- Radiation
- Quality
- Timing (frequency, duration)
- Severity
- Precipitating and aggravating factors
- Relieving factors
- Associated symptoms
- Effects on daily activities
- Previous diagnosis of similar episodes
- Previous treatments
- Efficacy of previous treatments

Directed Questions to Ask

- How long have the lesions been present?
- Do they come and go?
- Have you had any oral or dental procedure done lately?
- Any food triggers?
- Reaction to drugs?
- Stress level lately?
- Where is the location?
- Any other sores in/on the body?
- Is it single or in multiples?
- How big or how small?
- Increasing or decreasing in size?
- What is the color?
- Soft or hard?
- Is bleeding present?
- What precipitates bleeding?
- Is it painful?
- What is the pain rating on a scale of 0 to 10?
- What precipitates and aggravates the pain?
- What relieves the pain?
- Does it affect eating, swallowing, or taste?
- Do you know anyone who has had the same symptom?
- Any associated symptoms? Fevers? Malaise? Fatigue? Swollen nodes?
- Does it affect your daily activities?
- Have you been seen by a practitioner before for the same complaint?
- What was the diagnosis?
- What treatments were used?
- Did treatment relieve the sores?

Assessment: Cardinal Signs and Symptoms

- Mouth and throat
- Dental status
- Bleeding
- Discharge
- Presence of sores anywhere else
- Sore throat
- Aching tooth and gums
- Dysphagia
- Neck
- Swollen lymph nodes
- Pain
- Swelling
- Associated symptoms
- Fever
- Malaise
- Fatigue

Medical History: General

- Medical and surgical history
- Allergies
- List of all medications
- Herbal and traditional medications

Medical History: Specific to Complaint

- Frequent mouth sores
- Dental procedures
- Site of sore related to new denture or procedure
- Intake of food that precipitates mouth sores

PHYSICAL EXAMINATION

Vital Signs

- Temperature
- Pulse
- Respiration
- Oxygen saturation (SpO_2)
- Blood pressure (BP)

General Appearance

- Apparent state of health
- Appearance of comfort or distress
- Color
- Nutritional status
- State of hydration
- Hygiene
- Match between appearance and stated age

Mouth and Throat
- Lips: color, lesions, symmetry
- Oral cavity: breath odor, color, lesions of buccal mucosa
- Teeth and gums: redness, swelling, caries, bleeding
- Tongue: color, texture, lesions, tenderness of floor of mouth
- Throat and pharynx: color, exudates, uvula, tonsillar symmetry, and enlargement

Neck
- Symmetry
- Swelling
- Masses
- Active range of motion
- Thyroid enlargement

Palpation
- Tenderness, enlargement, mobility, contour, and consistency of nodes and masses
- Nodes: pre- and post-auricular, occipital, tonsillar, submandibular, submental, anterior and posterior cervical, supraclavicular
- Thyroid: size, consistency, contour, position, tenderness

CASE STUDY
History

Directed Question	Response
Was the onset sudden or gradual?	*It was sudden.*
Do you have any fever?	*Yes, it was 101 this morning.*
Do you have any aches?	*Yes, I am very achy.*
Is it hard to swallow?	*Yes, it is so painful.*
Are you able to drink fluids?	*Yes, I am drinking some fluids, but it hurts.*
If 10 is the worst pain you have ever had, what number is this pain?	*9 or 10.*
Do you have a headache?	*Mild headache here [points to front of head].*
Do you have a rash?	*No.*
Do you have fatigue?	*Yes, I am so tired.*
Do you have nasal congestion?	*No, I'm not stuffy.*
Do you have a cough?	*No, I'm not coughing.*
Do you have vomiting?	*No, my stomach is okay.*
Have you been exposed to anyone who has sore throat or strep throat?	*No, not that I know of.*

Physical Examination Findings

- VITAL SIGNS: temperature 100.4°F; respirations 20; pulse 82, regular; BP 128/88; SpO$_2$ 99%
- GENERAL APPEARANCE: anxious, uncomfortable, skin flushed, good skin turgor, unable to eat, can drink cool liquids and eat ice/popsicles, reports 3 lb weight loss, not sleeping
- MOUTH AND THROAT: lips clear, oral cavity; buccal mucosa with four lesions, two on upper palate, one under tongue, and one patient described as "lie bump" on top of tongue all with yellow centers, red, edematous, and painful; no geographic tongue, halitosis
- NECK: tracheal symmetry, good range of motion
- PALPATION: submental and submandibular lymph nodes soft, tender, and free moving bilaterally

DIFFERENTIAL DIAGNOSIS

Clinical Observations	Aphthous Ulcer	HSV	Oral Cancer
Onset	Abrupt	Abrupt	Gradual
Painful	Yes	Yes	No
Fever	Low	Either	No
Red halo	Yes	No	Either
White/yellow center	Yes	No	No
Vesicles	No	Yes	No
Nodes	Either	No	No

HSV, herpes simplex virus.

DIAGNOSTIC EXAMINATION

Exam	Code	Cost	Results
CBC with differential	85025	$75	<ul><li>Low WBC count: can be a sign of bone marrow disease or enlarged spleen</li><li>Agranulocytosis: failure of the bone marrow to produce enough neutrophils to fight infection; this causes an overgrowth of yeast, and can cause bacterial and viral infections</li><li>Neutropenia</li></ul>
Viral culture and PCR tests	87252	$75	<ul><li>Herpes simplex virus can be the cause of oral lesions</li><li>A positive viral culture can mean that the patient has been exposed to the virus</li><li>A negative result suggests absence of infection with HSV</li></ul>

CBC, complete blood count; HSV, herpes simplex virus; PCR, polymerase chain reaction; WBC, white blood cell.

CLINICAL DECISION MAKING

Case Study Analysis

- Lesions were in the upper palate, under tongue, presenting with yellow centers, redness, swelling along with pain followed by halitosis.
- Presents with a low-grade temperature of 100.8°F, complete blood count (CBC) was slightly elevated, +1 soft, mobile but tender submandibular and submental node, which suggests an inflammatory response.
- Abrupt onset rules out oral cancer. Absence of vesicles rules out HSV.

Patient provided with a prescription for Aphthasol and instructed on its use. Encouraged to avoid spicy foods and those hot in temperature. Reviewed the use of over-the-counter analgesics for systemic pain control and as an antipyretic. Discussed the importance of routine dental examinations. Scheduled a follow-up examination in 2 weeks and reviewed the importance of seeking medication attention sooner if symptoms do not subside or worsen prior to the scheduled appointment.

> **Diagnosis:** *Aphthous ulcer (canker sores)*

MUSCLE WEAKNESS

Case Presentation: A 40-year-old male presents with a complaint of muscle weakness.

INTRODUCTION TO COMPLAINT

- A decrease in strength in one or more muscles
- It is a common symptom of muscular, neurological, autoimmune, and metabolic disorders
- Muscular diseases include: muscular dystrophy and dermatomyositis
- Neurological disorders include: Guillain–Barré syndrome, amyotrophic lateral sclerosis (ALS), stroke, muscles that spasm, meningitis, pinched nerve (carpal tunnel syndrome), ruptured or herniated disk in the spine, concussion or pressure on the spinal cord
- Autoimmune neuromuscular disorders include: myasthenia gravis, multiple sclerosis, fibromyalgia, lupus
- Metabolic disorders include: Addison's disease and thyroid disease
- Decrease in physical fitness and loss of muscle tissue
- Side effect of illness/disease (such as flu, HIV, hepatitis, anemia, heart failure, atrial fibrillation, pyelonephritis, provoked vestibulodynia (PVD), diabetes mellitus (DM), pulmonary disease, and depression)
- Damage to nerves (caused by injury such as burns)
- Amyloidosis
- Hypokalemia/dehydration
- Vitamin D deficiency
- Food allergy
- Corticosteroid use
- Status poststroke
- Cancer (brain, leukemia, bone) and/or chemotherapy
- Medications (narcotics)
- Pregnancy
- Sleep disorders

HISTORY OF COMPLAINT

Symptomatology

Ask about the following characteristics of each symptom using open-ended questions:

- Onset
- Chronology
- Location
- Timing and duration
- Radiation

- Quality
- Severity
- Precipitating factors
- Relieving factors
- Associated symptoms
- Effects on daily activities
- Previous diagnosis of similar episodes
- Previous treatments and their efficacy

Directed Questions to Ask

- When does this tend to occur?
- How quick is the onset?
- How long does it last?
- Does anything seem to make it occur?
- Can you describe the weakness?
- Does it affect one muscle or group of muscles?
- What makes it worse?
- Does anything make it better?
- How long have you had the muscle weakness?
- Does it affect your daily activities?
- Does it cause pain? If so, rate your pain on a scale of 0 to 10.
- Have you ever been diagnosed with a neurological or muscular disease? Any family history of neurological or muscular diseases?
- Important past medical history (HIV, heart failure, anemia, stroke)?
- Any change in physical activities (increase or decrease)?
- Any change in medications (start or stop)?
- Any other symptoms associated with the weakness?
- Have you been sick recently?

Assessment: Cardinal Signs and Symptoms

General
- Fatigue

Head, Eyes, Ears, Nose, Throat (HEENT)
- Headache
- Neck pain
- Rash around eyes
- Dry eyes
- Dry mouth
- Facial droop
- Ptosis
- Dysphagia
- Facial weakness

Cardiac
- Chest pain

Respiratory
- Shortness of breath
- Crackles

Gastrointestinal
- Abdominal pain
- Diarrhea
- Constipation
- Vomiting
- Hepatomegaly

Genitourinary
- Dysuria
- Excessive urination
- Passing kidney stones

Musculoskeletal
- Pain
- Tenderness
- Neuropathy
- Joint swelling

Integumentary
- Bruising
- Skin bronzing
- Heliotrope rash

Other Associated Symptoms
- Memory loss
- Labile emotion
- Obesity

Medical History

Current Medical History
- Hyperlipidemia
- Hypertension (HTN)

Surgeries
- Tonsillectomy
- Appendectomy

Allergies
- Milk products

Medication
- Atorvastatin 20 mg daily
- Metoprolol 10 mg daily
- Ibuprofen 400 mg q4 prn for pain

Family History
- Mother and father: HTN

Social History
- Nonsmoker
- No drug/alcohol
- Works inside an office for 9 hours/day

Health Maintenance
- Received flu shot this year and is up to date on childhood vaccinations.

PHYSICAL EXAMINATION
Vital Signs

- Temperature
- Pulse
- Respiration
- Oxygen saturation (SpO_2)
- Blood pressure (BP)

General Appearance

- Minimal distress
- Lack of energy

HEENT
- Oral mucosa pink and moist
- No swelling, tenderness or drainage noted
- No adenopathy
- No facial rash

Cardiac
- Regular rate and rhythm (RRR)
- Absence of murmur, gallops, or rubs
- Capillary refill <2 seconds in all extremities
- No edema

Respiratory
- Clear to auscultation
- No shortness of breath

Gastrointestinal
- Abdomen soft and nontender

Genitourinary
- No pain with palpation

Musculoskeletal
- Pain in bilateral upper and lower joints and extremities
- Weakness in bilateral upper and lower extremities

Integumentary
- Pale
- Easily bruised

Psychology
- Depressed mood

CASE STUDY
History

Directed Question	Response
When does this tend to occur?	I experience throughout the day; morning, afternoon, and night.

Directed Question	Response
How quick is the onset?	*Gradual onset.*
How long does it last?	*All day.*
Does anything seem to make it occur?	*Lifting and turning, getting out of bed in the morning.*
Can you describe the weakness?	*It's all over and I can feel it in my joints especially.*
Does it affect one muscle or group of muscles?	*No, everything just feels weak.*
What makes it worse?	*Excessive movement and continuous movement.*
Does anything make it better?	*When I lie down and sometimes ibuprofen helps.*
How long have you had the muscle weakness?	*Over the past 3 months, it's gotten progressively worse.*
Does it affect your daily activities?	*Yes, I don't want to do anything because I'm weak and tired and have no interest in doing anything I used to.*
Does it cause you pain? If so, rate your pain on a scale of 0 to 10.	*Not really pain, just uncomfortable.*
Have you ever been diagnosed with a neurological or muscular disease? Any family history of neurological or muscular diseases?	*No, I've never been diagnosed and neither has my family.*
Important past medical history (HIV, heart failure, anemia, stroke)?	*No major past medical history that would cause the weakness.*
Any change in physical activities (increase or decrease)?	*Decreased activity, lack of sun exposure due to my job and I prefer to lie down inside.*
Any changes in medication (start or stop)?	*No changes in medication.*
Any other symptoms associated with the weakness?	*I'm feeling sadder and less interested in daily activities.*
Have you been sick recently?	*No.*

Physical Examination Findings

- VITAL SIGNS: temperature 98.5°F; respiratory rate (RR) 16; heart rate (HR) 86, regular; BP 136/70
- GENERAL APPEARANCE: weak, flat affect, appears exhausted
- EYES: pupils equal, round, and reactive to light and accommodation (PERRLA); extraocular movements intact

- NECK: no enlarged lymph nodes palpable. Neck is supple. Thyroid is not enlarged
- CHEST/CAVITY (CARDIOVASCULAR): lung sounds are clear in all fields. Heart S1, S2 no murmur, gallop, or rub
- ABDOMEN: soft, nontender without mass or organomegaly
- SKIN: pale
- EXTREMITIES: weakness in lower extremities and knee joints

DIFFERENTIAL DIAGNOSIS

Clinical Observations	Vitamin D Deficiency	Dehydration (Hypokalemia)	Pinched Nerve	Stroke
Onset	Gradual	Sudden	Gradual	Sudden
Pain	Yes	Yes/No	Yes	Yes/No
Vision impairment	None	None	Possible	Possible
Joint pain	Generalized	Generalized	Specific	Specific
Swelling of joint	None	Possible	Present	Possible
Weakness location	Generalized	Generalized	Specific	Specific
Fatigue	Present	Present	Specific to location	Present
Depression	Present	None	None	Possible
Other symptoms	Pale Milk allergy	Dry mucosa Abdominal pain	Symptoms specific to location	Unilateral symptoms

DIAGNOSTIC EXAMINATION

Exam	Code	Cost	Results
CBC without differential	D64.9	$25–$100	**CBC** **WBC count** • High WBC can be a sign of infection (can be bacterial or viral) • WBC count increased in certain types of leukemia • Low white counts can be a sign of bone marrow diseases, possible HIV infection, or an enlarged spleen **Hgb and Hct** • Hgb is the amount of oxygen-carrying protein contained within the red blood cells • Hct is the percentage of the blood volume occupied by red blood cells. • Low Hgb and Hct suggest an anemia • Anemia can be due to nutritional deficiencies, blood loss, destruction of blood cells internally, or failure to produce blood in the bone marrow

(continued)

Exam	Code	Cost	Results
			PLT • The number of cells that collect in blood vessels and prevent bleeding • High values can occur with bleeding • Low values can occur with anticoagulant use or forms of leukemia
Complete metabolic panel	I10	$28–$46	A comprehensive metabolic panel is a group of blood tests. They provide an overall picture of the body's chemical balance and metabolism **Normal Levels** • Albumin: 3.4–5.4 g/dL • Alkaline phosphatase: 44–147 IU/L • ALT: 10–40 IU/L • AST: 10–34 IU/L • BUN: 6–20 mg/dL • Calcium: 8.5–10.2 mg/dL • Chloride: 96–106 mEq/L • CO_2: 23–29 mEq/L • Creatinine: 0.6–1.3 mg/dL • Glucose: 70–100 mg/dL • Potassium: 3.5–5.0 mEq/L • Sodium: 135–145 mEq/L • Total bilirubin: 0.3–1.9 mg/dL • Total protein: 6.0–8.3 g/dL **Decreased potassium:** suggests dehydration **Elevated sodium:** suggests dehydration **Elevated BUN/creatinine:** suggests kidney damage/disease **Elevated ALT/AST:** suggests liver damage/disease
TSH level	Z13.29	$35–$500	**TSH level:** the pituitary gland located at the base of the brain secretes TSH. The amount of TSH that the pituitary sends into the blood stream depends on the amount of T4 that the pituitary sees. If the pituitary sees very little T4, then it produces more TSH to tell the thyroid gland to produce more T4. Once the T4 in the blood stream goes above a certain level, the pituitary's production of TSH is shut off **High TSH:** indicates that the thyroid gland is failing because of a problem that is directly affecting the thyroid (primary hypothyroidism) **Low TSH:** usually indicates an overactive thyroid that is producing too much thyroid hormone (hyperthyroidism). Occasionally, a low TSH may result from an abnormality in the pituitary gland, which prevents it from making enough TSH to stimulate the thyroid (secondary hypothyroidism) **Normal TSH:** (0.5 and 4.0 mIU/L) means that the thyroid is functioning normally
FREE T4 Level	Z13.29	$35–$500	**Free T4**, which does enter the various target tissues to exert its effects. The free T4 fraction is the most important to determine how the thyroid is functioning, and tests to measure this are called the free T4 **Elevated free T4:** suggests hyperthyroidism

(continued)

Exam	Code	Cost	Results
			Low free T4: suggests hypothyroidism Combining the TSH test with the FT4 or FTI results accurately determines how the thyroid gland is functioning
25-hydroxy vitamin D level	E55.9	$40–$70	**The 25-hydroxy vitamin D test:** is the most accurate way to measure how much vitamin D is in the body. In the kidney, 25-hydroxy vitamin D changes into an active form of the vitamin. The active form of vitamin D helps control calcium and phosphate levels in the body. **Normal vitamin D range:** between 20 and 40 ng/mL **Low vitamin D:** suggests Vitamin D deficiency **High vitamin D:** suggests hypervitaminosis D, an abnormally high storage levels of vitamin D, which can lead to toxic symptoms

ALT, alanine amino transferase; AST, aspartate amino transferase; BUN, blood urea nitrogen; CBC, complete blood count; Hct, hematocrit; Hgb, hemoglobin; PLT, platelet count; TSH, thyroid-stimulating hormone; WBC, white blood cell.

CLINICAL DECISION MAKING

Case Study Analysis

A history and examination were obtained and laboratory tests were ordered. After the office visit the patient continued to have generalized muscle weakness and decreased energy. CBC was normal, and no anemia or infection was suggested by the results. Complete metabolic panel (CMP) results suggest normal kidney and liver function, and no signs of dehydration or electrolyte imbalance. Thyroid-stimulating hormone (TSH)/free T4 were within normal limits, but 25-hydroxy vitamin D was low at 8 ng/mL. Patient denies any increased weakness, swelling of joints, or increased pain. Symptoms do not suggest a pinched nerve or stroke.

> *Diagnosis:* Vitamin D deficiency

The diagnosis is vitamin D deficiency. Patient has had a gradual increase in muscle weakness that is generalized. No signs of swelling of joints. Weakness is continuous throughout the day with relief coming from decreased activity and little relief from nonsteroidal anti-inflammatory drugs (NSAIDs). He has an allergy to milk products and has decreased exposure to sunlight related to his job. The patient is pale and has decreased energy. Increased fatigue and change in mood leading to depression. Extremely low vitamin D level at 8 ng/mL.

Discussed treatment options to include oral or parenteral vitamin D supplementation. Reviewed the availability of lactase tablets that can be taken by individuals with lactose intolerance. Discussed dietary choices that are high in calcium. Recommend a follow-up appointment in 1 month to reevaluate symptoms and vitamin D level.

NECK PAIN

Case Presentation: A 42-year-old construction worker presents to an urgent care clinic complaining of acute neck pain for 3 days.

INTRODUCTION TO COMPLAINT

Neck pain can be acute or chronic and can significantly disrupt activities of daily living (ADL).

Acute Pain

- Trauma (whiplash, strain, fracture)
- Overuse (strain)
- Infection (meningitis, lymphadenopathy from infection)
- Cardiac (angina)
- Systemic disease

Chronic Pain

- History of trauma
- Structural deformity
- Thoracic outlet syndrome
- Neurapraxia (peripheral nerve injury)
  - Entrapment of nerve (carpal tunnel syndrome [CTS])
  - Overuse syndrome
- Systemic disease

HISTORY OF COMPLAINT

Symptomatology

Ask about the following characteristics of each symptom using open-ended questions:

- Systemic disease (hypertension [HTN], cardiac disease, diabetes mellitus, osteoporosis)
- Surgical history
- Allergies (medication and seasonal)
- Medications currently used: daily and as needed (prescription and over-the-counter [OTC] drugs, including herbal and traditional therapies)
- Previous neck injury, trauma
- Severity of complaint
- Precipitating and aggravating factors
- Relieving factors
- Associated symptoms

- Effects on daily activities
- History of neck pain
- Previous diagnosis of similar episode:
  - When?
  - Frequency
- Previous treatments
  - Efficacy of previous treatments
- Was imaging done?
  - Findings

Directed Questions to Ask

Acute Neck Pain

- Was the onset sudden or gradual?
- What were you doing when it started?
- Was there any trauma prior to onset?
- What is your level of pain on a scale of 0 to 10?
  - When is the pain worse?
  - What makes the pain worse?
  - Does the pain keep you awake at night/awaken you from sleep?
- Does pain radiate to upper extremities?
- Describe the pain
- Do you have any associated chest pain or dyspnea?
- Do you have associated shoulder pain?
- Any recent upper respiratory symptoms (lymphadenopathy)?
- Do you have pain with range of motion (ROM)?
  - Is ROM limited?
- Is there associated upper extremity weakness?
  - Describe distribution of weakness
  - Is it constant or intermittent? If intermittent, describe what precipitates the pain.
- Do you have a headache (HA)?
  - Describe HA and where it is? Whole head, back of neck, right, or left?
- Do you have peripheral paresthesias (numbness, tingling)?
  - Where and what side? That is, the right fourth and fifth digits? Bilateral hands?
- Do you have dizziness or visual changes?
- Do you have fever or sign of infection?
  - Have you been exposed to anyone with meningitis?

Chronic Neck Pain

- Previous diagnosis of similar episode:
  - When?
  - Frequency (are episodes increasing)?
- Previous treatments
  - Efficacy of previous treatments
- Was imaging done?
  - Findings
- Is this episode similar?
- What were you doing when it started?
- Was there any trauma prior to onset?
- What is your level of pain on a scale of 0 to 10?
  - When is the pain worse?

- What makes pain worse?
- Does the pain keep you awake at night/awaken you from sleep?
- Do you have pain with ROM?
  - Is ROM limited?
- Is there associated upper extremity weakness?
  - Describe distribution of weakness.
  - Is it constant or intermittent? (If intermittent, describe what precipitates the pain)
- Do you have a HA?
  - Describe HA and where it is. Whole head, back of neck, right, or left?
- Do you have peripheral paresthesias (numbness, tingling)?
  - Where and what side? That is, the right fourth and fifth digits? Bilateral hands?
- Do you have dizziness or visual changes?

Assessment: Cardinal Signs and Symptoms

Head, Scalp, Eyes, Ears, Nose, Throat
- Upper respiratory symptoms
- Scalp and dental status (recent infections)
- Visual changes
- Lesions (herpes zoster)

Shoulders
- Shoulder pain
- History of shoulder trauma: recent or remote
- Pain with ROM
- Lesions (herpes zoster)

Chest
- Chest pain
- Shortness of breath
- Lesions (herpes zoster)

Back
- Thoracic or lumbar pain
- Pain with ROM
- Lesions (herpes zoster)

Other Associated Symptoms
- Fever
- Fatigue
- Dizziness

Medical History: General

- History: negative for systemic illness, cardiac disease, HTN, diabetes mellitus, previous neck pain/trauma/injury
- Past surgery: negative

Medical History: Specific to Complaint

- Medications: currently using OTC ibuprofen 400 mg two to three times per day without relief
- Allergies: no known drug allergies (NKDA)

PHYSICAL EXAMINATION

Vital Signs

- Temperature
- Pulse
- Respiration
- Blood pressure (BP)
- Oxygen saturation (SpO$_2$)

General Appearance

- Apparent state of health
- Appearance of comfort or distress
- Color and temperature of skin
- Nutritional status
- State of hydration
- Hygiene
- Match between appearance and stated age
- Difficulty with gait or balance

Head, Eyes, Ears, Nose, Throat (HEENT)
- General HEENT examination to rule out infection that may be causing lymphadenopathy

Neck
- Inspect
  - Position patient is holding head, neck, shoulders
  - Symmetry of neck and thyroid
    - Swelling
    - Visible spasm or mass
  - Compare sternocleidomastoid, trapezius, anterior and posterior triangles for symmetry
  - Presence of jugular venous distention
- Palpate
  - Bony tenderness: neck and shoulder
    - If localized cervical bony tenderness with history of trauma, *stop examination*, apply hard cervical collar, and get imaging as soon as possible
  - Localized muscle spasm and symmetry neck and shoulder
    - Sternocleidomastoid, trapezius, anterior and posterior triangles
    - Localized muscle tenderness neck and shoulder
    - Thyroid
    - Cervical lymph nodes: occipital, pre- and post-auricular, tonsillar, submaxillary, submental, superficial, and deep cervical chain anterior/posterior, infra- and supraclavicular
- Evaluate ROM of neck (after it has been determined there is no bony tenderness and cervical fracture has been ruled out). Observe for evidence of pain with ROM and if symmetrical right to left:
  - Flexion
  - Extension
  - Rotation
  - Lateral flexion
- Evaluate ROM of shoulders. Observe for evidence of pain with ROM and if symmetrical right to left:
  - Abduction

- Adduction
  - Internal and external rotation
- Evaluate distal neurological status if complaints of paresthesias

CASE STUDY
History

Directed Question	Response
Was the onset sudden or gradual?	Began 1 hour after a motor vehicle accident I had 3 days ago.
What were you doing when it started?	I was driving the car home.
Was there any trauma prior to onset?	No, it was a minor accident. I was rear-ended at a low speed. I did not hit my head.
What is your level of pain on a scale of 1 to 10?	Initially, 2 to 3 on 10, today 8/10.
When is the pain worse?	At work. I am a construction worker.
What makes pain worse?	Moving my neck in any position.
Describe pain	Feels very tight at back of neck and left upper back.
Does pain radiate to upper extremities?	No, just in back of my neck.
Does the pain keep you awake at night/ awaken you from sleep?	Yes.
Do you have any associated chest pain or dyspnea?	No.
Do you have associated shoulder pain?	No.
Any recent upper respiratory symptoms? (lymphadenopathy)	No.
Do you have pain with ROM?	Yes, with all movement.
Is ROM limited?	Yes.
Is there associated upper extremity weakness?	Not that I know of.
Do you have a headache?	Yes, worse in the morning.
Describe the headache and where it is.	At the back of my neck, top of my head.
Do you have peripheral paresthesias (numbness, tingling)?	No, my hands are okay.
Do you have dizziness or visual changes?	No visual change/dizziness.
Do you have a fever or sign of infection?	I feel okay other than my neck.

ROM, range of motion.

Physical Examination Findings

- VITAL SIGNS: temperature 98.8°F; respiratory rate (RR) 16; heart rate (HR) 108, regular; BP 142/84
- GENERAL APPEARANCE: well developed, appropriate for age; looks uncomfortable
- HEENT: no tenderness to palpation or evidence of upper respiratory infection
- NECK:
  - Holding head/neck to right with visible left trapezius spasm
  - No cervical bony tenderness to palpation
  - Left upper trapezius with palpable spasm and tenderness left of midline at base of neck
  - No cervical lymphadenopathy
  - Thyroid examination symmetrical, no tenderness or enlargement
  - Decreased and painful neck ROM with all movement
  - Full ROM of shoulder but complains of pain in neck with movements
  - Negative meningeal signs
- CHEST: lungs are clear in all fields; heart S1, S2 no murmur, gallop, or rub
- SKIN: no rashes
- EXTREMITIES: normal gait; sensation intact, distal digits

DIFFERENTIAL DIAGNOSIS

Clinical Observations	Neck Strain	Cervical Disc Displacement	Cervical Fracture	Meningitis
Pain	Yes	Yes/No	Yes	No
Headache	Yes/No	Yes/No	Yes/No	Yes
Decreased ROM	Yes	No	Yes	Yes
Paresthesias	No	Yes	Yes	No
Vision disturbances	No	No	No	Yes
Fever	No	No	No	Yes

ROM, range of motion.

DIAGNOSTIC EXAMINATION

Exam	Code	Cost	Results
Physical examination of the neck	92511	$100–$200	Evaluation of nose, nasopharynx, pharynx, and larynx Normal examination
CT scan: neck	70492	$1,000–$5,000	Visualized neck structures ruling out hematomas, fractures, soft tissue trauma Negative for fractures

(*continued*)

Exam	Code	Cost	Results
Lumbar puncture	62270	$3,000–$5,000	To test for bacterial meningitis: • Lumbar puncture tests collect spinal fluid from around the brain and spinal cord and analyze protein levels, glucose levels, cell counts, and the presence of infectious organisms Alerts for: • Cloudy spinal cord fluid • High spinal cord pressure • An increase in fluid antibodies • Abnormal glucose levels • Increased WBCs • Bacterial markers in fluid

WBC, white blood cell.

CLINICAL DECISION MAKING

Case Study Analysis

The advanced practice provider performs the history and physical examination on the patient and finds the following pertinent positives and negatives.

The pertinent positives are:

- History of low-speed rear-ended motor vehicle accident likely causing neck to move forward/backward
- Pain started about 1 hour after accident and has progressively worsened
- Describes pain as tightness that is worse in the morning
- Visible left trapezius spasm
- Tender to palpation
- Decreased and painful ROM of neck

The pertinent negatives are:

- Did not hit head and did not have neck pain at time of the accident
- No pain at the time of injury
- No radiating pain or paresthesias, which rules out cervical disc displacement and fracture
- Normal vital signs
- No evidence of acute infection (negative HEENT examination), which rules out meningitis
- No lymphadenopathy
- No cervical bony tenderness

No photophobia rules out meningitis. A series of neck x-rays confirmed a cervical fracture has not occurred.

> **Diagnosis:** *Cervical strain*

All findings reviewed with the patient. Discussed conservative treatment to include mild muscle relaxant, use of over-the-counter analgesics for pain control, application of heat/cold for 20 minutes several times a day, and possible referral to physical therapy for exercises and rehabilitation.

Follow-up appointment scheduled for 1 month. If symptoms persist or worsen, a referral to orthopedic or neurology clinic may be indicated.

NIGHT SWEATS

Case Presentation: A 51-year-old female reports to the clinic with a history of sudden onset of hot flushes and night sweats.

INTRODUCTION TO COMPLAINT

Night sweats are a symptom that can be observed in a variety of health imbalances. The following is a list of some of the more common ones.

- Hormonal changes (perimenopause/menopause)
- Effects of certain medications (antidepressants, steroids, aspirin)
- Stress and anxiety
- Infectious processes (abscesses, tuberculosis [TB], HIV/AIDS)
- Neurological problems (dysreflexia, autonomic neuropathy, stroke, Parkinson's)
- Hyperglycemia (medications are used to correct this and it results in hypoglycemia and spikes of epinephrine)
- Cancer (lymphoma most notably)
- Idiopathic hyperhidrosis

The vasomotor symptoms seen in perimenopause/menopausal women encompass both night sweats and hot flushes. In Western world cultures about 70% of women will experience these symptoms with varying frequency and varying levels of severity.

HISTORY OF COMPLAINT

Symptomatology

Ask about the following characteristics of each symptom using open-ended questions:

- Onset (sudden or gradual)
- Chronology
- Current situation (improving or deteriorating)
- Location
- Radiation
- Quality
- Timing (frequency, duration)
- Severity
- Precipitating and aggravating factors
- Relieving factors
- Associated symptoms
- Effects on daily activities

- Previous diagnosis of similar episodes
- Previous treatments
- Efficacy of previous treatments

Directed Questions to Ask

- When did you first start having the night sweats?
- How frequently are you having the night sweats?
- When was your last menstrual period?
- Have you had problems with inappropriate sweating previously?
- Have you noticed that you are running a fever?
- Do you have any known medical problems/diagnoses?
- Have you noticed any changes in your mobility? Muscle strength?
- Are you experiencing any numbness anywhere?
- Are you on any prescription medications, over-the-counter (OTC) medications, or supplements?
- Are you feeling overly stressed or anxious?

Assessment: Cardinal Signs and Symptoms

- Nocturnal sweating

Medical History: General

- Medical conditions and surgeries
- Allergies (seasonal as well as others)
- Medication currently used (prescription, birth control pill [BCP], and OTC)
- Herbal preparations and traditional therapies

Medical History: Specific to Complaint

- Onset of the night sweats
- Frequency of the night sweats
- Menstrual activity
- Known medical diagnoses

PHYSICAL EXAMINATION
Vital Signs

- Temperature
- Pulse
- Respiration
- Oxygen saturation (SpO_2)
- Blood pressure (BP)

General Appearance

- Apparent state of health
- Appearance of comfort or distress
- Color
- State of hydration

Neck
- Inspect for symmetry, swelling, masses
- Palpate for tenderness, thyroid enlargement, lymph node chain

Cardiovascular
- Inspect for capillary refill time
- Auscultate for heart sounds, check for murmurs, gallops, rubs
- Palpate for peripheral pulses

Respiratory
- Auscultate lungs for crackles, and wheezing

Abdomen
- Inspect for contour
- Auscultate for bowel sounds
- Palpate for pain, masses, organomegaly

Neurologic
- Orientation status
- Pupil reflexes/responses
- Test cranial nerves (CNs) II to XII
- Test fine and gross motor movements
- Test deep tendon reflexes (DTRs)
- Test motor and sensory capability

CASE STUDY

History

Directed Question	Response
When did you first start having the night sweats?	Last week when I was on vacation. I was on an Alaskan cruise and they hit me out of nowhere like a ton of bricks!
How frequently are you having the night sweats?	Nightly, sometimes have more than one episode a night.
When was your last menstrual period?	Three weeks ago.
Have you had problems with inappropriate sweating previously?	No.
Have you noticed that you are running a fever?	No.
Do you have any known medical problems/diagnoses?	No.
Have you noticed any changes in your mobility? Muscle strength?	No.
Are you experiencing any numbness anywhere?	No.

Directed Question	*Response*
Are you on any prescription medications, OTC medications, or supplements?	*I use some OTC micronized progesterone, a product called Progest-E. I have been on that for about the past 5 years. A 30-ml bottle of it usually lasts me about 5 months. I was at the bottom of that supply on my trip so that didn't help much. When I got home I opened a new bottle and I have almost emptied it in the past week just to try to get some relief from these hot flushes and the night sweats.*
Are you feeling overly stressed or anxious?	*I wasn't until I got hit with this mother lode of menopausal symptoms.*

OTC, over-the-counter.

Physical Examination Findings

- VITAL SIGNS: temperature 98.7°F; respiratory rate (RR) 16; heart rate (HR) 88, regular; BP 114/70; SpO$_2$ 99%
- GENERAL APPEARANCE: well-developed, healthy-appearing female who appears to be tired
- NECK: nontender, no thyroid enlargement or masses/nodules noted
- CARDIOVASCULAR: regular rate/rhythm without murmur or gallop
- RESPIRATORY: lungs clear
- ABDOMEN: soft, nontender, active bowel sounds, no masses or organomegaly
- NEUROLOGIC: alert and oriented X4, pupil reflexes/responses within normal limits (WNL), CNs II to XII grossly intact, fine and gross motor movements normal, DTRs WNL, no abnormality of motor or sensory capability noted on exam

DIFFERENTIAL DIAGNOSIS

Clinical Observations	Hormonal Changes	Infectious Processes	Neurologic Problems	Lymphoma	Medication Induced
CBC abnormalities	Not likely	Possibly elevated WBC	Not likely	Likely, secondary to the disease or the treatment for the disease	Not likely
Comprehensive metabolic panel abnormalities	Possibly related to glucose regulation	Possibly elevated glucose	Not likely	Possibly	Possibly, glucose impacted by steroids
Sensory testing abnormalities	Not likely	Not likely	Likely, depending on the type of neurologic problem	Not likely	Not likely

(continued)

Clinical Observations	Hormonal Changes	Infectious Processes	Neurologic Problems	Lymphoma	Medication Induced
Hormone testing abnormalities	Likely	Not likely	Not likely	Not likely	Not likely

CBC, complete blood count; WBC, white blood cell.

DIAGNOSTIC EXAMINATION

Exam	Code	Cost	Results
Complete blood count	85025	$49	To see if there is evidence of an infectious process
Comprehensive metabolic panel	80053	$49	For evaluation of metabolic problem contributors for the symptom profile
TSH	84443	$49	Hyperthyroidism can present with many of the same symptoms observed in "panic episodes"
FSH	83001	$49	To check for menopausal status

FSH, follicle-stimulating hormone; TSH, thyroid-stimulating hormone.

CLINICAL DECISION MAKING

Case Study Analysis

The advanced practice provider (APP) performs the assessment and physical examination on the patient and finds the following data: history of vasomotor symptoms consistent with perimenopausal/menopausal hormonal changes and no abnormal physical exam findings. A normal complete blood count (CBC) rules out an infection and lymphoma. No change in medications rules out a medication-induced cause. A normal neurologic examination rules out a neurologic cause for the symptoms.

The APP discusses hormone replacement therapy options with the patient. Suggested following up with OB/GYN provider.

Diagnosis: Night sweats/hot flushes, related to perimenopausal hormone changes

NIPPLE DISCHARGE

Case Presentation: A 32-year-old female reports to the clinic with a complaint of a "milky" looking discharge from her nipples.

INTRODUCTION TO COMPLAINT

Nipple discharge is the third most common breast-related complaint in female patients. Approximately 50% of women in their reproductive years experience physiologic nipple discharge. Physiologic discharge is characterized as bilateral, green, yellow, or milky fluid expressed from multiple duct openings and often associated with nipple stimulation.

Abnormalities in prolactin can result in galactorrhea (nonpuerperal lactation). These abnormalities can be secondary to pituitary tumors, primary hypothyroidism, or medications such as opiates, psychotropics, antihypertensives, prokinetics, and H_2 blockers.

Pathologic nipple discharge most typically is spontaneous and unilateral. The discharge can be bloody, serous, black, or green. The most common causes of pathologic nipple discharge are intraductal papilloma, ductal ectasia, and carcinoma.

HISTORY OF COMPLAINT

Symptomatology

Ask about the following characteristics of each symptom using open-ended questions:

- Onset (sudden or gradual)
- Chronology
- Current situation (improving or deteriorating)
- Location
- Radiation
- Quality
- Timing (frequency, duration)
- Severity
- Precipitating and aggravating factors
- Relieving factors
- Associated symptoms
- Effects on daily activities
- Previous diagnosis of similar episodes
- Previous treatments
- Efficacy of previous treatments

Directed Questions to Ask

- When did you first notice the nipple discharge?
- What color is the discharge?

- Is the discharge from one or both breasts?
- Have you noted any other breast changes associated with the discharge?
- Are you pregnant?
- Have you been told you have fibrocystic breast issues?
- Are you on any medications, prescribed, over the counter (OTC), or supplements?
- Have you experienced recent weight gain?
- What is your energy level like? Is that a change for you?
- Is your skin unusually dry? Is that a change for you?
- Are you experiencing unusual hair loss?
- Have you been having headaches? If yes, is that a change for you?
- Have you experienced any vision changes recently?
- Have you experienced any dizziness or "passing out" recently?
- Do you have any numbness in your face?

Assessment: Cardinal Signs and Symptoms

- Nipple discharge
- Any breast changes

Medical History: General

- Medical conditions and surgeries
- Allergies (seasonal, as well as others)
- Medication currently used (prescription, birth control pill [BCP], and OTC)
- Herbal preparations and traditional therapies

Medical History: Specific to Complaint

- Onset of discharge
- Unilateral or bilateral discharge
- Fibrocystic breast changes
- Weight gain, fatigue, dry skin, or hair loss

PHYSICAL EXAMINATION

Vital Signs

- Temperature
- Pulse
- Respiration
- Oxygen saturation (SpO_2)
- Blood pressure (BP)

General Appearance

- Apparent state of health
- Appearance of comfort or distress
- Color
- State of hydration

Face

- Inspect for symmetry

Neck
- Inspect for symmetry, swelling, masses
- Palpate for tenderness, thyroid size/shape; presence of nodules or cysts

Breasts
- Inspect for size, shape, symmetry
- Palpate for tenderness, presence of masses, nodules or cysts, expression of discharge

Neurologic
- Test for pupil reflexes and response to light; cranial nerves (CNs) II to XII, sensory function

CASE STUDY
History

Directed Question	Response
When did you first notice the nipple discharge?	*About a month ago. It seems to have increased over the past couple of weeks.*
What color is the discharge?	*Maybe sort of milky looking.*
Is the discharge from one or both breasts?	*Seems like I notice more from the left breast but I have had it from both breasts.*
Have you noted any other breast changes associated with the discharge?	*No, not noticed any breast changes.*
Have you been told you have fibrocystic breast issues?	*Never.*
Are you on any medications, prescribed, OTC, or supplements?	*A couple months ago I started taking OTC cimetidine for my heartburn issues. It was working so well at the recommended dose so about 6 weeks ago I increased the dose twofold because I know when a drug goes OTC they decrease the recommended dose from the prior prescription only dose recommendations.*
Have you experienced recent weight gain?	*No.*
What is your energy level like? Is that a change for you?	*Good . . . that is my typical.*
Is your skin unusually dry? Is that a change for you?	*Not really.*
Are you experiencing unusual hair loss?	*No more than usual for me.*
Have you been having headaches? If yes, is that a change for you?	*No, I am not a headache sort of person.*

Directed Question	*Response*
Have you experienced any vision changes recently?	*No.*
Have you experienced any dizziness or "passing out" recently?	*No.*
Do you have any numbness in your face?	*No.*

OTC, over the counter.

Physical Examination Findings

- VITAL SIGNS: temperature 98.0°F; respiratory rate (RR) 14; heart rate (HR) 80, regular; BP 111/70; SpO$_2$ 99%
- GENERAL APPEARANCE: well-developed, healthy female in no acute distress
- FACE: symmetrical, sensory capacity intact
- NECK: thyroid nontender, no thyromegaly, no thyroid nodules or cysts appreciated
- BREASTS: no masses palpable, nontender, small amount of milky discharge expressed from each breast
- NEUROLOGIC: pupil reflexes and responses within normal limits, CNs II to XII intact, sensory capacity intact

DIFFERENTIAL DIAGNOSIS

Clinical Observations	Physiologic Discharge	Pathologic Discharge	Medication Induced Discharge
Color of discharge	Green, yellow, milky	Bloody, serous, black, green	Milky
Unilateral/bilateral	Bilateral	Unilateral	Bilateral
Possible causes	Pituitary tumors, hypothyroidism	Intraductal papillomas, ductal ectasia, carcinoma	Opiates, psychotropics, antihypertensives, prokinetics, H$_2$ blockers

DIAGNOSTIC EXAMINATION

These are screening labs; more advanced studies of the discharge cytology and imaging ordered by a specialist if the nipple discharge is suspected to be pathologic.

Exam	Code	Cost	Results
TSH	84443	$49	To evaluate for TSH levels. If results indicate hypothyroidism, consider this as a possible etiology of the physiologic nipple discharge
Prolactin level	84146	$89	To evaluate for possible pituitary issues

TSH, thyroid-stimulating hormone.

CLINICAL DECISION MAKING

Case Study Analysis

The advanced practice provider (APP) performs the assessment and physical examination on the patient and finds the following data: expressed small amount of a milky discharge from nipple bilateral on exam, recent intake of high-dose cimetidine OTC. Symptoms do not support a physiologic or pathologic cause for the discharge. Nipple discharge is not yellow, green, black, or bloody.

The APP recommends to the patient that she discontinue the OTC cimetidine and trial use of OTC omeprazole. Discussed reason for using OTC stomach remedies. Suggested scheduling an appointment with the gastroenterology clinic to have chronic heartburn evaluated. Encouraged patient to return for further evaluation if nipple discharge does not subside or worsens after ending OTC cimetidine.

Diagnosis: *Nipple discharge, medication-induced*

PAINFUL INTERCOURSE

Case Presentation: *A 24-year-old female complained of painful intercourse. She states she has been experiencing painful intercourse for the past 6 months.*

INTRODUCTION TO COMPLAINT

- Recurrent or persistent genital pain that occurs just before, during, or after vaginal intercourse
- Causes include structural or physical causes, psychological or emotional factors

Physical Causes

- Insufficient lubrication
  - Insufficient foreplay
  - A drop in estrogen level (after childbirth, during breastfeeding)
  - Medication (antidepressants, blood pressure [BP] medications, sedatives, some anti-histamines, and certain birth control pills [BCPs])
- Injury, trauma
  - Traumatic injury to pelvis or peritoneum
  - Pelvic surgeries
  - Female circumcision
  - Episiotomy scars
  - Congenital abnormality
- Inflammation, infection, or skin disorders
  - Infection in the genital area or urinary tract
  - Eczema or other skin problems
- Certain illnesses or conditions
  - Endometriosis
  - Pelvic inflammatory disease
  - Uterine fibrosis
  - Retroverted uterus
  - Ovarian cysts
  - Cystitis
  - Uterine prolapse
  - Irritable bowel syndrome
- Surgical or medical treatments
  - Scarring from surgeries that involve the pelvic area
  - Hysterectomy, radiation, or chemotherapy for cancer treatments

Emotional Causes

- Psychological problems, such as anxiety, depression, concerns about physical appearance, fear of intimacy, or relationship

- Stress tightens pelvic floor muscles making intercourse painful
- History of sexual abuse

HISTORY OF COMPLAINT

Symptomatology

Ask about the following characteristics of each symptom using open-ended questions:

- Systemic disease (hypertension [HTN], cardiac disease, diabetes mellitus, osteoporosis)
- Surgical history
- Medications currently used: daily and as needed (prescription, BCP, and over-the-counter [OTC] drugs, including herbal and traditional therapies)
- Previous trauma
- Severity of complaint
- Precipitating and aggravating factors
- Relieving factors
- Associated symptoms
- Effects on daily activities

Directed Questions to Ask

- Do you have any sensation of burning?
- What are the circumstances that you think contributed to the painful intercourse?
- Do you have any redness or swelling?
- Do you have any lower abdominal pain?
- Do you have itching?
- Do you have any irritation or abrasions?
- Do you have any lesions?
- Do you have any warty growths?
- Do you have any dryness?
- Did you notice any unusual profuse discharge or malodorous discharge?
- Do you have any bleeding during or after intercourse?
- Do you have any voluntary or involuntary contraction of muscles around the vagina?
- Where are your injuries?

Assessment: Cardinal Signs and Symptoms

Vagina

- Sensation of burning
- Redness or swelling
- Lower abdominal pain
- Itching
- Irritation or abrasions
- Lesions
- Warty growths
- Dryness
- Presence of unusual profuse discharge or malodorous discharge
- Bleeding
- Voluntary or involuntary contraction of muscles around the vagina
- Where are your injuries?

Cervix
- Lower abdominal pain
- Foul smelling discharge
- Tenderness inside vagina

Other Associated Symptoms
- Fever
- Unusual fatigue
- Abdominal pain
- Rectal pain

Medical History: General
- Have you had any stomach or gastric problems in the past?
- Have you had any surgeries in the past?
- Are you allergic to anything like medication, food, or plants?
- Do you currently use any medications that include any prescription medications?
- Do you use any OTC medications?
- Did you use any herbal preparations or traditional therapies? Vitamins?

Medical History: Specific to Complaint
- When did you have your first menses? How old were you?
- When was your last menstrual period? Are they regular?
- Do you use tampons? Do you douche?
- Have you had a Pap smear? If so, when was it last done?
- When was the last time you had vaginal intercourse?
- Do you use contraceptives?
- Have you ever been pregnant? How many pregnancies?
- What are the outcomes of your pregnancies?
- Have you had any abortions?
- Do you have any history of infections like gonorrhea, syphilis, or herpes?

PHYSICAL EXAMINATION
Vital Signs
- Temperature
- Pulse
- Respiration
- Blood pressure (BP)
- Oxygen saturation (SpO_2)

General Appearance
Skin
- Note the condition of skin and observe for bruising or other signs of physical trauma

Abdomen
- Palpate all four quadrants

Pelvic
- External genitalia visualization; observe for bruises, lesions, swelling, lacerations

Internal Examination

- On speculum examination, observe for condition and color of vaginal mucosa; signs of inflammation, ulcers, and tears; observe color and position of the cervix, ulceration, nodules, cysts, or injury; observe the shape of the cervix and particularly for bleeding or discharge and, if present, its color, consistency, and odor

Bimanual Examination

- Palpate for nodules or tenderness in the vagina, including the region of the urethra and bladder; palpate the cervix and note mobility and presence of tenderness; palpate the ovaries and note any pain on palpation

Rectovaginal Examination

- During the rectovaginal exam, palpate for tenderness; palpate the uterus, and right and left adnexa for nodularity or thickening

Rectal Examination

- Observe and palpate the rectum for hemorrhoids, anal fissures, or other abnormalities

CASE STUDY

History

Directed Question	Response
Do you have a history of any medical conditions like diabetes, high blood pressure, or high cholesterol?	*No.*
Have you had any heart problems or history of cardiovascular disease?	*No.*
Do you have any breathing or respiratory problems?	*No.*
Have you had any stomach or gastric problems in the past?	*No.*
Have you had any surgeries in the past?	*I had episiotomies from my deliveries.*
Are you allergic to anything like medication, food, or plants?	*No.*
Do you have any history of infections like gonorrhea, syphilis, or herpes?	*I had a yeast infection once but never anything else.*
Do you currently use any medications that include any prescription medications?	*I take birth control pills, Tylenol for pain, and Alka-Seltzer for nausea.*
Do you use any over-the-counter medications?	*Yes, what I just told you.*
Do you use any herbal preparations or traditional therapies?	*Vitamins.*
When did you have your first menses?	*When I was 12 years old.*
How is your menstruation?	*I am regular.*

Directed Question	Response
When was your LMP?	*Two weeks ago.*
When was your last sexual activity?	*Last night.*
Do you use contraceptives, tampons, or douches?	*I use birth control pills, tampons, but no douches.*
Have you ever been pregnant? How many pregnancies?	*Two.*
What are the outcomes of your pregnancies?	*Two healthy little girls.*
Have you had any abortions?	*No.*
How many living children?	*Two.*
When was your last Pap smear test?	*One year ago.*
Do you have any redness or swelling?	*Yes.*
Do you have any sensation of burning?	*No.*
Can you tell me about your pain?	*I have pain in my vagina. It happened when my husband forced me to have sexual intercourse when I didn't want to.*
Is it a sudden pain or gradual pain?	*Sudden pain.*
Where is the pain? Is it near the outside, occurring at the start of the intercourse, or do you feel it farther in, when your partner is pushing deeper?	*The pain is in my vagina and it started when he shoved into me.*
Does it radiate to your pelvis, hips, or any part of your abdomen?	*No.*
On a scale of 0 to 10 with 0 no pain and 10 the worst pain you ever had, how do you rate your pain?	*10.*
When does the pain start? How long does the pain last? Does it hurt only during intercourse? Did this pain start only 6 months ago?	*The pain started when he forced himself into me! He doesn't give me time to adjust to his size. Yes, the pain has existed every time we have sex.*
What are the circumstances that you think contributed to the painful intercourse?	*When he forces me to have sex and I am not ready.*
Does your husband get angry with you when you complain of painful intercourse?	*Yes, he gets angry.*
Is there anything that makes it worse?	*When he drinks he is abusive. There is no talking to him.*
Is there some other discomfort that accompanies the painful intercourse?	*My legs hurt, my bottom hurts, and I can feel my insides shaking around.*

Directed Question	Response
How does this pain affect your daily activities?	I feel angry and sad.
Did you try to treat this pain with medications or other remedies?	I take Tylenol.
How effective was the treatment or remedies?	It helps.
Do you have any redness or swelling?	Yes.
Do you have any lower abdominal pain?	No.
Do you have itching?	No.
Do you have any irritation or abrasions?	Yes.
Do you have any lesions?	No.
Do you have any warty growths?	No.
Do you have any dryness?	Yes.
Did you notice any unusual profuse discharge or malodorous discharge?	No.
Do you have any bleeding?	Afterward.
Do you have any voluntary or involuntary contraction of muscles around the vagina?	Don't know what you mean? I feel tight and shaky.
Where are your injuries?	I have bruises on my legs, and down there.

LMP, last menstrual period.

Physical Examination Findings

- VITAL SIGNS: temperature 98.7°F (oral); respiration 18 breaths/min; pulse 72 beats/min; BP 120/72
- GENERAL APPEARANCE: well-developed healthy looking 24-year-old muscular female; admitted due to injuries sustained when her husband hit her; complaints of dyspareunia during sexual intercourse; in good state of health and presently not in distress; height: 5′6″ tall; weight 122 lb; well-groomed in tight jeans and blouse with heavy makeup but appears clean; appearance matches with her age; mood looks sad and depressed; skin clear without bruising, lesions, pale; nutritional status is good; no difficulty with gait or balance
- SKIN: warm; dry; no open lesions; color of the skin looks pale but no rashes, scarring, or warts; many bruises with finger imprints were noted on the inner aspect of thighs bilaterally, abdomen, and buttocks
- PELVIC EXAMINATION: external genitalia examination: bruises noted on the labia majora and labia minora; no lesions, swelling or ulcerations noted; no obvious signs of rectocele or cystocele; internal examination: on speculum examination, vaginal mucosa looks very dry, color pink, moist, no signs of inflammation, or ulcers; tear in vaginal orifice is noted; color and position of the cervix are normal, no ulceration, nodules, cysts, or injury; the shape of the cervix is slit-like, with no lesions noted; no bleeding or discharges evident within normal parameters; bimanual examination: no nodularity or tenderness in the vagina, including the region of the urethra and bladder; palpation of

the cervix was normal and mobile with no tenderness; head of the uterus was smooth and nontender; ovaries were mobile and no pain was evident upon exam; rectovaginal examination: rectovaginal examination was normal and nontender; uterus, right and left adnexa appear within normal limits; no nodularity or thickening of the uterosacral ligaments were noted; rectal examination: rectal examination revealed no abnormalities; no hemorrhoids, anal fissures were observed

DIFFERENTIAL DIAGNOSIS

Clinical Observations	Insufficient Lubrication	Atrophic Vaginitis	Pelvic Inflammatory Disease	Sexually Transmitted Infections	Endometriosis
Onset	Sudden, during insertion of penis	Well-defined coitus pain	During sex	During sex	During/after sex and menstruation
Quality of pain	Deep, during/after intercourse, rated 10/10	Difficulty and severe pain with penetration	Severe	Severe	Deep pelvic pain
Tenderness	Yes	Yes	Yes	Yes	Yes
Discharge	No	No	Severe	Yes	Yes/No
Itching	No	Yes	Yes	Yes	No
Burning	Yes	Yes	Yes	Yes	Yes
Abrasion	++	Yes	No	Yes	No
Bruises	+/−	No	No	No	No
Dryness/ friction	Severe	Severe	No	No	Yes/No
Erythema	Yes	Yes	Yes	Yes	No
Irritation/ rawness	Yes	Yes	No	No	No
Lesions	No	No	Yes	Yes	No
Abnormal bleeding	Spotting	Yes/No	Excessive	Yes	Yes
Fever	No	No	Yes	Yes	Yes
Palpable mass	No	No	Yes	No	Yes

DIAGNOSTIC EXAMINATION

Exam	Code	Cost	Results
External genitalia examination	88147	$150	• Vulva and labia: erythema, excoriations, and induration • Bruises noted on the labia majora and labia minora • Swelling/redness and abrasions
Internal vaginal examination	88141–88158	$150	• Using speculum: Can identify the presence of any foreign body like tampons, condom, etc., injury, or vaginal infections • Vaginal walls look dry with no lubrication • Can identify any pelvic dysfunctions • Can find any lesion or mass • Cotton swab test or Q tip test during a pelvic exam to diagnose PVD (vestibulitis)
Vaginal rectal examination	88141–88158	Part of office visit cost	• To determine pelvic/uterine dysfunctions • Identify pelvic mass • Identify retroverted uterus
Bimanual examination	88141–88158	Part of office visit cost	• Assess the status of uterus, fallopian tube, and cervical motion tenderness
Laboratory diagnostic studies	88150–88155	$55–$75	• Urine test for pregnancy is the first laboratory test • Test for pH >4.5 is consistent with bacterial vaginitis or atrophic vaginitis • Potassium hydroxide and wet mount preparation will show any bacterial vaginitis (clue cells) and yeast infection • Urine analysis and culture: Microscopic examination can rule out cystitis or PID • Serology for screening syphilis, e.g., VDRL • Blood test for complete blood count and ESR to check the infection
Pap smear	88150–88155	$35	• Send sample for culture (results can show any infection, STIs, PID)
Pelvic ultrasound or pelvic x-ray	76870	$525	• Determine pelvic organ dysfunction, injury and whether ectopic pregnancy • Identify presence of retroverted uterus

ESR, erythrocyte sedimentation rate; PID, pelvic inflammatory disease; PVD, provoked vestibulodynia; STI, sexually transmitted infection; VDRL, Venereal Disease Research Laboratory.

CLINICAL DECISION MAKING

Case Study Analysis

Results of pelvic examination and diagnostic study on a 24-year-old female reveal the diagnosis of insufficient lubrication of vagina. Evidence to support this is based on complaints of painful intercourse with dryness, friction, burning, tearing, and irritation. The absence of itching rules out atrophic vaginitis, pelvic inflammatory disease, sexually transmitted infections, and endometriosis. Further, the absence of pain during menstruation rules out endometriosis. The physical examination reveals abrasions, bruises, and a tear. Diagnostic tests included urine pregnancy test, Pap smear, and pelvic ultrasound and pelvic x-ray. The patient was scheduled to return in 1 week to review the results of diagnostic testing.

> **Diagnosis:** *Vaginal trauma due to insufficient lubrication because of inadequate arousal before sexual intercourse*

Follow-up appointment: The results of the pregnancy test were negative. The Pap smear showed no abnormal cells. The pelvic ultrasound and x-ray were negative for lesions or fractures. To reduce vaginal drying during intercourse it was recommended that the patient use an OTC lubricant.

The patient wanted to discuss actions to take when her spouse drinks and forces intercourse. The patient stated that the spouse can become abusive if sexual intercourse is denied. The patient has never been hospitalized for injuries sustained during episodes of abuse; however, she does have a fear of being injured. Patient did state that the spouse does not threaten or demonstrate harm to their children. Recommended talking with social services to discuss a personal safety plan and to return to the clinic if the symptoms do not subside.

PAINFUL URINATION

> **Case Presentation:** *A 45-year-old female reports to the clinic with a complaint of pain with urination, onset earlier this morning.*

INTRODUCTION TO COMPLAINT

Painful urination, or "dysuria," is generally more common in women than in men, with a reported prevalence of up to 25% of women in the United States.

Dysuria often signifies an infection of the lower urinary tract. The pain is typically described as burning, stinging, or itching. Pain sensation reported at the beginning or during micturition is suggestive of a urethral issue. Pain after micturition is suggestive of a problem in the bladder or prostate area. Some patients will report a history of "suprapubic" pain.

Common conditions that can manifest with dysuria include: urethritis, cystitis, pyelonephritis, urolithiasis, vulvovaginitis, balanitis, and acute prostatitis.

Less common conditions that can manifest with dysuria include: genital herpes, cervicitis, atrophic vaginitis, interstitial cystitis, and epididymitis.

HISTORY OF COMPLAINT
Symptomatology

Ask about the following characteristics of each symptom using open-ended questions:

- Onset (sudden or gradual)
- Chronology
- Current situation (improving or deteriorating)
- Location
- Radiation
- Quality
- Timing (frequency, duration)
- Severity
- Precipitating and aggravating factors
- Relieving factors
- Associated symptoms
- Effects on daily activities
- Previous diagnosis of similar episodes
- Previous treatments
- Efficacy of previous treatments

Directed Questions to Ask

- When did you start having pain with urinating?
- Is the sensation of the pain internal or external?
- Do you have pain in the suprapubic region?
- Do you have a fever?
- Have you had any chills?
- Have you had any nausea and/or vomiting?
- Have you had a sore throat recently?
- Have you changed personal hygiene products recently?
- Have you increased your vaginal penetration sexual activities recently?
- Have you noticed a vaginal discharge?
- Have you noted any changes in the color or odor of your urine?

Assessment: Cardinal Signs and Symptoms

- Urinary frequency
- Urinary urgency
- Pain with urination
- Burning with urination
- Fever
- Flank pain

Medical History: General

- Medical conditions and surgeries
- Allergies (seasonal, as well as others)
- Medication currently used (prescription, birth control pill [BCP], and over the counter [OTC])
- Herbal preparations and traditional therapies

Medical History: Specific to Complaint

- Onset of the pain with urination
- Changes in odor or color of urine
- Blood in urine
- Kidney stones
- Vaginal discharge

PHYSICAL EXAMINATION

Vital Signs

- Temperature
- Pulse
- Respiration
- Oxygen saturation (SpO_2)
- Blood pressure (BP)

General Appearance

- Apparent state of health
- Appearance of comfort or distress
- Color
- State of hydration

Mouth and Throat
- Inspect oral cavity for breath odor, color, lesions; throat and pharynx for color, exudates, tonsillar enlargement

Neck
- Inspect for symmetry, swelling, masses
- Palpate for tenderness, enlargement, lymph node chain

Abdomen
- Inspect for size and contour
- Auscultate for bowel sounds
- Palpate for pain, masses, bladder tenderness, costovertebral (CVA) angle tenderness

Pelvis
- Inspect for external genitalia, condition of vaginal tissues
- Palpate for cystocele, adnexal tenderness

CASE STUDY
History

Directed Question	Response
When did you start having pain with urinating?	*This morning—hit me like a "ton of bricks."*
Is the sensation of the pain internal or external?	*Feels deep inside.*
Do you have pain in the suprapubic region?	*You mean my lower abdomen, no.*
Do you have a fever?	*Don't think so.*
Have you had any chills?	*No.*
Have you had any nausea and/or vomiting?	*No.*
Have you had a sore throat recently?	*No.*
Have you changed personal hygiene products recently?	*No.*
Have you increased your vaginal penetration sexual activities recently?	*No.*
Have you noticed a vaginal discharge?	*No.*
Have you noted any changes in the color or odor of your urine?	*My urine looks "cloudy" to me today.*

Physical Examination Findings
- VITAL SIGNS: temperature 99.7°F; respiratory rate (RR) 18; heart rate (HR) 69, regular; BP 128/78; SpO$_2$ 98%
- GENERAL APPEARANCE: well-developed, healthy-appearing female in acute distress

- MOUTH: no oral lesions
- PHARYNX: no erythema, no tonsillar enlargement, no exudate
- NECK: no palpable lymph node
- ABDOMEN: soft, without mass or organomegaly; palpable tenderness suprapubic region; no CVA tenderness
- PELVIS: no problems noted external genitalia or vaginal tissue; no cystocele or adnexal tenderness

DIFFERENTIAL DIAGNOSIS

Clinical Observations	Lower Urinary Tract Infection	Kidney Infection	Kidney Stone	Vaginal Inflammation/Infection
Urinary frequency	Typical	Typical	Possible	Possible
Pain with urination	Typical	Typical	Typical	Possible
Fever	Not typical	Typical	Not typical but possible	Not typical

DIAGNOSTIC EXAMINATION

Exam	Code	Cost	Results
Urine dipstick	81000	$10	For presence of infection
Complete urinalysis, includes microscopy	81015	$49	For indicators of kidney problems

CLINICAL DECISION MAKING

Case Study Analysis

The advanced practice provider (APP) performs the assessment and physical examination on the patient and finds the following data: history of dysuria onset acutely this morning; urine dip reveals 2+ leukocytes and positive nitrates. The absence of a fever ruled out a kidney infection. The presence of urine leukocytes confirmed a lower urinary tract infection.

Appropriate antibiotic therapy is prescribed by the APP along with recommendations for the patient to take a daily dose of a high-quality probiotic product for the entire duration of antibiotic therapy and the two weeks following completion. It was also recommended that the patient drink 4 to 6 ounces of cranberry juice to help neutralize the urine and reduce burning. A review of toileting hygiene was conducted with the patient and symptoms that indicate the infection is worsening. The patient was reminded to complete the full course of antibiotics and to return for a follow-up appointment and possible further diagnostic testing if symptoms do not subside or worsen.

Diagnosis: Acute cystitis

PALPITATIONS

Case Presentation: A 35-year-old male presents with a complaint of spells of palpitations.

INTRODUCTION TO COMPLAINT

- A noticeably rapid, strong, or irregular heartbeat
- Possible etiologies:
  - Anxiety
  - Stress
  - Exercise
  - Caffeine
  - Nicotine
  - Alcohol/illegal drug use
  - Fever
  - Hormone changes
  - Medications that contain pseudoephedrine
  - Use of asthma inhalers that contain stimulants
  - Atrial fibrillation
  - Supraventricular tachycardia
  - Bradycardia
  - Thyroid diseases
  - Adrenal diseases
  - Sick sinus syndrome
  - Hypertension (HTN)
  - Cardiomyopathy
  - Aortic valve disease
  - Mitral valve prolapse
  - Septic shock
  - Hypoglycemia
  - Myocarditis
  - Alcohol withdrawal
  - Congestive heart failure (CHF)
  - Cardiac tamponade

HISTORY OF COMPLAINT

Symptomatology

Ask about the following characteristics of each symptom using open-ended questions:

- Onset
- Chronology

- Current situation
- Timing and duration
- Quality
- Severity
- Precipitating factors
- Relieving factors
- Associated symptoms
- Effects on daily activities
- Previous diagnosis of similar episodes
- Previous treatments and efficacy of previous treatments
- Family history

Directed Questions to Ask

- When does this tend to occur?
- How quick is the onset?
- How long does it last?
- Does anything seem to make it occur?
- Can you describe the palpitations?
- What makes it worse?
- What makes it better?
- How long have you had the palpitations?
- Does it affect your daily activities?
- Any family history of palpitations or cardiac arrhythmias or cardiac disease?
- Important past medical history (cardiac disease, HTN, adrenal/thyroid disease)?
- Any change in medications (start or stop)?
- Any other symptoms associated with the palpitations?
- Have you been sick recently?

Assessment: Cardinal Signs and Symptoms

General

- Fatigue
- Anxiety
- Sweating

Head, Eyes, Ears, Nose, Throat (HEENT)

- Headache
- Blurred vision

Cardiac

- Chest pain
- Tightening in chest
- HTN
- Hypotension

Respiratory

- Shortness of breath
- Feeling of fullness in lungs

Gastrointestinal/Genitourinary (GI/GU)

- Nausea
- Vomiting
- Epigastric pain

Musculoskeletal
- Weakness
- Tremor
- Flank pain

Neurologic
- Confusion
- Loss of consciousness
- Lightheadedness
- Fainting
- Dizziness

Medical History

- No current medical history till recently when the patient was admitted to the hospital 4 days ago after he experienced prolonged palpitations with extreme headache, confusion, and nausea/vomiting.
- Upon arrival to the hospital, the patient's blood pressure (BP) = 210/120, with no previous hypertensive issues.
- EKG was negative for ST elevation MI (STEMI) and was consistent with normal sinus rhythm (NSR).
- The patient was given 10 mg of labetalol and his BP was responsive with normalization to 130/80.
- Echocardiogram was negative for valvular disease or blockages, with ejection fraction (EF) = 55% to 60%.
- Last night the patient complained of palpitations with no sustained changes in heart rate/rhythm.
- Patient became diaphoretic with complaints of headache.
- During palpitations, the patient's pressure was noted to increase to 190/100.
- The patient was given 10 mg labetalol but BP was not responsive.

Surgeries
- Tonsillectomy
- Appendectomy

Allergies
- Penicillin

Medication
- No current medications

Family History
- Father: HTN, recently diagnosed with adrenal tumor
- Mother: coronary artery disease (CAD) and HTN

Social History
- Nonsmoker
- No drug/alcohol
- Married and currently working in the construction industry

Health Maintenance
- Received flu shot this year and is up to date on childhood vaccinations

PHYSICAL EXAMINATION
Vital Signs

- Temperature
- Pulse
- Respiration
- Oxygen saturation (SpO_2)
- BP

General Appearance

- State of health
- Any distress

HEENT
- Vision assessment
- Palpitation of neck (thyroid)

Cardiac
- Auscultate heart sounds
- Assess pulses

Respiratory
- Auscultate breath sounds

GI/GU
- Auscultate/percuss abdomen

Musculoskeletal
- Assess muscle strength (grips, gait, etc.)
- Assess flank pain

Neurologic
- Neurologic assessment (reflexes, cranial nerves)

Psychology
- Changes in mood

CASE STUDY
History

Directed Question	Response
When does this tend to occur?	*I experienced these palpitations a couple times a month over the past 3 months.*
How quick is the onset of the palpitations?	*Sudden onset.*
How long do the palpitations last?	*At first, they lasted a few seconds, but over the past month the palpitations have lasted longer than a minute.*
What aggravates it?	*When I get nervous or anxious sometimes, but I've noticed the palpitations start without any type of distress or movement.*

Directed Question	Response
What alleviates it?	*Usually it stops on its own.*
Does it affect your daily activities?	*Yes, recently it takes my breath away and I get dizzy and nauseous.*
Does it cause you pain? If so, rate your pain on a scale of 0 to 10.	*It doesn't cause me any pain, I just feel uncomfortable and sort of scared.*
Have you ever been diagnosed with palpitations? Any family history of palpitations?	*My father experienced palpitations but never got it treated.*
Important past medical history?	*No major past medical history that would cause the palpitations.*
What medication changes have you made recently (start or stop)?	*No changes in medication.*
Any other symptoms associated with the palpitations?	*Headache, nausea, and vomiting and sometimes I get very sweaty.*

Physical Examination Findings

- VITAL SIGNS: temperature 98.5°F; respiratory rate (RR) 15; heart rate (HR) 95, regular; BP 160/95
- GENERAL APPEARANCE: healthy, well-developed young male in no obvious distress
- EYES: pupils equal, round, and reactive to light and accommodation (PERRLA); extra ocular movements intact
- NECK: no enlarged lymph nodes palpable; neck is supple; thyroid is not enlarged
- CHEST/CARDIOVASCULAR: lung sounds are clear in all fields; regular rate and rhythm (RRR); heart S1, S2 no murmur, gallop, or rub
- GASTROINTESTINAL/GENITOURINARY: bowel sounds in all four quadrants, GU assessment within normal limits (WNL)
- MUSCULOSKELETAL: no weakness noted, left-sided costovertebral (CVA) tenderness noted
- NEUROLOGIC: cranial nerves intact, reflexes +2

DIFFERENTIAL DIAGNOSIS

Clinical Observations	Hyperthyroidism	Anxiety	Pheochromocytoma
Onset	Gradual	Gradual/sudden	Sudden
Chest pain	No	Yes/No	Yes/No
N/V	No	Yes/No	Yes
Confusion	No	Yes/No	Yes
Diaphoresis	Yes/No	Yes/No	Yes

(continued)

Clinical Observations	Hyperthyroidism	Anxiety	Pheochromocytoma
Paroxysmal hypertension	No	No	Yes
Flank pain	No	No	Yes/No
Headache	No	Yes/No	Yes

N/V, nausea and vomiting.

DIAGNOSTIC EXAMINATION

Exam	Code	Cost	Results
CBC without differential	D64.9	$25–$100	**CBC** **WBC count** • High WBC count can be a sign of infection (can be bacterial or viral) • WBC is also increased in certain types of leukemia • Low white counts can be a sign of bone marrow diseases, possible HIV infection, or an enlarged spleen **Hgb and Hct** • Hgb is the amount of oxygen-carrying protein contained within the red blood cells • Hct is the percentage of the blood volume occupied by red blood cells • Low Hgb and Hct suggest an anemia • Anemia can be due to nutritional deficiencies, blood loss, destruction of blood cells internally, or failure to produce blood in the bone marrow **PLT** • This is the number of cells that collect in blood vessels and prevent bleeding • High values can occur with bleeding • Low values can occur with anticoagulant use or forms of leukemia
Complete metabolic panel	I10	$28–$46	A comprehensive metabolic panel is a group of blood tests. They provide an overall picture of the body's chemical balance and metabolism **Normal levels** • Albumin: 3.4–5.4 g/dL • Alkaline phosphatase: 44–147 IU/L • ALT: 10–40 IU/L • AST: 10–34 IU/L • BUN: 6–20 mg/dL • Calcium: 8.5–10.2 mg/dL • Chloride: 96–106 mEq/L • CO_2: 23–29 mEq/L • Creatinine: 0.6–1.3 mg/dL • Glucose: 70–100 mg/dL

(*continued*)

Exam	Code	Cost	Results
			• Potassium: 3.5–5.0 mEq/L • Sodium: 135–145 mEq/L • Total bilirubin: 0.3–1.9 mg/dL • Total protein: 6.0–8.3 g/dL **Decreased potassium:** suggests dehydration **Elevated sodium:** suggests dehydration **Elevated BUN/creatinine:** suggests kidney damage/disease **Elevated ALT/AST:** suggests liver damage/disease
CT of abdomen	R93.5	$1,200	CT images of internal organs, bones, soft tissue, and blood vessels typically provide greater detail than traditional x-rays, particularly of soft tissues and blood vessels CT scanning of the abdomen is typically used to detect: • Infections • Inflammatory bowel disease • cancers of the liver, kidneys, pancreas, and bladder • Trauma
MRI	B030ZZZ	$600–$1,550	MRI of the body uses a powerful magnetic field, radio waves, and a computer to produce detailed pictures of the inside of your body Unlike conventional x-ray examinations and CT scans, MRI does not utilize ionizing radiation. Instead, radio waves redirect alignment of hydrogen atoms that naturally exist within the body while you are in the scanner without causing any chemical changes in the tissues. As the hydrogen atoms return to their usual alignment, they emit energy that varies according to the type of body tissue from which they come. The magnetic resonance scanner captures this energy and creates a picture of the tissues scanned based on this information **Abdominal MRI** Assesses: • Blood flow in the abdomen • Blood vessels in the abdomen • The cause of abdominal pain or swelling • The cause of abnormal blood test results, such as liver or kidney problems • Lymph nodes in the abdomen • Masses in the liver, kidneys, adrenals, pancreas, or spleen
Free metanephrine level	R82.5	$100 or greater	The plasma free metanephrines test is used to help diagnose or rule out the presence of a rare tumor called a pheochromocytoma or a paraganglioma that releases excess metanephrines. Testing also may be used when a tumor has been treated or removed to monitor for recurrence. Normal: 12–60 pg/mL

(*continued*)

Exam	Code	Cost	Results
24-hour CATU	R791.9	$350 or greater	CATU is used to diagnose certain diseases that increase catecholamine production. Levels can fluctuate, so testing generally is not recommended if you are not showing symptoms. The chance of a false positive test is high.
			Epinephrine: 16 years or older = 0.0–20.0 mcg/24 hours
			Norepinephrine: 10 years or older = 15–80 mcg/24 hours
			Dopamine: 4 years or older = 65–400 mcg/24 hours

ALT, alanine amino transferase; AST, aspartate amino transferase; BUN, blood urea nitrogen; CATU, catecholamine urine testing; CBC, complete blood count; Hct, hematocrit; Hgb, hemoglobin; PLT, platelet count; WBC, white blood cell.

CLINICAL DECISION MAKING

Case Study Analysis

- An abdominal/pelvic CT was performed and a small mass was noted on the left adrenal gland.
- MRI was also performed, which confirmed adrenal mass.
- Complete blood count (CBC) and basic metabolic panel (BMP) were unremarkable.

The sudden onset and associated HTN ruled out hyperthyroidism and anxiety as possible causes. The presence of a headache ruled out the possibility of hyperthyroidism. Since his father never sought treatment for a similar symptom, a genetic association is unknown.

After adrenal mass was found, the following tests were performed:

- Free metanephrine serum test: 105 pg/mL (high)
- 24-hour urine (with catecholamine testing)
  - Epinephrine: 32 mcg/24 hours (high)
  - Dopamine: 435 mcg/24 hours (high)
  - Norepinephrine: 95 mcg/24 hours (high)

Diagnosis: Pheochromocytoma

The patient was referred to a renal specialist to discuss further treatment including medication and surgery. Additional follow-up will be through the renal clinic.

PANIC EPISODES

Case Presentation: *A 20-year-old female reports to the clinic seeking assistance for her recent onset of panic episodes.*

INTRODUCTION TO COMPLAINT

A panic episode is characterized by a sudden onset of an intense fear when there is no real danger or apparent cause. This fear triggers severe physical symptoms and cause a great deal of "fright" for the person having the episode.

It is not uncommon for an individual to experience a panic "episode" a few times in their lifetime. For individuals who have recurrent episodes over a long period of time, they likely have a condition called panic disorder. Common symptoms experienced with a panic episode include:

- Sense of impending doom or death
- Pounding rapid heart rate (HR) and/or chest pain
- Tightness in the throat and/or shortness of breath
- Shaking/trembling
- Sweating, chills, hot flashes
- Nausea and/or abdominal cramping
- Faintness, lightheadedness or dizziness

Panic episodes often manifest in the late teens or early adulthood, and are experienced by females more than males.

HISTORY OF COMPLAINT

Symptomatology

Ask about the following characteristics of each symptom using open-ended questions:

- Onset (sudden or gradual)
- Chronology
- Current situation (improving or deteriorating)
- Location
- Radiation
- Quality
- Timing (frequency, duration)
- Severity
- Precipitating and aggravating factors
- Relieving factors
- Associated symptoms

- Effects on daily activities
- Previous diagnosis of similar episodes
- Previous treatments
- Efficacy of previous treatments

Directed Questions to Ask

- When did you first experience a panic episode?
- How often are you having panic episodes?
- How long do the panic episodes typically last?
- Have you had any major traumatic events (loss of loved one, abuse, accident, injury, etc.)?
- Have you had major life changes recently?
- Do you smoke?
- Do you drink alcohol?
- Do you use recreational drugs?
- Do you have any known medical problems?

Assessment: Cardinal Signs and Symptoms

- Intense fear, feeling of doom or death
- Sensation of rapid, pounding heart rate and/or chest pain
- Throat tightness and/or shortness of breath
- Shaking/trembling

Medical History: General

- Medical conditions and surgeries
- Allergies (seasonal, as well as others)
  Medication currently used (prescription, birth control pill [BCP], and over the counter [OTC])
- Herbal preparations and traditional therapies

Medical History: Specific to Complaint

- Onset of panic episodes
- Frequency of panic episodes
- Major trauma(s)
- Addictive habits

PHYSICAL EXAMINATION
Vital Signs

- Temperature
- Pulse
- Respiration
- Oxygen saturation (SpO_2)
- Blood pressure (BP)

General Appearance

- Apparent state of health
- Appearance of comfort or distress

- Color
- State of hydration

Neck
- Inspect for symmetry, swelling, masses
- Palpate for tenderness, thyroid enlargement, lymph node chain

Cardiovascular
- Inspect for capillary refill time
- Auscultate for heart sounds, check for murmurs, gallops, rubs
- Palpate for peripheral pulses

Respiratory
- Auscultate lungs for crackles, and wheezing

Abdomen
- Inspect for contour
- Auscultate for bowel sounds
- Palpate for pain, masses, organomegaly

Neurologic
- Orientation status
- Pupil reflexes/responses
- Test cranial nerves (CNs) II to XII
- Test fine and gross motor movements
- Test deep tendon reflexes (DTRs)

CASE STUDY

History

Directed Question	Response
When did you first experience a panic episode?	*About 2 months ago.*
How often are you having panic episodes?	*At first once every couple weeks but now maybe once or twice a week.*
How long do the panic episodes typically last?	*About 10 minutes.*
Have you had any major traumatic events (loss of loved one, abuse, accident, injury, etc.)?	*Umh, yes . . . about 3 months ago I ended an abusive relationship.*
Have you had major life changes recently?	*Had been living with my boyfriend who was abusive. Had to move back in with my parents.*
Do you smoke?	*No.*
Do you drink alcohol?	*Occasional wine.*
Do you use recreational drugs?	*No.*
Do you have any known medical problems?	*No.*

Physical Examination Findings

- VITAL SIGNS: temperature 96.4°F; respiratory rate (RR) 20; heart rate (HR) 96, regular; BP 111/60; SpO$_2$ 98%
- GENERAL APPEARANCE: well-developed, healthy female who is mildly anxious
- NECK: no masses or asymmetry noted, no thyromegaly, thyroid nontender without nodules or cysts
- CARDIOVASCULAR: normal rate/rhythm without murmur or gallop
- RESPIRATORY: lungs clear
- ABDOMEN: soft, nontender without mass or organomegaly
- NEUROLOGIC: alert and oriented four times, pupils equal, round, and reactive to light and accommodation (PERRLA), CNs II to XII grossly intact, DTRs within normal limits (WNL), extremity strength WNL, sensory and motor function intact

DIFFERENTIAL DIAGNOSIS

Clinical Observations	Panic Episode	Panic Disorder
Sudden onset	Yes	Yes/No
Frequency of panic experience	Infrequent, episodic	Frequent, negatively impacts life activities
History of trauma	Yes/No	Yes/No, not uncommon

DIAGNOSTIC EXAMINATION

Exam	Code	Cost	Results
TSH	84443	$49	Evaluates TSH levels; hyperthyroidism can present with many of the same symptoms observed in "panic episodes"
Comprehensive metabolic panel	80053	$49	For evaluation of metabolic problem contributors for the symptom profile

TSH, thyroid-stimulating hormone.

CLINICAL DECISION MAKING

Case Study Analysis

The advanced practice provider (APP) performs the assessment and physical examination on the patient and finds the following data: recent history of the end of an abusive relationship, no abnormal physical exam findings. Since the episodes are not impacting activities of daily living, a panic disorder can be ruled out. Thyroid-stimulating hormone (TSH) level was within normal limits. Results from the complete metabolic panel (CMP) were all within normal limits. Based upon these findings, the patient most likely is experiencing panic episodes.

The APP educates the patient on the use of Emotional Freedom Technique (EFT) at the first sign of increasing anxiety or onset of panic sensations. EFT is a form of counseling intervention that draws on various theories of alternative medicine, including acupuncture, neuro-linguistic programming, energy medicine, and Thought Field Therapy (TFT). The patient is counseled to return for a follow-up examination in 2 weeks. Further consultation with a mental health professional may be required if episodes continue.

Diagnosis: *Panic episodes, triggered by emotional trauma*

PELVIC PAIN

Case Presentation: A 43-year-old female reports with a complaint of pain in pelvic region.

INTRODUCTION TO COMPLAINT

Pelvic pain is the terminology given to describe the pain that is typically experienced in the lowest part of the abdomen, the lower back region, and the pelvis. The pain may radiate into the thighs.

The pain may have an acute, self-limiting presentation or it may be experienced chronically (intermittent or constant pain over at least a 6-month period of time).

Pelvic pain can arise from problems in the reproductive system, the urinary system, the digestive system, or the musculoskeletal system. Identified mediators of pelvic pain include:

- Endometriosis
- Pelvic inflammatory disease (PID)
- Uterine fibroids
- Irritable bowel syndrome (IBS)
- Interstitial cystitis
- Ovarian remnant (after total hysterectomy with bilateral salpingectomy with oophorectomy)
- Pelvic congestion syndrome
- Tension in the pelvic floor muscles
- Nerve entrapment
- Prostatitis or epididymitis in the male patient
- Psychological factors

Chronic pelvic pain is a complex issue. Chronic pelvic pain can be mediated by a single factor or multiple factors. This makes it challenging to identify the etiology of the condition.

HISTORY OF COMPLAINT

Symptomatology

Ask about the following characteristics of each symptom using open-ended questions:

- Onset (sudden or gradual)
- Chronology
- Current situation (improving or deteriorating)
- Location
- Radiation

- Quality
- Timing (frequency, duration)
- Severity
- Precipitating and aggravating factors
- Relieving factors
- Associated symptoms
- Effects on daily activities
- Previous diagnosis of similar episodes
- Previous treatments
- Efficacy of previous treatments

Directed Questions to Ask

- When did you first notice the pain?
- Where are you feeling the pain?
- What is the intensity of the pain?
- Is the pain intermittent or constant?
- Can you describe the type of pain (dull/sharp, aching/throbbing, stabbing/burning, etc.)?
- Can you identify any possible cause of the pain?
- Does anything alleviate or exacerbate the pain?
- When was your last menstrual period? Or have you had a hysterectomy?
- Do you have severe pain with your periods?
- Do you have uterine fibroids?
- Do you have IBS? Tell me about your daily bowel activity.
- Do you have interstitial cystitis? Tell me about your daily urinary activity.
- Do you have sexual intercourse? If yes, do you have one or more sexual partners?
- Have you ever had a sexually transmitted disease (STD)?
- Are you experiencing any psychological or emotional stress?

Assessment: Cardinal Signs and Symptoms

- Pain in the lower abdomen
- Pain in the low back
- Pain in the pelvic region
- Pain in the upper thighs

Medical History: General

- Medical conditions and surgeries
- Allergies (seasonal as well as others)
- Medication currently used (prescription, birth control pill [BCP], and over the counter [OTC])
- Herbal preparations and traditional therapies

Medical History: Specific to Complaint

- Endometriosis
- IBS
- STD
- Interstitial cystitis
- Uterine fibroids

PHYSICAL EXAMINATION

Vital Signs

- Temperature
- Pulse
- Respiration
- Oxygen saturation (SpO_2)
- Blood pressure (BP)

General Appearance

- Apparent state of health
- Appearance of comfort or distress
- Color
- State of hydration

Abdomen

- Inspect for size and contour
- Auscultate for bowel sounds
- Palpate for pain, masses, bladder tenderness

Pelvis

- Inspect external genitalia, condition of vaginal tissues, appearance of cervix
- Palpate for cervical motion tenderness, adnexal tenderness, size/shape/position of uterus, height of anterior superior iliac crests

CASE STUDY

History

Directed Question	Response
When did you first notice the pain?	A few weeks ago.
Where are you feeling the pain?	In my pelvic area, groin area, and sometimes in my upper thighs.
What is the intensity of the pain?	Anywhere from a 2/10 to a 7/10.
Is the pain intermittent or constant?	Intermittent.
Can you describe the type of pain (dull/sharp, aching/throbbing, stabbing/burning, etc.)?	It is sort of throbbing.
Can you identify any possible cause of the pain?	No.
Does anything alleviate or exacerbate the pain?	I take ibuprofen when it gets bad and that helps.
When was your last menstrual period? Or have you had a hysterectomy?	My last period was about 2 weeks ago.
Do you have severe pain with your periods?	I didn't use to but for the past several months the pain can get really bad.

Directed Question	*Response*
Do you have uterine fibroids?	*No.*
Do you have IBS? Tell me about your daily bowel activity.	*No. I have a couple bowel movements a day.*
Do you have interstitial cystitis? Tell me about your daily urinary activity.	*No. I pee about three to four times a day.*
Do you have sexual intercourse? If yes, do you have one or more sexual partners?	*I do. I am in a stable relationship with one sexual partner right now.*
Have you ever had a sexually transmitted disease?	*No.*
Are you experiencing any psychological or emotional stress?	*No.*

IBS, irritable bowel syndrome.

Physical Examination Findings

- VITAL SIGNS: temperature 98.1°F; respiratory rate (RR) 16; heart rate (HR) 62, regular; BP 119/69; SpO$_2$ 99%
- GENERAL APPEARANCE: well-developed, healthy-appearing female in no acute distress
- ABDOMEN: soft, nontender without mass or organomegaly
- PELVIS: no cervical motion tenderness, uterus fundus palpable above the pubis symphysis; anterior superior iliac crests are at the same height

DIFFERENTIAL DIAGNOSIS

Clinical Observations	Endometriosis	Uterine Fibroids	PID	Interstitial Cystitis	IBS
Pelvic pain	Yes/No	Yes/No	Yes/No	Yes/No	Yes/No
Changes in menstrual cycle	Yes	Yes	Yes/No	Yes/No	No

IBS, irritable bowel syndrome; PID, pelvic inflammatory disease.

DIAGNOSTIC EXAMINATION

Exam	Code	Cost	Results
Complete blood count	85025	$49	To see if there is evidence of an infectious process
Chlamydia, DNA urine	87491	$89	To evaluate if STD is present
Gonorrhea, DNA urine	87591	$89	To evaluate if STD is present

(continued)

Exam	Code	Cost	Results
Transvaginal ultrasound	76830	$525 average	To evaluate uterus for presence of fibroid
MRI of abdomen and pelvis	74177	Range $1,000–$5,000	To evaluate gastrointestinal system and to diagnose adenomyosis

STD, sexually transmitted disease.

CLINICAL DECISION MAKING

Case Study Analysis

The advanced practice provider performs the assessment and physical examination on the patient and finds the following data: history of changes in menstrual pain pattern and on examination an enlarged uterus. Since the patient's last menstrual period was 2 weeks earlier, pregnancy as a cause for uterine enlargement is unlikely. Since an enlarged uterus is not associated with endometriosis, PID, IBS, or interstitial cystitis, additional diagnostic testing will focus on uterine fibroids as a cause.

A transvaginal ultrasound is prescribed for further evaluation. In addition, the patient will have testing for sexually transmitted infections (STIs). Depending on the results, an MRI of the abdomen and pelvis may be required.

A follow-up appointment is made for 1 week at which time the results of the ultrasound and laboratory tests will be reviewed.

> ***Diagnosis:*** *Enlarged uterus, possible uterine fibroids*

RECTAL BLEEDING

Case Presentation: A 60-year-old male presents with complaints of intermittent rectal bleeding over the past 2 weeks.

INTRODUCTION TO COMPLAINT

- Hematochezia, also known as rectal bleeding, is characterized by the passage of bright red blood from the rectum
- It may be attributed to a number of conditions such as hemorrhoids, anal fissures, diverticular disease, inflammatory bowel disease (irritable bowel syndrome [IBS], Crohn's, or ulcerative colitis), and colorectal cancer
- Other causes include upper gastrointestinal (GI) bleeding, radiation proctitis, anal ulcer, or angiodysplasia
- Originates from anal lesions or other benign colorectal conditions; however, rectal bleeding may be a symptom of colorectal cancer or premalignant polyps within the colon
- Rectal bleeding is common in American adults with as high as 19% of patients
- Colon cancer is the third leading cause of cancer-related deaths within the United States
- Colorectal cancer screening via colonoscopy is recommended for all adults 40 years and older
- Asymptomatic colonoscopy screening is the most cost-effective way to detect, diagnosis, and begin early treatment of colorectal disease in adults older than 40 years

HISTORY OF COMPLAINT

Symptomatology

Ask about the following characteristics of each symptom using open-ended questions:

- Onset
- Chronology
- Current situation
- Timing (frequency, duration)
- Severity
- Precipitating/aggravating factors
- Alleviating factors
- Associated symptoms
- Effects on daily activities
- Previous diagnosis of similar episodes
- Previous treatments and their effectiveness in symptom relief

Directed Questions to Ask

- Describe how you feel when it happens, do you feel pain with the bleeding?
- How long does the bleeding last?
- Does the bleeding occur after eating certain foods?
- Have you had any injuries or trauma to your belly or back recently?
- Have you noticed any changes in your overall health since the bleeding started, can you describe them?
- Have you experienced any changes in the amount of food you eat or how often you go to the bathroom?
- How frequently does it happen?
- Can you describe any changes in your energy?
- When was your last colonoscopy? Did they find any issues?
- Describe how your daily routine has changed with the bleeding? Are you nauseous or experiencing diarrhea or any fever?
- Do you feel like you are able to complete a bowel movement or do you feel like you still have to go sometimes?

Assessment: Cardinal Signs and Symptoms

General

- Fatigue
- Weakness, or malaise

Cardiac

- May experience tachycardia with fever or arrhythmias with severe blood loss

GI

- Nausea
- Vomiting
- Diarrhea
- Constipation
- Loss of appetite

Respiratory

- Shortness of breath (SOB) or tachypnea with severe blood loss

Musculoskeletal

- Pallor
- Generalized weakness

Genitourinary (GU)

- Hemorrhoids
- Changes in bowel or bladder continence

Medical History

- Medical conditions: hyperlipidemia, diabetes mellitus type 2, season allergies
- Surgical history: right femoral stent, 2009; three cardiac stents, 2010
- Patient denies history of heart attack although he has had multiple cardiac stents, denies stroke, personal or family history of cancer
- Psychiatric: denies depression, anxiety, suicidal ideation, or domestic violence
- Patient has never had a colonoscopy, sees his provider only when he is sick at the Veterans Administration clinic
- Medications: metformin 1,000 mg twice a day with meals, clopidogrel 75 mg daily, aspirin 81 mg daily, simvastatin 40 mg HS, loratadine 10 mg daily as needed for allergies

- Allergies: no known drug allergies (NKDA)
- Patient denies illicit drugs, smokes one pack per day, drinks three to six beers every weekend
- Diet/exercise: He is a long-distance truck driver and leads a sedentary lifestyle. He exercises sporadically and infrequently, continues to eat fast food while he is on a contract but tries to eat fresh fruits and a salad every day.

PHYSICAL EXAMINATION

Vital Signs

- Temperature
- Blood pressure
- Respiration
- Oxygen saturation at room temperature

General Appearance

- Patient is well-groomed
- Age-appropriate in appearance
- No apparent distress

Cardiovascular

- S1, S2
- Denies chest pain, SOB, or heartburn symptoms

Gastrointestinal

- Denies nausea, vomiting, complains of constipation and straining to have bowel movement

Genitourinary

- No issues with incontinence

Musculoskeletal

- Normal, active range of motion (ROM) in all extremities, no weakness

Skin

- Appropriate for ethnicity, no pallor or cyanosis

CASE STUDY

History

Directed Question	Response
Describe how you feel when it happens, do you feel pain with the bleeding?	I have a lot of cramping sometimes after I eat, I just think some foods don't agree with me. I feel a lot of pressure when I'm trying to have a bowel movement, and I do have pain while straining. I've been having a lot of lower belly pain on my left side for the past few weeks. Then I notice blood on the toilet paper when I'm finished.
How long does the bleeding last?	It usually lasts for a few hours, but it's just a few spots of blood on my underwear after I'm finished wiping.

Directed Question	*Response*
Does the bleeding occur after eating certain foods?	*I notice I don't bleed as much when I'm consistently eating my salads. But I definitely have some more cramping and bleeding after I eat popcorn or trail mix.*
Describe any injuries or trauma to your belly or back recently.	*I haven't had any injuries but I do have a sore low back after sitting in my truck for hours and hours at a time.*
Have you noticed any changes in your overall health since the bleeding started, can you describe them?	*Just that constipation and cramping, but I still have a good appetite and I'm not nauseous. I have been trying to eat better and stick to good heart foods like veggies, trail mix, fruit, and low-salt popcorn.*
Have you experienced any changes in the amount of food you eat or how often you go to the bathroom?	*No, I notice that I'm hungrier if I'm sticking to my heart healthy diet.*
How frequently does it happen?	*I have noticed the blood with every bowel movement in these past few weeks, but before that I didn't ever notice blood on the toilet paper.*
Can you describe any changes in your energy?	*I feel like I have less energy the past few days, but I thought that was because I wasn't sleeping well and have been putting in some extra hours at work.*
When was your last colonoscopy? Did they find any issues?	*I have never had a colonoscopy, I didn't want to go through that if I didn't need to. Besides, that's for people who have stomach problems.*
Describe how your daily routine has changed with the bleeding? Are you nauseous or experiencing diarrhea or fevers?	*I have been feeling a little piqued in the past week, but like I said I've been working a lot. I have this bellyache in my lower belly that just won't go away no matter how many TUMS I take.*
Do you feel like you are able to complete a bowel movement or do you feel like you still have to go sometimes?	*Actually, I feel like I strain a lot because I don't always feel like I'm finished. But eventually the sensation either passes or I have to get on with my day so I just tell myself I'll try again later.*

PHYSICAL EXAMINATION FINDINGS

- VITAL SIGNS: temperature 100°F; RR 16; HR 90/regular; blood pressure 120/80
- GENERAL APPEARANCE: well-developed, healthy appearing male with apparent acute distress.

- EYES: no injection; anicteric; PERRLA; extra ocular movements intact
- NOSE: nares are patient; no edema or exudate of turbinates
- MOUTH: no oral lesions; teeth and gums in good repair
- PHARYNX: tonsils are moderately enlarged, red with pockets of white exudate
- NECK: Tonsillar nodes are 1.5 cm, round, mobile, tender bilaterally; no other cervical nodes palpable; neck is supple; thyroid is not enlarged
- CHEST: Lungs are clear in all fields; heart S1 S2 no murmur, gallop, or rub
- ABDOMEN: soft, nontender without mass or organomegaly
- SKIN: no rashes
- EXTREMITIES: no joint pain or swelling

DIFFERENTIAL DIAGNOSIS

Clinical Observations	GI Bleed	Hemorrhoids	Diverticulitis	Colorectal Cancer	Inflammatory Bowel Disease (IBS, Crohn's, UC)
Onset	Sudden	Gradual	Intermittent with irritating foods	Gradual	Gradual
Pain	Yes/No	Yes	Yes	Yes/No	Yes/No
Duration	Acute	Chronic	Intermittent	Until treatment succeeds	Chronic
Fatigue	Yes/No	No	No	Yes/No	No
Weight changes	Yes/No	No	Yes	Yes/No	Yes
Constipation/ diarrhea	No	No	Yes	Yes/No	Yes
Nausea	Varies	No	No	Varies	Varies
Fever	Yes/No	None	Yes/No	Yes	None

GI, gastrointestinal; IBS, irritable bowel syndrome; UC, ulcerative colitis.

DIAGNOSTIC EXAMINATION

Exam	Code	Cost	Results
CMP	I10	$28	Normal results: Glucose 70–99 mg/dL (fasting), 70–125 mg/dL (nonfasting) Sodium 136–144 mEq/L Potassium 3.7–5.2 mEq/L Chloride 96–106 mmol/L CO_2 20–29 mmol/L

(continued)

Exam	Code	Cost	Results
			BUN 7–20 mg/dL Creatinine 0.8–1.4 mg/dL BUN/creatinine ratio 10:1–20:1 Calcium 8.5–10.9 mg/dL Magnesium 1.8–2.6 mEq/L Protein 6.3–7.9 g/dL Albumin 3.9–5.0 d/dL Globulin 2.0–3.5 g/dL Albumin/globulin ratio 1.7–2.2 Bilirubin 0.3–1.9 mg/dL ALP 44–147 IU/L ALT 8–37 IU/L AST 10–34 IU/L Glomerular filtration rate 90–120 mL/min/1.73 m^2 Abnormal results: values outside of normal range can be indications of dehydration, kidney/liver dysfunction, malnutrition, or malignant disease process
CBC	R68.69	$29	Measures the different blood cell components and assists in diagnosis of nutrient/oxygen delivery dysfunction, infective process, and further blood cell production Hemoglobin is responsible for delivering oxygen to cells (normal male 13.5–17.5 g/dL). A decrease in this number is indicative of anemia and can result in impaired oxygen delivery to tissues Hematocrit is the total percentage of blood composed of red blood cells (normal female 40%–55%). A decrease in this number can indicate anemia or dilution of blood with fluid WBCs attach themselves to foreign cells, infected tissues and wounds to promote phagocytosis and removal of dangerous products. A decrease in WBCs can be a sign of bone marrow damage, dysfunctional cell production, or leukemia; an elevated WBC count is a sign of an active infection process within the body Normal 5,000–10,000/mL Platelets are the cells that aid in clotting, whether it be helpful (tissue damage and cuts) or malignant (thrombi formation). Decreased platelets indicate the potential to have uncontrolled bleeding in response to an assault, while increased can indicate the patient is at increased risk for DVT/PE/clots. Normal 150k–400k/mL
Colonoscopy	V76.51	$2,006	Normal: normal colon mucosa and tissue without polyps, ulceration, outpouching Abnormal: polyps, diverticulosis (outpouching of mucosa), ulcers, hemorrhoids, chronic inflammatory changes, carcinomas, hemorrhaging
Abdominal CT	R93.5	$411	Normal: organs presenting without inflammatory process, normal size/structure, lack of tortuous vasculature, no evidence of free air in peritoneal cavity, no fistula or growths on organs Abnormal: noted fistula, wall thickening on structures or organs, free air in abdominal cavity, expanding bowel loops with gas or excessive stool impaction, masses or irregular growth

ALP, alkaline phosphatase; ALT, alanine amino transferase; AST, aspartate amino transferase; BUN, blood urea nitrogen; CBC, complete blood count; CMP, complete metabolic panel; DVT, deep vein thrombosis; PE, pulmonary embolism; WBC, white blood cell.

CLINICAL DECISION MAKING
Case Study Analysis

After physical assessment and detailed history of onset, the patient had blood work (complete metabolic panel [CMP], complete blood count [CBC]), which revealed a hemoglobin of 10.5 mL and elevated white blood cells (WBCs) at 14.5×10^9/L. A digital rectal exam was performed, which indicated internal hemorrhoids. The patient presented with a low-grade fever, lower left quadrant tenderness, and some symptomatic abdominal cramping after foods, known to exacerbate diverticulitis, such as popcorn and seeds.

The patient was sent for a colonoscopy as he has never had one and currently presents with hematochezia. His colonoscopy revealed diverticulitis in his sigmoid colon with diffuse areas of inflammation and irritation. No evidence of bleeding, polyps, or diverticulosis was noted on colonoscopy beyond the colon. Internal hemorrhoids were visualized on colonoscopy with moderate irritation and friable tissue. It is recommended to confirm diagnosis with abdominal CT when inflammation is found on colonoscopy. The colonoscopy ruled out colorectal cancer as a cause for the rectal bleeding. The patient's overall symptoms did not support the diagnosis of GI bleed or inflammatory bowel disease.

> **Diagnosis:** *Diverticulitis with internal hemorrhoids*

- Common symptoms of diverticulitis are left lower abdominal pain, cramping, constipation, and blood in stool. It is similar to inflammatory bowel disease and requires specific diagnosis for appropriate treatment.
- Diverticulitis is a diagnosis of exclusion based on physical assessment and medical history. Colonoscopy is the diagnostic tool of choice, and if an inflammatory process is found then confirmation with abdominal CT with contrast is recommended to determine extent of tissue involvement and to rule out bowel perforation.
- Classic signs on abdominal CT confirming diverticulitis are pericolic fat infiltration, thickened fascia, muscular hypertrophy, and the focal thickening of the colonic wall with arrowhead shaped lumen pointed to the inflamed diverticula ("arrowhead sign").
- Blood work usually presents with elevated WBCs, immature band formation, and a left shift in patients with an active infectious process.
- Studies have found an inverse relationship in patient's intake of insoluble fiber and incidence of disease.
- Mayo Clinic and American Academy of Family Physicians recommend hospitalization and inpatient treatment of diverticulitis for patients with significant infectious process, who are unable to tolerate oral intake, are older than 85 years old, or have potentially complicating comorbidities.
- This patient, having the ability to tolerate oral intake was prescribed amoxicillin–clavulanate 875/125 mg orally twice daily for 7 days. He was advised to take Tylenol 500 mg every 6 hours as needed for pain. Additionally, he was prescribed a clear liquid diet for 48 hours to allow for bowel rest, after which he can progress to a full liquid diet for the next 24 hours and resume regular foods thereafter, provided his abdominal pain has resolved. He was provided education on which foods to avoid (nuts, pumpkin seeds, popcorn, sunflower seeds, and sesame seeds) and given a booklet with high-fiber diet information. He was advised to consume 20 to 35 g of fiber a day and avoid fast foods. Instructions were provided for the patient to follow up with his family physician within 2 weeks or sooner if his symptoms persist or worsen.

RECTAL PAIN

Case Presentation: A 38-year-old Caucasian female presents to the acute care office with complaints of rectal pain (proctalgia).

INTRODUCTION TO COMPLAINT

- Pain is subjective and needs to be assessed by asking about the severity of the pain
- Could be from hemorrhoids, which would present as a discomfort type of pain with fullness
- Could be from anal fissures, which would present as severe, tearing pain followed by throbbing discomfort after a bowel movement
- Could be from rectal cancer, which would present similar to hemorrhoids
- Could be from proctitis, which would present as discomfort type pain with tenesmus
- Could be from a sexually transmitted disease (STD), which would present as perianal discomfort with discharge
- Could be from an abscess, which would present with a throbbing, continuous pain

HISTORY OF THE COMPLAINT

Symptomatology

Ask about the following characteristics of each symptom using open-ended questions:

- Onset sudden or gradual
- Exact location
- Current situation improving or worsening
- Duration
- Character
- Associated symptoms
- Alleviating factors
- Timing
- Severity
- Previous diagnosis of similar episodes
- Efficacy of previous treatments

Directed Questions to Ask

- Was the pain sudden or gradual?
- How often is the pain occurring?
- Where is the pain exactly? In the rectum, around the rectum, or elsewhere?
- How long has the pain been occurring?
- Can you describe the pain?
- Are you having bleeding or bloody stools?

- Have you noticed any masses in the anal area?
- Does having a bowel movement make the pain worse?
- Have you ever had this happen before? If so, what were you told at that time?
- Are you having diarrhea or constipation?
- Do you feel like you are completely emptying your bowels?
- Have you tried any treatments for the pain?
- Are you sedentary? Would you say you sit a lot during the day?
- Have you been doing any heavy lifting or strenuous exercising?
- Has anyone in your family ever been diagnosed with cancer?

Assessment: Cardinal Signs and Symptoms

General
- Assess for fatigue
- Weight loss

Abdomen
- Assess for abnormal abdomen
- nausea
- vomiting, or constipation

Genitourinary (GU)
- Assess the rectal area for masses
- Overt signs of bleeding
- Discharge

Medical History: General

Past Medical History
- Allergies: no known drug allergies (NKDA)
- Medical: insomnia and anxiety
- Surgical: wisdom teeth removal in 2000
- Psychosocial: never been hospitalized for psych issues; sees a therapist for anxiety
- OB/GYN: gravida 1, para 1
- Medication: Ambien 10 mg PO every HS for insomnia, buspirone 15 mg PO twice a day, and etonogestrel contraceptive implant in left upper arm

Family History
- Mother: hypertension
- Father: hypertension and benign prostatic hyperplasia (BPH)
- Brother: alive and well, no current history

Social History
- Tobacco: never smoked
- Alcohol: glass of wine about once a month
- Sexual: sexually active with her husband of 14 years
- Illicit drugs: she denies
- Diet: she eats a healthy balanced diet using the food pyramid; she avoids red meat
- Family: she lives with her husband and their daughter who is 10 years old
- Occupational: Mrs. Walker is a school teacher for first grade; she goes to work regularly and enjoys her summers off
- Health maintenance: she sees her OB/GYN annually and her therapist once every two months; she sees her regular primary MD once a year unless issues arise

- Vaccinations: flu shot this year and Tdap in 2012
- Exercise: she walks 30 minutes three times a week and wears her Fitbit to help keep track of steps taken during the day

Medical History: Specific to Complaint

- Denies ever being diagnosed with a sexually transmitted infection (STI). She had hemorrhoids after the birth of her child, but they have not bothered her since. She has not traveled to any foreign countries.

PHYSICAL EXAMINATION

Vital Signs

- Temperature
- Heart rate (HR)
- Respiration
- Blood pressure (BP)
- Height
- Weight
- BMI

General Appearance

- State of health
- Appearance of comfort or distress
- Hygiene

Abdomen
- Palpate for tenderness
- Masses
- Distention

GU
- Assess for masses, bleeding, discharge
- Digital rectal examination (DRE) for rectal tone, bleeding, masses

CASE STUDY

History

Directed Question	Response
Was the pain sudden or gradual?	*The pain was gradual, the worst being today.*
How often is the pain occurring?	*The pain is constant.*
Where is the pain exactly? In the rectum, around the rectum, or elsewhere?	*It feels as if the pain is around the rectum.*
How long has the pain been occurring?	*This has been going on for 4 days.*
Can you describe the pain?	*It is a throbbing pain.*
Are you having bleeding or bloody stools?	*No.*

Directed Question	*Response*
Have you noticed any masses in the anal area?	*I feel some swelling back there, not sure if it is a mass.*
Does having a bowel movement make the pain worse?	*Yes, the strain makes the pain worse.*
Have you ever had this happen before? If so, what were you told at that time?	*No. I had hemorrhoids after the birth of my child. This does not feel like a hemorrhoid.*
Are you having diarrhea or constipation?	*No.*
When you use the bathroom do you feel like you are completely emptying your bowels?	*Yes.*
Have you tried any treatments for the pain?	*I used some preparation H, but it did not help.*
Are you sedentary? Would you say you sit a lot during the day?	*No. I teach first grade so I am on my feet a lot during the day.*
Have you been doing any heavy lifting or strenuous exercising?	*No.*
Has anyone in your family ever been diagnosed with cancer?	*No.*

Physical Examination Findings

- VITAL SIGNS: temperature 98.7°F; heart rate (HR) 72; BP 110/68; weight 140 lb, height 6′5″, body mass index (BMI) 23.29
- GENERAL APPEARANCE: well-groomed, well-developed, healthy-appearing female in no acute distress.
- CHEST/CARDIOVASCULAR: lung sounds clear; heart regular rate and rhythm; no murmurs, rubs, or gallops
- ABDOMEN: soft, nontender without mass or organomegaly
- GENITOURINARY/RECTAL: erythematous mass noted in perianal area; no overt bleeding noted. DRE reveals negative occult blood; no lymphadenopathy in the groin area

DIFFERENTIAL DIAGNOSIS

Clinical Observations	Hemorrhoid	Anal Fissure	Anal Abscess	Anal Cancer
Onset	Either	Sudden	Either	Gradual
Pain	Yes	Yes	Yes	Yes
Associated bleeding	Yes	Yes	No	Yes
Mass present	Yes	No	Yes	Yes

(continued)

Clinical Observations	Hemorrhoid	Anal Fissure	Anal Abscess	Anal Cancer
Discharge	Yes	No	No	No
Worsened by bowel movement	Yes	Yes	Possible	No

DIAGNOSTIC EXAMINATION

Exam	Code	Cost	Results
CBC	R69.89	$12	Assess WBC count for infection
Urinalysis	R82.90	$25	Any woman of childbearing age should be assessed for pregnancy
DRE	Z12.5	$0, can be done while examining patient	Assess for masses, occult blood in stool
Wound culture	S81.802A	$45	Determine what infection is present, sensitivities for antibiotic selection

DRE, digital rectal examination; CBC, complete blood count; WBC, white blood cell.

CLINICAL DECISION MAKING

Case Study Analysis

Gradual pain worsening in nature. The pain is constant and throbbing occurring around the rectum. An erythematous mass is present in the perianal area. White blood cell (WBC) count on the complete blood count (CBC) is slightly elevated; however, the patient is afebrile. The absence of bleeding ruled out an anal fissure, cancer, or hemorrhoids.

> **Diagnosis:** *Perianal abscess*

- Incision and drainage of the abscess is performed and wound is cultured
- Broad-spectrum antibiotics started until results are returned
- Sitz baths prescribed and education provided on keeping the wound clean until it is healed
- Prescribed Ultram 50 mg orally every 4 to 6 hours for moderate to severe pain not relieved by Tylenol (not to exceed 400 mg/day)

The patient is to return for a follow-up appointment in 1 week at which time the results from the wound culture will be reviewed and antibiotics adjusted if necessary.

RINGING IN THE EARS (TINNITUS)

Case Presentation: *A 77-year-old patient complains of "ringing in his ears" and states his hearing has gotten progressively worse.*

INTRODUCTION TO COMPLAINT

Tinnitus is not a condition itself—it is a symptom of an underlying condition, such as age-related hearing loss, ear injury, or a circulatory system disorder. Causes are:

- Presbycusis: occurs with aging
- Acoustic trauma: long exposure to loud noise
- Ear infections: bacterial or viral infections
- Earwax blockage: causes hearing loss or irritation of the eardrum, which can lead to tinnitus
- Bony structure changes: otosclerosis
- Temporomandibular joint (TMJ) disorders: TMJ impairment
- Head injuries or neck injuries: head or neck trauma, hearing nerves, or brain function linked to hearing
- Acoustic neuroma: This noncancerous (benign) tumor develops on the cranial nerve that runs from the brain to the inner ear and controls balance and hearing; condition generally causes tinnitus in only one ear
- Ototoxicity: a side effect of certain medications or alcohol
- Ménière's disease: inner ear disorder that may be caused by abnormal inner ear fluid pressure
- Pulsatile tinnitus: head and neck tumors, atherosclerosis, high blood pressure (BP), turbulent blood flow, and malformation of capillaries

HISTORY OF COMPLAINT

Symptomatology

Ask about the following characteristics of each symptom using open-ended questions:

- Onset (sudden or gradual)
- Chronology
- Current situation (improving or deteriorating)
- Timing (frequency, duration)
- Severity
- Precipitating and aggravating factors
- Relieving factors
- Associated symptoms
- Effects on daily activities

- Previous diagnosis of similar episodes
- Previous treatments
- Efficacy of previous treatments

Directed Questions to Ask

- Was the onset sudden or gradual?
- Is it a continuous problem or does it get better or worse at times?
- Is there any pain associated with the ringing in the ears?
- Have you been feeling fatigued?
- Have you experienced vertigo (a sensation that the room is spinning)?
- Have you experienced any dizziness?
- Have you any difficulty in hearing?
- Have you been feeling confused and falling down; losing your balance?
- Have you been having nausea and vomiting?
- Have you experienced a "full" sensation in the ear?
- Have you experienced any abnormal movements of the eye that can't be controlled?
- Have you had other related symptoms?
- Have any ear drainage?

Assessment: Cardinal Signs and Symptoms

Ears
- Hearing loss
- Ear drainage
- Pain

Neck
- Pain
- Swelling
- Enlarged lymph nodes

Other Associated Symptoms
- Fever
- Malaise
- Nausea or vomiting
- Dizziness

Medical History: General

- Medical conditions and surgeries
- Allergies (seasonal, as well as others)
- Medication currently used, including over-the-counter (OTC) medication
- Herbal preparations and traditional therapies

Medical History: Specific to Complaint

- Past ringing in the ears
- Recurrent ear infections
- Recent viral infection or other infections of the respiratory tract
- Recent trauma to the ear

PHYSICAL EXAMINATION
Vital Signs

- Temperature
- Pulse
- Respiration
- Oxygen saturation (SpO_2)
- BP

General Appearance

- Apparent state of health
- Appearance of comfort or distress
- Color
- Nutritional status
- State of hydration
- Hygiene
- Match between appearance and stated age
- Difficulty with gait or balance

Ears
- Visual ear exam with otoscope looking for drainage, red edematous tympanic membrane and mobility, ear wax, and structural changes
- Use tuning fork to assess basic hearing: perform Rinne and Weber tests

Eyes
- Vision examination
- Examine pupils of the eyes with pen light
- Extraocular muscles (EOMs)

Nose
- Inspect nasal passage for drainage, redness, and edema
- Illuminate sinuses

Throat
- Inspect throat for redness, swollen tonsils, drainage, or exudate

Neck
- Symmetry
- Swelling
- Masses
- Active range of motion
- Thyroid enlargement

Neurologic

- Testing strength of extremities
- Watching patient walk

Cardiac

- Check heart sounds, check for murmurs, gallops, and rubs

Respiratory

- Check lung sounds for crackles, rales, and wheezing

Palpation

- Palpate sinuses for tenderness; palpate lymph nodes for tenderness, enlargement, mobility, contour, and consistency of nodes and masses
- Nodes: pre- and post-auricular, occipital, tonsillar, submandibular, submental, anterior and posterior cervical, and supraclavicular
- Palpate carotid arteries

Auscultation

- Place stethoscope over the ear, temporal area, or neck to hear any pulsating sound (if audible, evaluation of vascular system of head and neck to detect vascular tumors). Auscultate for heart sounds.

CASE STUDY

History

Directed Question	Response
Was the onset sudden or gradual?	*Gradual.*
Is it a continuous problem or does it get better or worse at times?	*Continuous.*
Is there any pain associated with the ringing in the ears?	*No.*
Have you been feeling fatigued?	*No.*
Have you experienced vertigo (a sensation that the room is spinning)?	*Yes.*
Have you experienced any dizziness?	*Yes.*
Have you any difficulty in hearing?	*Yes.*
Have you been feeling confused and falling down; losing your balance?	*Yes.*
Have you been having nausea and vomiting?	*No.*
Have you experienced a "full" sensation in the ear?	*No.*
Have you experienced any abnormal movements of the eye that can't be controlled?	*No.*
Have you had other related symptoms?	*No.*
Having any ear drainage?	*No.*

Physical Examination Findings

- VITAL SIGNS: temperature 98.6°F; respiration rate 20; pulse 72; BP 120/80; oxygen saturation 96% room air
- GENERAL APPEARANCE: healthy-appearing, no apparent distress, pleasant
- EARS: abnormal Weber, abnormal Rinne, cannot hear out of left ear, can hear out of right ear, ringing in left ear only, high-pitched ringing in ears
- EYES: no injection, anicteric, pupils equal, round, and reactive to light and accommodation (PERRLA), and extraocular movements intact
- NOSE: no injection, anicteric, PERRLA, extraocular movements intact
- MOUTH: no oral lesions; teeth and gums in good repair
- PHARYNX: tonsils are moderately enlarged, red with pockets of white exudate
- NECK: tonsillar nodes are 1.5 cm, round, mobile, and tender bilaterally; no other cervical nodes palpable; neck is supple; thyroid is not enlarged
- CHEST: lungs are clear in all fields; heart S1 and S2 no murmur, gallop, or rub
- SKIN: good skin color

DIFFERENTIAL DIAGNOSIS

Clinical Observations	Hearing Loss	Ringing in Ears	Dizziness	Ear Drainage	Ear Pain	Fever	Ear Fullness
Presbycusis	Yes	Yes/No	No	No	No	No	No
Acoustic trauma	Common	Common	No	No	No	No	No
Ear infections	Yes/No	Yes/No	No	Common	Common	Common	Yes/No
Earwax blockage	Common	Yes/No	No	No	Yes/No	No	Yes/No
Ear bone changes	Yes/No	Yes/No	Yes/No	No	No	No	No
TMJ disorders	No	Yes/No	Yes/No	No	Yes/No	No	No
Acoustic neuroma	Common	Yes/No	Yes/No	No	No	No	No
Ototoxicity	Common	Common	Common	No	No	No	No
Ménière's disease	Common	Common	Common	No	No	No	Yes/No

TMJ, temporomandibular.

DIAGNOSTIC EXAMINATION

Exam	Code	Cost	Results
CT scan of head with contrast	70470	$750–$950	CT yields cross-sectional images of a part of the head through computerized axial tomography
CBC	85025	$75	CBC • The CBC typically has several parameters that are created from an automated cell counter. The most relevant are: WBC count: • The number of white cells • High WBC count can be a sign of infection • WBC count is also increased in certain types of leukemia • Low WBC count can be a sign of bone marrow diseases or an enlarged spleen • Low WBC count is also found in HIV infection, in some cases Hgb and Hct • Hgb is the amount of oxygen-carrying protein contained within the RBC • Hct is the percentage of the blood volume occupied by RBCs MCV • Identify cause of an anemia: Low values suggest iron deficiency; high values suggest deficiencies of either vitamin B_{12} or folate, ineffective production in the bone marrow, or recent blood loss Platelet count • High values can occur with bleeding, cigarette smoking. Low values can occur from premature destruction or excess production by the bone marrowStates such as immune thrombocytopenia, acute blood loss, drug effects (such as heparin), infections with sepsis, entrapment of platelets in an enlarged spleen, or bone marrow failure from diseases such as myelofibrosis or leukemia
BMP	80047	$160	The BMP includes the following tests: • Glucose: Abnormal levels can indicate diabetes or hypoglycemia; glucose normal range: 64–128 mg/dL • Calcium: Essential for the proper functioning of muscles, nerves, and the heart and is required in blood clotting and in the formation of bones Elevated or decreased calcium levels may indicate a hormone imbalance or problems with the kidneys, bones, or pancreas. Serum calcium normal range: 8.5–10.2 mg/dL • Sodium: Vital nerve and muscle function; serum sodium: 136–144 mEq/L • Potassium: Cell metabolism and muscle function; serum potassium normal range: 3.7–5.2 mEq/L • CO_2 (carbon dioxide, bicarbonate): Maintains the body's acid–base balance (pH). CO_2 normal range: 20–29 mmol/L • Chloride: Regulates the amount of fluid in the body and maintains the acid–base balance. Serum chloride normal range: 101–111 mmol/L • BUN: Conditions that affect the kidney have the potential to affect the amount of urea in the blood. BUN normal range: 7–20 mg/dL • Creatinine: Waste product produced in the muscles; filtered out of the blood by the kidneys so blood levels are a good indication of how well the kidneys are working. Creatinine normal range: 0.8–1.4 mg/dL

(*continued*)

Exam	Code	Cost	Results
EKG	93000	$800	An EKG records the electrical activity of the heart. It is used to measure: • Heart rate • The effects of drugs or devices used to control the heart (such as a pacemaker) • The size and position of heart • Abnormal heart rhythms • Damage or changes to the heart muscle • Changes in the amount of sodium or potassium in the blood • Congenital heart defect • Enlargement of the heart • Fluid or swelling around the heart • Myocarditis • Past or current MI

BMP, basic metabolic panel; BUN, blood urea nitrogen; CBC, complete blood count; CO_2, carbon dioxide; Hct, hematocrit; Hgb, hemoglobin; MCV, mean corpuscular volume; MI, myocardial infarction; RBC, red blood cell; WBC, white blood cell.

CLINICAL DECISION MAKING

Case Study Analysis

Patient has had a recent fall that resulted in a fractured clavicle and progressive hearing loss. Patient has experienced dizziness and loss of balance. Physical examination reveals an abnormal Rinne and Weber tests, and abnormal EKG with frequent premature atrial contractions and premature ventricular contractions noted. The absence of ear drainage, pain, fever, and ear fullness rules out an ear infection. Additional information about the patient's medications is required to determine if ototoxicity is causing the symptom. It is possible that the fall might have precipitated the symptom, so trauma cannot be ruled out. It is unclear if the abnormal EKG findings precipitated the dizziness and subsequent fall.

> *Diagnosis:* *Alteration in hearing related to hearing loss and tinnitus confirmed by physical examination and assessment with positive Rinne and Weber test. Diagnostic examinations will determine further issues.*

Although the symptom that caused the patient to seek medical attention is tinnitus, a cardiac cause cannot be ruled out. Recommend following up with ear, nose, and throat (ENT) specialist first and then schedule an appointment with the cardiology clinic for further evaluation of cardiac dysrhythmia. Patient counseled to change positions slowly, ambulate with care, and avoid using hazardous equipment, including driving. Will await report from the ENT.

RUNNY NOSE

Case Presentation: *A 30-year-old computer programmer presents to the clinic complaining of a 12-day history of a runny nose.*

INTRODUCTION TO COMPLAINT

- Rhinorrhea (nasal discharge) is a common complaint in family practice
- The most frequent etiologies include common viral upper respiratory infections (URIs), acute bacterial rhinosinusitis (ABRS), allergic rhinitis, and nonallergic rhinitis

Acute Viral Rhinosinusitis (AVRS)

- The most common upper respiratory viruses causing the "common cold" are rhinoviruses (30%–50%), coronaviruses (10%–15%), and other viruses (5%)
- Symptoms typically start with a sore throat, which then progresses to include nasal congestion, rhinorrhea, sneezing, cough, and mild malaise
- If there is a fever, it tends to resolve after 24 to 48 hours
- Nasal purulence, which is defined as nasal discharge with color, can occur with a viral respiratory rhinitis, particularly in the later stages of the illness

Acute Bacterial Rhinosinusitis

- It is a complication of a viral URI in only 0.5% to 2% of cases
- Symptoms of AVRS and ABRS are similar
- During the first 10 days, many cases of acute ABRS resolve spontaneously
- Both ABRS and AVRS can produce purulent nasal discharge
- Consider bacterial sinusitis if there is unilateral sinus pain or maxillary tooth pain that tends to worsen when bending over
- Another sign of ABRS is when a presumed viral URI initially improves and then worsens after 5 to 6 days ("double sickening")
- If symptoms are severe, including fever >39°C or 102°F with purulent nasal discharge and a headache for 3 or more days, this is consistent with ABRS that requires consideration of immediate antibiotic treatment
- Red-flag symptoms requiring emergent referral include persistent high fever, meningeal signs, or visual disturbances

Allergic Rhinitis

- Affects 10% to 30% of adults in the United States
- Common symptoms include rhinorrhea, sneezing, nasal pruritus, and congestion
- Frequently accompanied by conjunctivitis symptoms, such as increased lacrimation, irritation, and pruritus of the eyes
- Can appear seasonally in which case it is usually associated with outdoor allergens, which are primarily pollens

- Perennial allergic rhinitis is more frequently caused by indoor allergens, such as dust mites, mold spores, pet dander, and cockroaches
- Objective findings in allergic rhinitis can include a pale and boggy nasal mucosa, watery rhinorrhea, and injected conjunctiva
- Patients can develop dark circles under the eyes, called allergic shiners, secondary to nasal congestion
- A nasal crease is also a common finding caused by patients pushing up on the tip of the nose ("allergic salute") in an attempt to relieve nasal pruritus

Nonallergic Rhinitis

- Fifty percent of patients presenting with rhinitis may have either nonallergic rhinitis or a combination of nonallergic and allergic rhinitis, which is termed "mixed rhinitis"
- Symptoms of nonallergic rhinitis as compared to allergic rhinitis more frequently include nasal congestion, postnasal drainage (PND), and later age of onset (>20 years)
- Conjunctivitis symptoms are not present
- Tends to be exacerbated by weather changes and irritant odors
- Except in the mixed variety, it is associated with negative allergen testing by either an immunoassay blood test or skin testing

HISTORY OF COMPLAINT

Symptomatology

Ask about the following characteristics of each symptom using open-ended questions:

- Onset
- Duration, timing, frequency
- Character of the discharge, color
- Location of discharge, from nose only or also in throat
- Pain in the sinus areas
  - What makes it worse?
  - What makes it better?
- Treatments or medications

Directed Questions to Ask

Head, Eyes, Ears, Nose, Throat (HEENT)

- Do your ears hurt or feel congested? Does your face hurt? If so, where is the pain? What would you rate the pain on a scale of 0 to 10?
- Do you have a headache? If you do, rate the pain on a scale of 0 to 10.
- Is your nose congested?
- Do you have a runny nose? If so, what color is it?
- Does your nose itch?
- Does your throat hurt?
- Do your upper teeth hurt?
- Do the glands in your neck seem swollen or painful?
- Does any nasal drainage drip down into your throat?
- Have you had any change in your vision?
- Do you have a stiff neck?
- Are your eyes bothering you?

Respiratory

- Are you coughing?
- If so, are you coughing up any phlegm?
- If the patient has a cough productive of sputum, inquire as to the quantity, color, and whether there is any hemoptysis. It also can be helpful to ask the patient whether the sputum seems to be coming from the nose/throat (PND) versus the chest.
- Are you wheezing?
- Do you feel short of breath?

Gastrointestinal

- Have you had any stomach symptoms, such as nausea, vomiting, or diarrhea?
- Are you taking any medication? Are you allergic to any medications?
- Do your symptoms seem to be improving, staying the same, or getting worse?

Assessment: Cardinal Signs and Symptoms

- Runny nose
- Sinus pressure
- Headache
- Dizziness

Medical History: General

- Past medical history
- Past surgical history
- Current medications
- Allergies to medications
- Social history
- Family history

Medical History: Specific to Complaint

- Sinus infection
- Allergies
- Nasal or sinus surgery
- Exposure to anyone with similar symptoms

PHYSICAL EXAMINATION

Vital Signs

- Temperature
- Pulse
- Respiration
- SpO_2
- Blood pressure (BP)

General Appearance

- Any signs of acute distress?
- Does the voice sound normal or do you hear signs of nasal congestion and/or hoarseness?
- Any obvious difficulty breathing, such as mouth breathing, wheezing, or increased respiratory effort?

Ears
- Are the ear canals normal?
- Are the tympanic membranes normal?

Eyes
- Has there been any change in your vision?
- Are your eyes bothering you?
- Are your eyes itchy?

Nose
- Is there mucosal swelling? Is it unilateral or bilateral?
- What is the color of the mucosa, such as pale, red, or normal?
- Is there any drainage? If so, what color is it?

Throat
- Is there any redness?
- Is there any exudate?
- If the tonsils are present, are they enlarged?
- Is there any PND?
- Is there a cobblestone appearance to the posterior pharynx?

Neck
- Is there any submental, submandibular, tonsillar, anterior, or posterior cervical adenopathy?
- Test for nuchal rigidity by having the patient touch chin to chest; if able to there is no nuchal rigidity or meningeal signs

Lungs
- Are the lungs clear bilaterally?
- Is there good air exchange?
- Is patient breathing easily?

Heart
- Is there a regular rate and rhythm?
- Is there a murmur or abnormal heart sounds?

Skin
- Is there a rash?

CASE STUDY

History

Directed Question	Response
When did your symptoms begin?	*They began 12 days ago.*
Do your symptoms seem to be improving, staying the same, or getting worse?	*At first, it seemed like I just had a cold, which after 5 or 6 days seemed to be improving. Then, I suddenly felt worse.*
How much do your symptoms affect you?	*I am so tired that it is difficult for me to work.*
Have you been able to work or exercise?	*I stayed home yesterday and today. I have not gone to the gym since my symptoms got worse. I do not seem to have the energy.*

Directed Question	**Response**
Does anything seem to make your symptoms better or worse?	*When I lean over, my face becomes more painful, especially on the right side.*
Have you tried any medications or home remedies for your symptoms?	*I tried using my Neti pot. It makes my nose feel a little better for a short time.*
Are your symptoms worse at a certain time of day, when you are indoors versus outdoors or in any certain positions, such as supine versus standing?	*When I am lying flat at night, I cough more.*
Have you had a fever, chills, or fatigue?	*I may have had a fever the past few days.*
Have you ever had similar symptoms?	*Yes, I did about 3 years ago.*
Have you ever been diagnosed with a sinus infection?	*Yes, when I had similar symptoms 3 years ago.*
Do you have a history of allergies?	*Yes, I tend to get a runny nose during the spring-time pollen season. However, this time of year (winter), my allergies are not a problem.*
Do your ears hurt or feel congested?	*Initially, they felt a little full. Now, they are feeling better.*
Does your face hurt? If so, where would you rate the pain on a scale of 0 to 10?	*Yes, my cheekbones and forehead hurt, particularly on the right side. I would rate the pain as 5/10.*
Do you have a headache?	*Only my forehead and cheeks hurt.*
Is your nose congested?	*Yes, it feels very congested.*
Do you have a runny nose? If so, what color is the drainage?	*Yes, I have a runny nose. The drainage varies between clear and yellow. It particularly tends to be yellow on the right side.*
Does your nose itch?	*No, it does not.*
Does your throat hurt?	*It feels irritated.*
Do your upper teeth hurt?	*Yes, they are mildly painful.*
Do the glands in your neck seem swollen or painful?	*They are a little tender.*
Does any nasal drainage drip down into your throat?	*Yes, it particularly bothers me at night when I am lying flat.*
Has there been any change in your vision?	*No, my vision is normal.*
Are your eyes bothering you?	*My eyes are fine.*
Is your neck stiff?	*No, it feels normal.*

Directed Question	*Response*
Are you coughing?	*Sometimes, the drainage in my throat causes me to cough, particularly when I lie down.*
If so, are you coughing up any phlegm?	*Yes, occasionally I am.*
Do you have a cough productive of sputum and, if so, what is the quantity, color, and is there hemoptysis? Also, does the sputum seem to be coming from the nose/throat [postnasal drainage] or the chest?	*It is a small amount of yellowish phlegm, which seems to be coming from the back of my throat.*
Are you wheezing?	*No, I am not.*
Do you feel short of breath?	*No, I do not.*
Have you had any stomach symptoms, such as nausea, vomiting, or diarrhea?	*No, my stomach is fine.*

Physical Examination Findings

- VITAL SIGNS: temperature 100.4°F (38°C); respiratory rate (RR) 16; pulse (P) 88; blood pressure (BP) 110/70; oxygen saturation (SpO$_2$) 99% on room air
- GENERAL APPEARANCE: no signs of acute distress; patient appears mildly fatigued; she is breathing through her mouth; voice has a nasal quality to it
- EARS: ear canals, normal
- TYMPANIC MEMBRANES: normal
- EYES: conjunctiva, no injection, no increase in lacrimation or purulent drainage
- NOSE: bilateral erythema and edema of turbinates with significant yellow drainage on the right; nares, obstructed air passages
- THROAT: posterior pharynx: mildly injected, scant PND, no exudate, tonsils 1+, no cobblestoning (common in allergic disease secondary to enlargement of lymphoid tissue)
- NECK: anterior cervical lymph nodes: tender but not enlarged; no posterior cervical chain or submental lymph node enlargement or tenderness; easily touches chin to her chest (no nuchal rigidity)
- LUNGS: breathing easily. Clear to auscultation bilaterally with good aeration
- HEART: regular rate and rhythm, no murmur, S3, or S4

DIFFERENTIAL DIAGNOSIS

Clinical Observations	Acute Viral Rhinosinusitis	Acute Bacterial Rhinosinusitis	Allergic Rhinitis	Nonallergic Rhinitis
Fever	<24–48 hours	*>48 hours	Afebrile	Afebrile
Purulent drainage	Yes/No	Yes (often unilateral)	Usually clear	Usually clear
Congestion	Yes	Yes	Yes/No	Yes

(continued)

Clinical Observations	Acute Viral Rhinosinusitis	Acute Bacterial Rhinosinusitis	Allergic Rhinitis	Nonallergic Rhinitis
Nasal pruritus	No	No	Yes	Yes/No
Postnasal drainage	Yes/No	Yes	Yes/No	Yes/No
Duration until symptom improvement	<10 days	≥10 days	Seasonal vs. perennial	Perennial
Triggers	None	None	Allergens	**Nonallergic
Sinus pain	If present: bilateral	Unilateral and worse with bending over	If present: bilateral	None
***Nasal mucosa	Red, swollen turbinates, purulent drainage less common, if present is bilateral	Red with purulent drainage, which is often unilateral	Pale/boggy	Possibly boggy
Eye symptoms	Possible increased lacrimation	None	Frequently increased lacrimation and pruritus	Absent
Nasal pruritus	Absent	Absent	Frequently present	Yes/No

*Bacterial sinusitis can also present without fever; temperature ≥39°C with severe symptoms, consider immediate antibiotic treatment.
**Examples of common triggers are weather changes (cold), spicy or hot food, scents.
***Typical appearance with frequent exceptions.

DIAGNOSTIC EXAMINATION

Viral URI versus acute bacterial sinusitis: Differentiating ABRS versus AVRS is primarily a clinical diagnosis. Currently, there is no diagnostic testing in the primary care setting that has a high sensitivity and specificity. Both sinus x-rays and CT scans can have false positives. They can show air/fluid levels and mucosal thickening of the sinuses in both viral and bacterial sinusitis. Forty-two percent of sinus CT scans show abnormalities in healthy sample populations. Furthermore, sinus CT scans are associated with significant radiation exposure.

Allergy testing is not routinely done for differentiating ABRS versus AVRS. In more chronic conditions, if underlying allergies are suspected, allergy testing can be done. Skin testing is the most accurate and least expensive diagnostic available. Immunoassay tests (a blood test) can also be performed. Their highest sensitivity is for airborne allergens. However, they are less accurate than skin tests and more costly. Nurse practitioners may choose to use immunoassay tests if skin testing is not readily available, patients prefer a blood draw to a visit with a specialist, or if patients are not able or willing to stop antihistamine use prior to skin testing.

Exam	Code	Cost	Results
IgE level	82785	Approximately $100	An elevated IgE is not a sensitive marker for allergic rhinitis. A level of >100 is present in only 44% of patients with allergic rhinitis.
Allergen-specific immunoassay tests	Varies depending on which test is ordered. Geographically appropriate panels of tests are frequently available. An example would be the Northwest Allergen Panel, which tests for common allergens in the Pacific Northwest.	Approximately $200–$800 depending on the number of tests ordered	Tests for the presence of IgE to specific allergens, such as dust or ragweed. If there is a positive result for a specific allergen, it is important to correlate it with the patient's symptoms before diagnosing this specific allergen as the cause of the patient's symptoms.

IgE, immunoglobulin E.

CLINICAL DECISION MAKING

Case Study Analysis

Through a thorough history and physical the advanced practice provider has found the following pertinent positives:

- The patient has had a "double sickening" with what likely began as AVRS, which then progressed to ABRS.
- She has unilateral sinus pain.
- She has unilateral purulent nasal discharge.
- Her upper teeth are painful.
- She has increased sinus pain when she bends over.
- She has a history of seasonal allergies.
- She is not taking any medications, nor does she have any allergies to medications.

Pertinent negatives: Does not have symptoms typical of a more allergic presentation, such as nasal pruritus, clear watery rhinorrhea, or conjunctival symptoms. The presence of a temperature rules out acute viral rhinosinusitis, allergic rhinitis, and nonallergic rhinitis. Assessment findings indicate acute bacterial rhinosinusitis.

> **Diagnosis:** *Although your patient does have a history of seasonal allergic rhinitis, you determine that your patient's current symptoms and physical examination are consistent with a diagnosis of acute bacterial rhinosinusitis*

A broad-spectrum antibiotic is prescribed. The patient is directed to use over-the-counter analgesics for pain management. Warm soaks to the forehead/nasal region are encouraged to enhance comfort. The patient is reminded to complete the entire course of antibiotics and to return if the symptoms do not subside or worsen after 2 weeks.

SHORTNESS OF BREATH

Case Presentation: A 50-year-old Caucasian female presents to the clinic with a complaint of shortness of breath (SOB) for the past 3 days.

INTRODUCTION TO COMPLAINT

- Shortness of breath, otherwise known as "dyspnea," is the subjective feeling of an uncomfortable sensation of breathing discomfort and labored breathing
- It is common, usually occurs as a result of cardiac or respiratory function disorders, may represent conditions from psychiatric to nonurgent to life-threatening, and can be acute or chronic
- Immediate attention is necessary to determine whether the cause is life-threatening and to address the airway, breathing, and circulation and stabilize prior to further evaluation and treatment

Life-Threatening Causes

Upper Airway

- **Tracheal foreign objects (food, coins, bones, dentures, pills)**—uncommon in adults
- **Angioedema**—swelling of the lips, tongue, posterior pharynx, larynx over days to hours; causes are allergic, nonsteroidal anti-inflammatory drugs (NSAIDs), or angiotensin-converting enzyme (ACE)-inhibitor induced
- **Anaphylaxis**—severe swelling of upper airway, tongue; triggered by allergens; progresses to airway occlusion over a period of a few minutes to hours
- Infections of the pharynx and neck cause swelling and pain (epiglottitis, peritonsillar abscess, retropharyngeal abscess)
- **Airway trauma/burns**—hemorrhage and swelling

Pulmonary

- **Pulmonary embolism (PE):** dyspnea at rest, tachypnea, pleuritic chest pain; history of deep vein thrombosis; prolonged bed rest due to illness, surgery (orthopedic), trauma; prolonged sitting after a long car, bus, train, or airplane trip; women who are pregnant, postpartum, or taking oral contraceptives; smoking; bleeding abnormalities causing blood to be hypercoagulable; obstruction of pulmonary arterial vasculature usually from an embolus (clot) from deep venous system of lower extremities; may occur from a clot in upper extremities; may present as acute or chronic
- **Pneumothorax:** trauma; spontaneous, can happen to anyone

Cardiac

- **Acute coronary syndrome (STEMI/NONSTEMI, UNSTABLE ANGINA):** dyspnea may be the only presentation in females, older adults, and diabetics; caused by the lack of blood supply to a coronary artery by inflammation within the vessel walls and/or clot; history of coronary artery disease

- **Cardiac arrhythmia:** dyspnea can be a result of cardiac conduction abnormalities (atrial flutter, atrial fibrillation, heart block, tachyarrhythmias); may be due to myocardial ischemia
- **Cardiac tamponade:** acute dyspnea; classic triad of hypotension, distended neck veins, and muffled heart tomes may be absent; and causes are trauma, malignancy, drugs, infection

Causes of Acute Dyspnea

Chronic Obstructive Pulmonary Disease (COPD) Exacerbation
- Viral
- Bacterial infection
- Inadequate medication management
- Can be chronic
- Consider PE if the patient does not improve with COPD treatment

Asthma Exacerbation
- Dyspnea with wheezing
- Severe if using accessory muscles, diaphoresis, fragmented speech, fatigue
- Viral
- Allergens
- Exercise
- Bacterial infection
- Environmental precipitants
- Inadequate medication management
- Can be chronic

Lung Infections
- Productive cough, fever, pleuritic chest pain
- Not acute unless underlying COPD or asthma
- Bronchitis
- Pneumonia

Congestive Heart Failure (CHF)
- New onset (acute) or chronic
- Dyspnea on exertion (DOE), orthopnea, paroxysmal nocturnal dyspnea (PND), and cough to severe pulmonary edema
- Tachypnea, pulmonary crackles, + jugular vein distention (JVD), S3 gallop, peripheral edema
- Can follow myocardial ischemia and arrhythmia
- Pump failure (systolic or diastolic)
- Volume overload

Valvular Dysfunction
- Dyspnea may be a symptom of aortic stenosis or mitral regurgitation

Severe Anemia
- Dyspnea due to lack of oxygen-carrying capacity
- Acute (hemorrhage) or chronic

Anxiety
- Dyspnea, chest pain, palpitations, dizziness with anxiety
- Underlying anxiety or depression
- Diagnosis of exclusion as common with other medical conditions

Viral Infections
- Caused by a viral illness, such as the common cold, the most common type of viral illness (mild)

HISTORY OF COMPLAINT

Symptomatology

Ask about the following characteristics of each symptom using open-ended questions:

- Onset (sudden, gradual, or chronic)
- Character
- Duration
- Current situation (improving or deteriorating)
- Pain and location
- Quality
- Radiation
- Severity
- Timing (onset, frequency, duration)
- Exacerbating and relieving factors
- Medication usage
- Associated symptoms
- Effects on daily activities
- Previous diagnosis of similar episodes
- Previous treatments
- Efficacy of previous treatments

Directed Questions to Ask

- Was the onset sudden or gradual?
- Can you describe it?
- How long has this been going on?
- Have you had any recent trauma or falls?
- On a scale of 0 to 10 how bad is it?
- What seemed to trigger it?
- Is it getting better or worse?
- What makes it worse?
- What have you tried to relieve it?
- Has this ever happened before?
- What has worked in the past to relieve it?
- Do you have asthma, COPD, hypertension (HTN), heart disease, or diabetes?
- What medications are you on?
- Have you been taking your medications?
- Do you have a cough?
- If yes to cough, is it dry and hacking or productive?
- If dry and hacking, are you wheezing?
- If productive, what color is the sputum?
- Has the sputum changed in color?
- Is the SOB worse after coughing?
- Is the SOB worse with lying down?
- Is the SOB worse with exertion?
- How far can you walk before SOB? Is this worse than before?

- How many stairs can you climb before SOB? Is this worsening?
- Does the SOB awaken you at night?
- What relieves the SOB?
- Do you have any fevers or chills?
- Do you have any body aches?
- Do you have nausea, vomiting, or diaphoresis?
- Does your chest hurt?
- Have you had chest pain before?
- Is this like chest pain you have had before?
- If yes, point to where your chest hurts and does it radiate?
- On a scale of 0 to 10 rate your chest pain.
- Describe your chest pain—is it sharp, stabbing, one side, or dull and aching, with a heaviness?
- Is your chest pain worse with deep breaths?
- Is your chest pain worse with movement?
- Does it hurt to touch your chest?
- Does your arm, shoulder, back, or neck hurt?
- What makes your chest pain worse or better?
- Do you have weakness?
- Do you have palpitations, dizziness, or syncope?
- Do you have fatigue?
- Do you smoke?
- Have you had any recent surgeries or travel?
- Have you ever had a blood clot before?
- Could you be pregnant?
- Does one side hurt worse than the other?
- Do you use cocaine?
- Are you under a great deal of stress?

Assessment: Cardinal Signs and Symptoms

Head, Eyes, Ears, Nose, Throat (HEENT)
- Headache
- Sinus congestion
- Postnasal drip
- Dental status
- Oral lesions
- Sore throat
- Dysphagia

Neck
- Pain
- Swelling
- Enlarged glands

Respiratory
- Productive cough
- Chest tightness
- Wheezing
- Unilateral leg swelling
- Environmental exposure
- History of intubation

Cardiac
- Chest pain
- Pink, frothy sputum
- Extremity swelling
- Orthopnea, DOE

Gastroenterology
- Nausea and vomiting

Psychiatric
- Stress
- Medication overdose

Neurologic
- Headaches
- Trauma

Other Associated Symptoms
- Fever
- Malaise
- Weakness
- Fatigue

Medical History: General

- Medical conditions and surgeries
- Allergies (seasonal as well as others)
- Medications currently used (inhalers, antihypertensive medications, birth control pills [BCPs], antibiotics, diuretics, pain medications, and over-the-counter [OTC] drugs)
- Herbal preparations and traditional therapies

Medical History: Specific to Complaint

- Asthma
- COPD
- Cardiac history
- Surgeries
- Pregnancy
- Smoker

PHYSICAL EXAMINATION
Vital Signs

- Temperature
- Pulse
- Respiration
- Pulse oximetry
- Blood pressure (BP)

General Appearance

- Apparent state of health
- Appearance of comfort or distress
- Color
- Nutritional status

- State of hydration
- Hygiene
- Match between appearance and stated age
- Difficulty with gait or balance

HEENT

- HEAD: trauma, tenderness to palpation
- EYES: conjunctiva and sclera, pupils, equal, round, and reactive to light and accommodation (PERRLA), extraocular muscles (EOMs)
- NOSE: discharge at nares, inflammation, turbinates, discharge/congestion
- FACE: facial swelling, maxillary/frontal tenderness
- THROAT: airway obstruction
- LIPS: color, lesions, symmetry, swelling
- TONGUE: color, texture, lesions, tenderness of floor of mouth, swelling
- THROAT AND PHARYNX: color, exudates, uvula, tonsillar symmetry, and enlargement

Neck

- Symmetry, swelling, masses
- Active range of motion
- Thyroid enlargement
- JVD
- Trachea midline

Palpation

- Tenderness, enlargement, mobility, contour, and consistency of nodes and masses
- NODES: pre- and post-auricular, occipital, tonsillar, submandibular, submental, anterior and posterior cervical, supraclavicular
- THYROID: size, consistency, contour, position, tenderness

Lungs

- INSPECTION: intercostal, subcostal, and supraclavicular retractions; abnormalities of chest wall with inspiration/expiration; prolongation of expiratory phase; rash or tenderness
- AUSCULTATION: equal breath sounds, wheezes, rhonchi, rales
- PALPATION: tenderness
- PERCUSSION: dullness secondary to effusion or consolidation; hyperresonance of a pneumothorax

Cardiovascular

- AUSCULTATION: size, rhythm, gallops, murmurs, clicks, or rubs
- JVD
- Extremities for edema

Gastroenterology

- Bowel tones
- Tenderness
- Masses or organomegaly

Vascular

- Femoral and extremity pulses
- Capillary refill
- Clubbing, edema, calf tenderness or swelling, erythema
- Unilateral lower extremity swelling

CASE STUDY
History

Directed Question	Response
Was the onset sudden or gradual?	It came on gradually over 3 days.
Can you describe it?	I feel like I can't get enough air.
How long has this been going on?	Three days.
Have you had any recent trauma or falls?	No.
On a scale of 0 to 10 how bad is it?	About a 6.
What seemed to trigger it?	My kids are sick with colds.
Is it getting better or worse?	Worse, that's why I came in.
What makes it worse?	Coughing.
What have you tried to relieve it?	My inhaler—but it's not working anymore. I think it's empty.
Has this ever happened before?	Yes, always after a cold.
What has worked in the past to relieve it?	My inhaler and steroids.
Do you have asthma, COPD, HTN, heart disease, or diabetes?	Asthma.
Have you ever been intubated?	No.
Have you ever been to the emergency department for your asthma?	No, I come to the clinic.
What medications are you on?	Albuterol.
Have you been taking your medications?	Yes, too much and it ran out last night. It didn't help anyway.
Do you have a peak flow meter at home?	I can't find it.
Do you have a cough?	Yes, hacking and wheezing all the time.
If yes to cough, is it dry and hacking or productive?	Yes.
If dry and hacking, are you wheezing?	Yes.
If productive, what color is the sputum?	No sputum.
Has the sputum changed in color? Is the SOB worse after coughing?	Yes, I cough so hard I vomit.
Is the SOB worse with lying down?	Yes, my nose is plugged and worse in the morning.
Is the SOB worse with exertion?	I've been home resting.
How far can you walk before SOB? Is this worse than before?	I cough with any walking.

Directed Question	*Response*
How many stairs can you climb before SOB? Is this worsening?	*Yes.*
Does the SOB awaken you at night?	*Yes, it did last night.*
What relieves the SOB?	*Not coughing.*
Do you have any fevers or chills?	*Yes, mild.*
Do you have any body aches?	*Yes.*
Do you have nausea, vomiting, or diaphoresis?	*Vomit after coughing.*
Does your chest hurt?	*Yes, from coughing.*
Have you had chest pain before?	*My chest gets sore from coughing. Same as before.*
Is this like chest pain you have had before?	*Yes.*
If yes, point to where your chest hurts and does it radiate?	*My chest is sore all across the top from coughing.*
On a scale of 0 to 10 rate your chest pain.	*6.*
Describe your chest pain—is it sharp, stabbing, one side, or dull?	*It is sore from coughing.*
Do you feel a heaviness?	*No.*
Is your chest pain worse with deep breaths?	*Yes, I can't take a deep breath or I cough.*
Is your chest pain worse with movement?	*No.*
Does it hurt to touch your chest?	*Yes, across the top.*
Does your arm, shoulder, back, or neck hurt?	*No.*
What makes your chest pain worse or better?	*Not coughing.*
Do you have weakness?	*No.*
Do you have palpitations, dizziness, or syncope?	*No.*
Do you have fatigue?	*Yes.*
Do you smoke?	*No.*
Have you had any recent surgeries or travel?	*No.*
Have you ever had a blood clot before?	*No.*
Could you be pregnant?	*No.*

Directed Question	Response
Does one side hurt worse than the other?	No.
Do you use cocaine?	No.
Are you under a great deal of stress?	No.

COPD, chronic obstructive pulmonary disease; HTN, hypertension; SOB, shortness of breath.

Physical Examination Findings

- VITAL SIGNS: temperature 99°F; respiratory rate (RR) 30; heart rate (HR) 110, regular; BP 130/60; pulse oximetry 97%
- GENERAL APPEARANCE: well-developed, healthy-appearing female with labored breathing at 30 beats per minute, leaning forward "tripod" position, sweating, coughing, in moderate distress; color is good; able to speak in short sentences; alert and oriented in time, place, and person
- EYES: no injection, anicteric, PERRLA, extraocular movements intact
- NOSE: nares are patent; no nasal discharge; turbinates not swollen; no congestion
- MOUTH: no oral lesions; teeth and gums in good repair; no swelling
- PHARYNX: pink; tonsils normal without exudate; airway is patent; no stridor; no drooling
- FACE: no facial swelling
- NECK: no neck swelling or tenderness with palpation; neck is supple; no JVD; thyroid is not enlarged; trachea midline
- HEART: regular rhythm, rate; S1 and S2 no murmur, gallop, or rub; capillary refill adequate
- LUNGS: breath sounds are equal and symmetrical throughout; chest with expansion; RR labored; tachypneic at 30; expiratory wheezes present throughout all fields; no rhonchi or bibasilar crackles
- ABDOMEN: soft, nontender without masses or organomegaly
- SKIN: no rashes
- EXTREMITIES: no joint pain or swelling; no calf tenderness/swelling; no ankle edema
- NEUROLOGIC: without neurological deficits

DIFFERENTIAL DIAGNOSIS

Clinical Observations	CHF	Asthma/ COPD	PE	ACS	PNA
Onset	Either	Either	Sudden	Either	Gradual
Cough	Yes/No	Yes	No	No	Yes
Fever	No	Yes/No	No	No	Yes
Chills	No	No	No	No	Yes
Sweats	No	Yes/No	Yes/No	Yes/No	Yes/No
Chest tightness	No	Yes/No	Yes	Yes/No	No

(continued)

Clinical Observations	CHF	Asthma/ COPD	PE	ACS	PNA
Orthopnea	Yes	Yes/No	No	Yes/No	No
Wheezing	Yes/No	Common	Not common	Not common	Not common
Pleuritic chest pain	No	No	Yes	Yes/No	No
Calf pain/ swelling	Yes	No	Yes, one leg	No	No
Anxiety	Yes	Yes	Yes	Yes	Yes
Fatigue	Yes	Yes	Yes	Yes	Yes
Malaise	Yes	No	No	Yes	Yes
Weakness	No	No	No	Yes/No	No

ACS, acute coronary syndrome; CHF, congestive heart failure; COPD, chronic obstructive pulmonary disease; PE, pulmonary embolism; PNA, pneumonia.

DIAGNOSTIC EXAMINATION

Exam	Code	Cost	Results
EKG	93000	$150	An EKG with dyspnea may reveal: • Ischemia and or infarction (ST segment changes) • Arrhythmias/rhythm abnormalities • Enlarged ventricles • Heart valve abnormalities • Global and regional left ventricular function (normal contraction) • Estimate of the ejection fraction or amount of blood pumped out by each • Ventricular contraction • A mural thrombosis (blood clot in the ventricle wall) • Normal EKG cannot rule out cardiac disease Compare with previous EKG
Posterior–anterior and lateral chest radiograph	71020	$517	An anterior–posterior and lateral CXR will reveal: • Acute heart failure (cardiomegaly, interstitial edema, and vascular congestion) • Pneumonia—infiltrate considered "gold standard" (may be nondiagnostic if early and/or dehydrated) • Pneumothorax • Pleural effusion • COPD/asthma—large lung volumes and flattened diaphragm suggest air trapping; however, CXR may be normal • Foreign body—consider with unilateral air trapping Compare with previous CXR

(*continued*)

Exam	Code	Cost	Results
Cardiac biomarkers (troponin I)	84484	$11	• Cardiac troponin I is specific for cardiac tissue and is detected in the serum only if myocardial injury has occurred • Diagnostic level for increased cardiac risk with the new assay is troponin I >0.25 ng/mL. A level of 0.1–0.25 ng/mL is considered intermediate. A level of < 0.1 ng/mL is considered negative • By 6 hours after symptom onset using troponin I screening, there is a 95%–99% detection rate of patients who are ultimately shown to have had a myocardial infarction • The assay identifies patients who are at higher risk for cardiac events and mortality • Each increase of 1.0 ng/mL in the cardiac troponin I level is associated with an increase in the relative risk of mortality • The troponin I assay allows early identification and stratification of patients with chest pain suggestive of ischemia, allows identification of patients who present 48 hours to 6 days after infarction, and identifies patients with false-positive elevations in CK-MB (such as in rhabdomyolysis) • A negative troponin I assay does not exclude the diagnosis of unstable angina and does not exclude myocardial infarction if time of testing is less than 6 hours after myocardial infarction • Serial measurements are necessary to rule out acute coronary syndrome • Repeat troponin assay after initial testing in 6 hours • May be elevated with PE, sepsis, pericarditis, myocarditis, warfarin use
BMP	80048	$119	The BMP typically has several parameters that are created from an automated cell counter. The most relevant are: • Glucose: energy source for the body; a steady supply must be available for use, and a relatively constant level of glucose must be maintained in the blood (hypoglycemia, hyperglycemia) • Na (sodium): electrolyte imbalance (hyponatremia, especially in elderly fragile females) • K (potassium): electrolyte abnormality (hyperkalemia or hypokalemia, especially due to medications or recent illnesses with vomiting and diarrhea) • BUN: waste products filtered out of the blood by the kidneys; conditions that affect the kidney have the potential to affect the amount of urea in the blood (dehydration) • Creatinine: waste product produced in the muscles; filtered out of the blood by the kidneys, so blood levels are a good indication of how well the kidneys are working (acute/chronic renal insufficiency)
CBC with differential	85025	$75	The CBC typically has several parameters that are created from an automated cell counter. The most relevant are: WBC count • The number of white blood cells • High WBC count can be a sign of infection • WBC count is also increased in certain types of leukemia • Low WBC counts can be a sign of bone marrow diseases or an enlarged spleen • Low WBC count is also found in HIV infection in some cases

(continued)

Exam	Code	Cost	Results
			Hgb and Hct • Hgb is the amount of oxygen-carrying protein contained within the RBCs • Hct is the percentage of the blood volume occupied by RBCs • In most laboratories Hgb is actually measured, whereas the Hct is computed using the RBC measurement and the MCV measurement • Purists prefer to use the Hgb measurement as it is more reliable. Low Hgb or Hct suggests an anemia • Anemia can be due to nutritional deficiencies, blood loss, destruction of blood cells internally, or failure to produce blood in the bone marrow • High Hgb can occur due to lung disease, living at high altitudes, or excessive bone marrow production of blood cells MCV • This helps diagnose a cause of anemia. Low values suggest iron deficiency; high values suggest deficiencies of either vitamin B_{12} or folate, ineffective production in the bone marrow, or recent blood loss with replacement by newer (and larger) cells from the bone marrow Platelet count • This is the number of cells that plug up holes in your blood vessels and prevent bleeding • High values can occur with bleeding, cigarette smoking, or excess production by the bone marrow • Low values can occur from premature destruction states, such as immune thrombocytopenia, acute blood loss, drug effects (such as heparin), infections with sepsis, entrapment of platelets in an enlarged spleen, or bone marrow failure from diseases such as myelofibrosis or leukemia • Low platelets also can occur from clumping of the platelets in a lavender-colored tube. You may need to repeat the test with a green-top tube in that case
D-dimer	85379	$20.92	• Use of test depends on patient's pretest probability for PE • Limitations: In patients with low or moderate probability of clots in the deep veins of the leg, a negative D-dimer result generally rules out DVT. Some patients with blood clots will have false negatives. This is most common among older patients, those who have undergone prolonged hospitalization, and those with markedly elevated C-reactive protein levels. • Reference range(s) • <0.50 mcg/mL • Clinical significance • D-dimer is one of the measurable by-products of activation of the fibrinolytic system. Quantitation of D-dimer assesses fibrinolytic activation and intravascular thrombosis. D-dimer is of particular value in excluding the diagnosis of venous thromboembolism among patients at high risk.
BNP	83880	$50	• BNP may assist with assessing whether acute decompensated heart failure is the contributing cause of dyspnea (SOB) • BNP is a hormone that is secreted by the ventricular cells in response to high ventricular filling pressures and is a useful indicator of left ventricular dysfunction • Use caution when interpreting values in patients with chronic heart failure

(*continued*)

Exam	Code	Cost	Results
Peak-flow meter with nebulizer treatment	94640	$30	<ul><li>PEFR can be useful in differentiating between cardiac and pulmonary causes of dyspnea</li><li>Information about presence and severity of airflow obstruction</li><li>Determine severity of bronchoconstriction in asthma</li><li>Compare to personal best</li><li>Assess improvement with nebulizer treatments</li></ul>
Arterial blood gas	82803	$80	<ul><li>Limited</li><li>Oxygenation assessed with transcutaneous pulse oximetry</li><li>Provides a more accurate assessment of oxygenation</li><li>Provides ability to calculate an alveolar/arterial oxygen gradient</li><li>Patients at risk for cardiac or neurologic compromise secondary to hypoxia can be identified</li><li>Measures carbon dioxide, which indicates severity of airflow obstruction</li></ul>
Lower extremity duplex venous ultrasound	93971	$100	<ul><li>Evaluate DVT with high sensitivity (95%) and specificity (95%) for lower extremity DVT</li><li>May be a cost-effective first test for evaluating possible PE in patients with signs/symptoms of PE and in those with contraindications to chest CTA (pregnant, renal insufficiency, contrast dye allergy)</li></ul>
Oximetry	94760	$414	<ul><li>At rest or with exercise is helpful in detecting hypoxia, but not hypercarbia</li></ul>
CTA chest	71275	$1,000	<ul><li>Indicated in patients with a high pretest probability of venous thromboembolism, + D-dimer (patients in whom D-dimer is likely to be positive)</li><li>Test of choice to rule out PE</li><li>CTA will identify a clot as a filling defect in a contrast-enhanced pulmonary artery</li><li>Sensitivity 83%–90% and specificity is 95%</li><li>May also be helpful in diagnosis of other problems, such as malignancy, pneumonia, and pulmonary edema</li></ul>
Ventilation/perfusion (V/Q) scan	78588	$1,200	<ul><li>Compares emission of radioisotope that is injected into pulmonary arteries with emission of radioisotope that is inhaled into the alveoli</li><li>V/Q scan can rule out PE in 96%–100% of cases when homogeneous scintillation is demonstrated through the lung in the perfusion portion</li><li>Usefulness is limited as only one third of V/Q scans will demonstrate findings sufficient to diagnose or rule out PE with certainty</li><li>For patients in whom a CTA is contraindicated</li></ul>

BMP, basic metabolic panel; BNP, brain natriuretic peptide; BUN, blood urea nitrogen; CBC, complete blood count; CK-MB, creatinine kinase isoenzyme MB; CTA, computed tomography angiography; CXR, chest x-ray; COPD, chronic obstructive pulmonary disease; DVT, deep vein thrombosis; Hct, hematocrit; Hgb, hemoglobin; MCV, mean corpuscular volume; PE, pulmonary embolism; PEFR, peak expiratory flow rate; RBC, red blood cell; SOB, shortness of breath; V/Q, ventilation/perfusion; WBC, white blood cell.

CLINICAL DECISION MAKING

Case Study Analysis

The advanced practice provider performs the assessment and physical examination on the patient and finds the following pertinent positives: gradual onset of worsening dyspnea for 3 days after being exposed to sick children not relieved with inhaler, hacking spasmodic cough with clear sputum, vomit after coughing, RR 30 beats per minute, in moderate distress, unable to speak in full sentences, respirations labored with audible wheezing. Bilateral breath sounds present with end expiratory wheezes. Diagnostic testing reveals peak flows below personal best at 150%. Pertinent negatives are absence of fever, pleuritic chest pain, of cough with blood, or purulent sputum. The complete blood count, laboratory test results, and chest x-ray are normal. The EKG is normal.

Absence of calf pain/swelling and malaise rules out CHF or a PE. Wheezing is not associated with CHF, PE, acute coronary syndrome, or pneumonia. Based on these findings, the patient most likely is experiencing an exacerbation of asthma.

> **Diagnosis:** *Asthma exacerbation—mild to moderate with viral upper respiratory infection*

Current medications for asthma need to be evaluated and possibly changed. A rescue inhaler should be prescribed along with a long-acting bronchodilator. Corticosteroids may also be indicated. The patient should be encouraged to schedule an appointment with a pulmonologist for ongoing treatment and evaluation of asthma.

SHOULDER PAIN

Case Presentation: A 45-year-old male presents to the clinic with right shoulder pain.

INTRODUCTION TO THE COMPLAINT

- Shoulder pain is a very common musculoskeletal complaint. The pain can be intrinsic (in the shoulder joint, tendons, and surrounding ligaments) or referred pain from the neck, chest, or abdomen.
- The shoulder joint is the most complex joint in the human body. Due to this complex network of a number of anatomic structures, the shoulder has tremendous mobility.

Acute Shoulder Pain

- Defined as pain experienced for less than 2 weeks
- Blunt trauma is a common cause of acute shoulder pain. Examples include falls directly on the shoulder, falls onto an outstretched arm
- Fractures: clavicle, proximal humerus, and scapula
- Dislocations: 25% of all shoulder injuries; 95% being anterior glenohumeral dislocations
- Younger patients tend to experience sports injuries due to overuse (muscular strain), as well as fractures and dislocations

Chronic Shoulder Pain

- Involves injury to the rotator cuff. These injuries generally occur in middle-aged or older patients.
- Rotator cuff injuries result from poor athletic technique, poor muscular conditioning, poor posture, and failure of the subacromial bursa to protect the supporting tendons, which results in an injury from acute inflammation to degenerative thinning and calcification and then finally to a tendon tear.
- Impingement syndrome is used to describe symptoms that occur from the compression of the rotator cuff tendons and the subacromial bursa between the greater tubercle of the humeral head and the lateral edge of the acromion process.
- Older adults tend to present with frozen shoulder (adhesive capsulitis) and symptomatic osteoarthritis.
- Adhesive capsulitis is a stiffened glenohumeral joint that has lost significant range of motion (ROM).
- Any shoulder pain that causes a patient not to use his or her shoulder can lead to decreased mobility and ultimately adhesive capsulitis.
- Osteoarthritis of the glenohumeral joint represents wear and tear of the articular cartilage. It is a problem that arises as a result of trauma that occurred years earlier.
- Osteoarthritis is quite rare and could be due to a secondary cause.

Referred Shoulder Pain

- Generally it is poorly localized or vaguely described
- Neural impingement at the level of the cervical spine
- Peripheral nerve entrapment distal to the spinal column
- Diaphragmatic irritation due to splenic laceration, perforated viscous, ruptured ectopic pregnancy, intrathoracic tumors, and distention from hepatic capsule can produce ipsilateral pain
- Myocardial ischemia associated with left shoulder pain

Anatomy of the Shoulder Joint

- This mobility is enhanced by a girdle of three bones, the clavicle, scapula, and proximal humerus.
- There are four articular surfaces (joints): sternoclavicular, acromioclavicular, glenohumeral, and scapulothoracic.
- The glenohumeral joint, commonly called the shoulder joint, is the principal articular surface.
- Intrinsic pain is located in either the glenohumeral structures or the extraglenohumeral structures.
- The glenohumeral structures involved in acute or chronic shoulder pain are the glenohumeral joint and the rotator cuff.
- The rotator cuff is composed of four muscles (supraspinatus, infraspinatus, subscapularis, and teres minor and a cuff around the head of the humerus to which all four muscles attach).
- The glenohumeral ligaments serve as stabilizers; they include the superior, middle, and inferior glenohumeral ligaments.
- Extraglenohumeral structures involved in a shoulder pain complaint are acromioclavicular and sternoclavicular joints and the scapulothoracic articulation.
- Anterior shoulder pain can involve the biceps tendon.
- Three muscles provide additional stability to the glenohumeral joint.
- These muscles include the teres major, latissimus dorsi, and pectoralis major.
- The neural networks of the brachial plexus are formed proximal to the glenohumeral joint; an injury to the brachial plexus can present as shoulder pain.

HISTORY OF COMPLAINT

Symptomatology

Ask about the following characteristics of each symptom using open-ended questions:

- Onset (sudden or gradual)
- Chronology
- Current situation (improving or deteriorating)
- Location
- Radiation
- Quality
- Timing (frequency, duration)
- Severity
- Precipitating and aggravating factors
- Relieving factors
- Associated symptoms

- Effects on daily activities
- Previous diagnosis of similar episodes
- Previous treatments
- Efficacy of previous treatments

Directed Questions to Ask

- What is your age?
- Which is your dominant hand?
- What are your work or sports activities?
- Was the onset of shoulder pain sudden or gradual?
- Was there an injury you can recall?
- Describe the injury.
- Can you point to exactly where the pain is?
- Does your shoulder joint feel loose or unstable?
- Do you notice muscle weakness, catching, stiffness?
- What activities were being done at the time of injury? Were you lifting overhead, pulling, throwing, or is there no apparent cause for injury or reinjury?
- Does the pain awake you from sleep, especially when lying on the affected side?
- Does the pain occur only after activity?
- Does the pain occur during activity but does not restrict performance?
- Does the pain occur during activity and restrict performance?
- Is the pain chronic and unremitting?

Assessment: Cardinal Signs and Symptoms

Neck
- Any neck pain
- Sharp pain radiating from neck to shoulder

Elbow
- Pain
- Decreased ROM

Neurologic (Upper Extremity)
- Numbness
- Paresthesia
- Weakness

Respiratory
- Cough
- Wheezing
- Pleuritic chest pain

Cardiac
- Dyspnea
- Chest pain or discomfort
- Palpitations

Other Associated Symptoms
- Fever
- Night sweats
- Weight loss

Medical History: General

- Past and current medical conditions, especially diabetes (risk factor for "frozen shoulder")
- Previous orthopedic treatments and surgeries
- Any history of prolonged immobility
- Allergies (seasonal, as well as others)
- Medication currently used (prescription, birth control pill [BCP], and over-the-counter [OTC] drugs)
- Herbal preparations and traditional therapies

Medical History: Specific to Complaint

- Previous shoulder treatments—diagnostic testing, hospitalizations, surgeries, and pain management

PHYSICAL EXAMINATION

Vital Signs

- Temperature
- Pulse
- Respiration
- Oxygen saturation (SpO_2)
- Blood pressure (BP)

General Appearance

- Apparent state of health
- Appearance of comfort or distress
- Color
- Nutritional status
- State of hydration
- Hygiene
- Match between appearance and stated age

Neck

- Swelling
- Tenderness upon palpation
- Active ROM
- Special test: head compression test (with patient sitting on a low stool, stand behind the patient, lock hands together, and then apply gentle but firm downward pressure on head, using both hands locked together)

Elbow

- Swelling
- Tenderness upon palpation
- Active ROM

Shoulder

- INSPECTION: observe how the patient moves and carries shoulders; inspect front and back of shoulders for any swelling, discoloration, symmetry, muscle atrophy, scars, abrasions, lacerations, and venous distention; observe the height of the shoulders and scapulae

- PALPATE: palpate the acromioclavicular joint, sternoclavicular joint, cervical spine, biceps tendon, anterior glenohumeral joint, coracoid process, acromion, and scapula; palpate for point tenderness, snapping, grinding and bony crepitus; palpate the area distal and proximal to the pain location
- ROM: assess passive and active ROM—forward elevation, abduction, external rotation, internal rotation
- SPECIAL TESTS: maneuvers to test for rotator cuff problems—empty can test and Neer's test; maneuver to test for acromioclavicular joint disease—cross-arm test; maneuver to test for glenohumeral joint stability—apprehension test; maneuver to test ROM—scratch test and painful arc test

Associated Systems for Assessment

A complete assessment of cardiac, respiratory, gastrointestinal, and upper extremity neurology, if concerned about referred pain.

- Assess for nerve injury
- Sensation in the arm and hand on the affected side
- Motor function should be evaluated by the major nerves of the extremity
- Assess for arterial blood flow
- Evaluate for circulatory compromise on the affected side
- Capillary refill should be assessed in each finger
- Pulses, radial, ulnar, and brachial, need to be evaluated

CASE STUDY
History

Directed Question	Response
Was the onset sudden or gradual?	It was gradual.
How long have you had the pain?	Around 2 weeks or so.
Is the pain improving or deteriorating?	Getting worse.
Where is the pain located?	Really in the front of my shoulder but does wake me up at night when I roll on my shoulder.
What does the pain feel like?	Achy but when I roll on it, it throbs.
How often does the pain occur?	When I reach over my head and at night. Otherwise a dull ache that is always there.
How severe is the pain on a scale of 0 to 10?	It is usually about 2 to 3 but with certain movements it can go to a 6 to 7.
What aggravates or makes the pain worse?	Overhead movement and rolling on my shoulder at night.
What relieves the pain?	I have used muscle rub such as Icy Heat, which helped, putting heat on it. Ibuprofen did not help very much.
Any associated symptoms?	Not really.

Directed Question	*Response*
What effects does this pain have on your daily activities?	*I feel like I am not moving my shoulder as much.*
Have you had similar episodes of pain?	*Back in my 20s, I experienced shoulder pain when I was playing basketball.*
Do you remember what the diagnosis was of this episode?	*I had some sort of tendonitis but I do not remember the name.*
What previous treatments have you tried?	*I think pain killers and rest.*
Were the previous treatments effective?	*Yes, it went away.*
What is your age?	*45 years old.*
Which is your dominant hand?	*Right hand.*
What are your work or sports activities?	*I have been playing more tennis with my wife lately and a couple weekends ago I wallpapered our bathroom.*
Was there an injury you can recall?	*No real injury but did hurt a lot worse after our weekend of wallpapering.*
Does your shoulder joint feel loose or unstable?	*No.*
Do you notice muscle weakness, catching, stiffness?	*Shoulder definitely feels stiff in the morning.*
What activities were being done at the time of injury? Were you lifting overhead, pulling, throwing, or no apparent cause for injury or reinjury?	*Was playing more tennis as well as wallpapering in the bathroom.*
Does the pain awake you from sleep, especially when lying on the affected side?	*Rolling over on the affected side does worsen the pain.*
Does the pain only occur after activity?	*Pain is worse with overhead lifting, otherwise a general dull ache in shoulder.*
Does the pain occur during activity?	*Yes, but does not restrict performance.*
Does the pain occur during activity and restrict performance?	*Worried about moving shoulder too much and causing increasing pain.*
Is the pain chronic and unremitting?	*Pain is a chronic ache.*

Physical Examination Findings

- VITAL SIGNS: temperature 98.71°F; respiratory rate (RR) 16; heart rate (HR) 78, regular; BP 132/80
- GENERAL APPEARANCE: well-developed, healthy-appearing male in no acute distress
- NECK: no tenderness on palpation, full ROM, negative head compression test
- ELBOW: normal appearance bilaterally, no tenderness on palpation, fully active and passive ROM

- SHOULDERS: normal appearance bilaterally, normal strength bilaterally; right shoulder: + tenderness at the subacromion process; normal passive ROM; increased pain with midarc abduction and external pain with impingement testing (Neer and Hawkins tests), + crepitus noted with abduction greater than 60°
- NEUROLOGIC: sensation and strength equal bilaterally
- EXTREMITIES PERIPHERAL CIRCULATION: radial, ulnar, and brachial pulses equal bilaterally

DIFFERENTIAL DIAGNOSIS

Clinical Observations	ROM	Pain	Loss of Muscle Strength	Numbness
Impingement (tendinopathy, bursitis)	Yes	Yes	Yes	Yes
Rotator cuff tears	Yes	Yes	Yes	No
Ligament tears	Yes	Yes	Yes	No
Arthritis	No	Yes	No	No
Gout	No	Yes	No	No
Glenohumeral joint degenerative joint disease	Yes	Yes	Yes	Yes

ROM, range of motion.

DIAGNOSTIC EXAMINATION

Exam	Code	Cost	Results
Lidocaine injection test (in office procedure)	96372	Price varies; billable	Can be used to confirm the diagnosis of rotator cuff tendonitis Can help exclude a diagnosis of frozen shoulder The point of entry is 1–1.5 inches below the midpoint of the acromion The angle of entry parallels the acromion. A 1.5-inch (4 cm) 22-gauge needle is inserted to a depth of 1–1.5 inches. And 1 mL of lidocaine is injected into the deltoid and 1–2 mL into the subacromial bursa
Shoulder radiograph: complete, minimum of two views	73030	$150–$200	Overall, radiographic studies are inexpensive, readily available, and easily interpreted. The disadvantages are exposure to radiation, poor tissue, requires radiology technician for high-quality images, two-dimensional view Anterior–posterior and axillary views of shoulder (two views) are necessary to evaluate patients who have experienced trauma, lost ROM, or experienced severe trauma:

(continued)

Exam	Code	Cost	Results
			<ul><li>Fractures of the proximal humerus, clavicle, and scapula</li><li>Glenohumeral dislocations</li><li>Glenohumeral osteoarthritis</li><li>Acromioclavicular joint arthritis</li><li>Sternoclavicular joint arthritis</li></ul>Beneficial in osteoarthritis; axillary view demonstrates the joint space narrowing that indicates cartilage destruction
Shoulder MRI without contrast Shoulder MRI with contrast	73221 73222	$1,000– $1,500	The advantage of an MRI is its superior contrast resolution; its disadvantages are: it is a costly diagnostic test and it interacts with metals in the body. MRI is the preferred imaging study for patients with suspected impingement and rotator cuff injury. A normal MRI indicates that the likelihood of a rotator cuff tear is less than 10% MRI findings for rotator cuff tears are not highly specific, especially in older patients. The sensitivity and specificity for impingement diagnosis are 93% and 87%, respectively. This diagnostic tool is useful in the evaluation of avascular necrosis, biceps tendinopathy, and rupture.
Ultrasound of shoulder	76881	$150– $300	The diagnostic accuracy of an ultrasound in the hands of skilled operators is equal to that of an MRI in identifying a number of conditions, including rotator cuff tears, labral tears, biceps tendon tears, and dislocations. It is helpful in detecting complete rotator cuff tears but less helpful in identifying partial tears. Decreased cost and being preferred by a majority of patients are some of the other benefits.

CLINICAL DECISION MAKING

Case Study Analysis

The advanced practice provider performs the assessment and physical examination on the patient and finds the following pertinent positives. Right shoulder pain for 2 weeks due to increase of tennis playing and one weekend of wallpapering. The patient's physical examination reveals positive tenderness at the subacromion process. Increased pain with midarc abduction and external pain with impingement testing (Neer and Hawkins tests) + crepitus noted with abduction greater than 60°. Pertinent negatives are absence of trauma, neck pain, and radiation of pain and normal passive ROM. A lidocaine injection test relieved the patient's symptoms, which confirmed the diagnosis of rotator cuff tendonitis.

Diagnosis: *Rotator cuff tendonitis*

The patient was counseled to avoid playing tennis until the symptoms subside. OTC analgesics were suggested for pain control in addition to application of ice or heat. The patient was encouraged to continue with routine activities, however not to unnecessarily strain the limb or affected shoulder for 2 to 4 weeks. A follow-up appointment is recommended for 1 month at which time consultation with an orthopedic surgeon may be required if symptoms persist.

SKIN LESION

Case Presentation: *A 70-year-old White retired photographer presents to the clinic with a complaint of a skin lesion.*

INTRODUCTION TO THE COMPLAINT

Skin complaints are some of the most common reasons for seeking care. They can be benign or represent an underlying medical condition. Many skin lesions look similar and so making an accurate diagnosis can be a challenge. Besides a thorough history, assessing the skin in a systematic way is essential to making an accurate diagnosis. Knowing the type of lesion, size, and distribution of the lesion, associated findings, and the patient (child, adult, child starting puberty, older adult, or pregnant female) all aid in sorting out the diagnosis.

HISTORY OF THE COMPLAINT

Symptomatology

Ask about the following characteristics of each symptom using open-ended questions:

- Onset (sudden or gradual)
- Chronology
- Current situation (improving or deteriorating)
- Location
- Radiation
- Quality
- Timing (frequency, duration)
- Severity
- Precipitating and aggravating factors
- Relieving factors
- Associated symptoms
- Effects on daily activities
- Previous diagnosis of similar episodes
- Previous treatments
- Efficacy of previous treatments

Directed Questions to Ask

- Did the lesion start suddenly or come on slowly?
- How long have you had the lesion?
- Do you have only one lesion and where is it located?
- If you have more than one lesion where are they located?
- Can you describe the color, size, and shape of the lesion?
- Is the lesion raised?

- Is the lesion painful?
- Does the lesion have any drainage? Or, is it crusted or scaling?
- Has the appearance of the lesion changed since it appeared?
- Have you had any fevers, chills, itching, fatigue, or decreased appetite?
- Have you ever had a cancer?
- Have you had any recent injury to your skin or trauma?
- Have you traveled recently?
- Have you been exposed to any chemicals in your home or your work?
- Have you been camping, hiking, or working outdoors?
- Are you taking any medications or drugs?
- Have you started any new medications recently?
- Have you had a change in diet or skin care products?
- What makes your lesion better and what makes it worse?
- Have you applied any creams, lotions, or gels?
- How often do you bathe and what products do you use?
- Do you have any itching?
- Was the itching immediate or gradual?
- Can you describe the intensity of the itching and the location?
- Is the itching worse at night or at a certain time of the year?
- What makes the itching better and what makes it worse?
- Have you applied heat or cold and has that helped?

Assessment: Cardinal Signs and Symptoms

General
- Fever
- Malaise
- Anorexia
- Headache

Head, Eyes, Ears, Nose, Throat (HEENT)
- Red eyes
- Conjunctivitis
- Upper respiratory infection (URI)

Respiratory
- Asthma
- Allergies
- Cough

Cardiovascular
- Varicosities
- Pedal edema

Gastrointestinal
- Anorexia
- Abdominal pain

Musculoskeletal
- Arthritis
- Joint stiffness

Medical History: General

- Medical conditions, surgeries, and blood transfusions
- Allergies (seasonal, as well as others)

- Medication currently used: prescription, birth control pill (BCP), and over-the-counter (OTC) drug
- Herbal preparations and traditional therapies

Medical History: Specific to Complaint

- Childhood asthma or allergies
- Skin cancers or precancers
- Varicella as a child
- Use of sunscreen
- Diabetes
- Psoriasis
- Thyroid or other endocrine disorders
- HIV

Family History

- Atopic dermatitis
- Psoriasis
- Seborrheic dermatitis
- Asthma
- Hay fever
- Environmental allergens
- Persistent rashes inherited skin disorder

Social History

- Occupation
- Drug and alcohol use
- Outdoor activities, hobbies, or sports
- Military service with focus on type of military occupation

PHYSICAL EXAMINATION

Vital Signs

- Temperature
- Pulse
- Respiration
- Blood pressure (BP)

General Appearance

- Apparent state of health
- Color
- Nutritional status
- State of hydration
- Hygiene
- Older or younger than stated age

Skin, Hair, and Nails

Inspection

- Overall inspection of the skin
- Note skin color
- Inspect the lesion. Is it primary or secondary?
- Identify the size, shape, and elevation of the lesion
- Inspect for the color and arrangement of the lesion

- Note the distribution of the lesion
- Inspect the hair for color, distribution, texture
- Inspect for lesions or infestations in the scalp
- Inspect the nails for color
- Inspect the nails for smoothness and consistency

Palpation
- Palpate the skin for temperature, texture, and moisture
- Assess skin turgor
- Palpate the skin lesion, squeeze, or scrape the lesion
- Palpate the nails for texture, temperature, and tenderness

CASE STUDY
History

Directed Question	Response
Did it start suddenly or come on slowly?	*It was slow.*
How long have you had the lesion?	*Probably 9 months.*
Do you have only one lesion and where is it located?	*One on my head.*
If you have more than one lesion where are they located?	*No.*
Can you describe the color, size, and shape of the lesion?	*It is yellow, round, and one inch.*
Is the lesion raised?	*I cannot tell.*
Is the lesion painful?	*No.*
Does the lesion have any drainage? Or, is it crusted or scaling?	*I think scaling, it feels rough.*
Has the appearance of the lesion changed since it appeared?	*I think it is worse.*
Have you had any fevers, chills, itching, fatigue, or decreased appetite?	*No.*
Have you ever had a cancer?	*No.*
Have you had any recent injury to your skin or trauma?	*No.*
Have you traveled recently?	*No.*
Have you been exposed to any chemicals in your home or work?	*No.*
Have you been camping, hiking, or working outdoors?	*I sail almost every day.*
Are you taking any medications or drugs?	*Yes, I take BP and diabetes pills.*

Directed Question	Response
Have you started any new medications recently?	*No.*
Have you had a change in diet or skin care products?	*No.*
What makes your lesion better and what makes it worse?	*Nothing.*
Have you applied any creams, lotions, or gels?	*Jergens lotion after I shower.*
How often do you bathe and what products do you use?	*Daily, and I use Dove soap.*
Do you have any itching?	*A little.*
Was the itching immediate or gradual?	*Gradual.*
Can you describe the intensity of the itching and the location?	*Not bad.*
Is the itching worse at night or at a certain time of the year?	*No.*
What makes the itching better and what makes it worse?	*Using lotion after I shower.*
Have you applied heat or cold and has that helped?	*No.*

BP, blood pressure.

Physical Examination Findings

- VITAL SIGNS: temperature 98.6°F; respiratory rate (RR) 16; heart rate (HR) 82, regular; BP 128/74
- GENERAL APPEARANCE: well-developed, healthy-appearing tanned male in no acute distress; appears to be stated age and in good health
- SKIN: tanned, dry skin; scalp—one lesion, 0.5 cm, central scalp, yellow/tan, firm with irregular edge and scaling; proximal to this lesion is another lesion, 0.5 cm, yellow/tan, firm with irregular edge and scaling
- HAIR: male-patterned baldness with white hair
- NAILS: nail and nail fold intact, and adhered to the bed; nails translucent with longitudinal ridging but without grooves or pitting

DIFFERENTIAL DIAGNOSIS

Clinical Observations	Seborrhea	Rosacea	Cancer	Actinic Keratoses
Color	Red edematous	Dull red	Pale	Pale
Scale	Yes	None	No	No

(*continued*)

Clinical Observations	Seborrhea	Rosacea	Cancer	Actinic Keratoses
Smoothness of skin	Yes	Yes	Irregular edges	Scaly irregular surface
Pustules	No	Yes	None	No
Scarring	None	No	None	Yes
Border of lesion	None	No borders	Irregular	Irregular

DIAGNOSTIC EXAMINATION

Exam	Code	Cost	Results
Scraping	87220	$35–$50	Identification of nonspecific fungal, nail scrape, or skin using a #15 scalpel blade. Place on slide with a cover slip and apply potassium hydroxide. Direct examination with low light. You may see spores or hyphae. Tzanck smear for herpes virus infection, scrape base of vesicle and place on slide. Apply Giemsa or Wright's stain. Multinucleated giant cells confirm diagnosis. Confirm with viral cultures. Scraping for mites at burrows and place scraping on slide with mineral oil to see the parasite, eggs, or mite feces.
Cultures	87070	$55–$75	Allows correct identification of microbial organisms of a wound or draining tissue. Collect and grow bacterial, viral, or fungal cultures in appropriate media.
Patch test	95044	$35–$45	Exposes patient to the most common allergens in patches with 20 of the most common allergens. Apply to skin and removed 2 days later. A positive reaction is eruption at the site of the allergen.
Biopsy	11100	$75–$95	Shave biopsy is for papular, pedunculated, or exophytic lesions. For inflammatory skin lesions use punch biopsy. Excisional biopsy is used to remove an entire lesion and provides a deeper specimen.

All lesions should be biopsied if there is any doubt.

CLINICAL DECISION MAKING

Case Study Analysis

The advanced practice provider performs the assessment and physical examination on the patient and finds the following data: a gradual onset of two scalp lesions, 0.5 cm, firm, yellow/tan, and with irregular edges and scaling in an older adult with a history of frequent sun exposure. Since the lesion is not red and pustules are absent, seborrhea and rosacea can be ruled out. Cancerous lesions are not typically scaly.

Diagnosis: *Actinic keratosis*

The patient was counseled to use topical sunscreen with a sun protection factor (SPF) of at least 50 when out of doors. To confirm the diagnosis, the patient was encouraged to make an appointment with a dermatologist to have the lesions examined further with possible biopsy.

SKIN PAIN

Case Presentation: *A 43-year-old female reports to the clinic with a complaint of "pain" wherever her skin is touched.*

INTRODUCTION TO COMPLAINT

- Skin pain is the result of altered functioning of the nerves in the skin. The altered function can be secondary to a neurologic injury or a disease state.
- Depending on the causative factor, the skin pain can be in a single location or it can be in multiple locations. The skin pain can be accompanied by other symptoms such as swelling, redness, and/or itching.
- Common causes of skin pain include burns (sun, heat, radiation, chemicals), and injuries such as bruises, abrasions, and lacerations. Impaired blood flow can also be a causative factor for skin pain.

HISTORY OF COMPLAINT

Symptomatology

Ask about the following characteristics of each symptom using open-ended questions:

- Onset (sudden or gradual)
- Chronology
- Current situation (improving or deteriorating)
- Location
- Radiation
- Quality
- Timing (frequency, duration)
- Severity
- Precipitating and aggravating factors
- Relieving factors
- Associated symptoms
- Effects on daily activities
- Previous diagnosis of similar episodes
- Previous treatments
- Efficacy of previous treatments

Directed Questions to Ask

- When did you first notice the skin pain?
- Where are you experiencing the skin pain?

- Do you have any other symptoms associated with the skin pain?
- Have you recently been exposed to any new chemical products?
- Have you recently been exposed to any sources of extreme heat in that area of the body?
- Have you had any recent injury to that area of your body?
- Have you noticed any changes in the color of your skin lately?

Assessment: Cardinal Signs and Symptoms

- Pain in the affected area of the skin when touched

Medical History: General

- Medical conditions and surgeries
- Allergies (seasonal as well as others)
- Medication currently used (prescription, birth control pill [BCP], and over the counter [OTC])
- Herbal preparations and traditional therapies

Medical History: Specific to Complaint

- Onset of skin pain
- Location of the skin pain
- Injury
- Exposure to extreme heat or new chemical agents
- Changes in the color of the skin in the affected and surrounding area

PHYSICAL EXAMINATION

Vital Signs

- Temperature
- Pulse
- Respiration
- Oxygen saturation (SpO_2)
- Blood pressure (BP)

General Appearance

- Apparent state of health
- Appearance of comfort or distress
- Nutritional status
- State of hydration

Skin

- Inspect for color changes, evidence of injury
- Palpate for tenderness with touch

Cardiovascular

- Inspect for capillary refill time
- Auscultate for heart sounds, check for murmurs, gallops, rubs
- Palpate for peripheral pulses

Respiratory

- Auscultate lungs for crackles, and wheezing

Abdomen
- Inspect for contour, heaves, scars, bruising
- Auscultate for bowel sounds, bruits
- Palpate for pain, masses

CASE STUDY
History

Directed Question	Response
When did you first notice the skin pain?	*About a year ago.*
Where are you experiencing the skin pain?	*Almost anywhere I am touched on my arms and legs.*
Do you have any other symptoms associated with the skin pain?	*I am tired and I ache all over.*
Have you recently been exposed to any new chemical products?	*No.*
Have you recently been exposed to any sources of extreme heat in that area of the body?	*No.*
Have you had any recent injury to that area of your body?	*No.*
Have you noticed any changes in the color of your skin lately?	*No.*

Physical Examination Findings
- VITAL SIGNS: temperature 96.7°F; respiratory rate (RR) 18; heart rate (HR) 60, regular; BP 98/65; SpO$_2$ 99%
- GENERAL APPEARANCE: well-developed, healthy-appearing female demonstrating a look of despair
- SKIN: warn, pink, tender to light touch over extremity skin surfaces, no evidence of injury
- CARDIOVASCULAR: heart regular rate and rhythm, peripheral pulses palpable, no delay in capillary refill time noted
- RESPIRATORY: bilateral breath sound clear and equal
- ABDOMEN: soft, nontender without mass or organomegaly

DIFFERENTIAL DIAGNOSIS

Clinical Observations	Mechanical Injury	Heat/Chemical Injury	Circulation Issue	Other Etiologies
Pain when skin touched	Yes	Yes	Yes	Yes

(*continued*)

Clinical Observations	Mechanical Injury	Heat/Chemical Injury	Circulation Issue	Other Etiologies
Skin color changes	Yes/No; depending on extent of injury—likely	Yes/No; depending on the nature of the injury—likely	Yes/No; depending on the extent of the issue—possible	Yes/No
Associated swelling	Yes/No; depending on the mechanism of injury—possible	Yes/No; depending on the nature of the injury—possible	Yes/No; depending on the impairment—possible	Yes/No
Associated itching	Yes/No	Yes/No	Yes/No	Yes/No

DIAGNOSTIC EXAMINATION

Exam	Code	Cost	Results
Comprehensive metabolic panel	80053	$49	For screening evaluation of potential metabolic disturbances, creatinine, BUN, and electrolytes

BUN, blood urea nitrogen.

CLINICAL DECISION MAKING

Case Study Analysis

The patient experiences pain when skin is touched, most prominently over the extremities—especially over the anterior tibial region. (*Note*: An evaluation was conducted of the "tender points" included in the diagnostic criteria for fibromyalgia—findings reveal eight positive points; screening complete metabolic panel [CMP] did not demonstrate any abnormal findings.) The patient has no history of recent injury. There is no evidence of altered circulation. Skin is warm and pink. No ecchymosis or areas of skin breakdown noted. Edema not present and no evidence of itching.

> *Diagnosis*: *Skin pain, etiology unknown, clinical diagnosis of fibromyalgia is considered*

The patient was encouraged to avoid using harsh soaps or chemicals on the skin, to avoid extremes in temperature, to protect the skin when out of doors, and to not alter currently used items such as soap and detergent. Further treatment will depend on the findings after the rheumatology appointment scheduled in 2 weeks.

SKIN RASHES

Case Presentation: A 45-year-old female presents with a complaint of an itchy red rash on her arms and legs.

INTRODUCTION TO COMPLAINT

- Skin complaints are very common in primary care settings; it is estimated that 7% of all outpatient visits are for a primary skin complaint.
- Patients with common chronic medical conditions, such as diabetes and obesity, frequently have skin complaints. Yet for primary care clinicians accurately diagnosing skin conditions is challenging.
- With skin complaints it is important to be able to accurately identify and describe the characteristics of the skin lesions.
- With skin lesions, the objective findings present in locations are detectable on physical exam.
- With your differential diagnosis of skin lesion, you need to learn how to describe the primary lesion, examine the distribution of the lesions, and be able to describe secondary lesions.

Terms used to describe primary lesions are as follows:

- **Macules** are nonpalpable lesions that vary in pigmentation from the surrounding skin. There are no elevations or depressions of the skin.
- **Papules** are palpable discrete lesions that measure less than 5 mm, presenting as isolated or grouped.
- **Plaques** are larger superficial flat lesions, often forming a confluence of papules.
- **Nodules** are palpable, discrete lesions measuring more than 6 mm, presenting as either an isolated or a grouped lesion. Tumors are considered large nodules.
- **Cysts** are enclosed cavities with a lining that contains a liquid or semisolid material.
- **Pustules** are well-circumscribed papules containing purulent material.
- **Vesicles** are small, less than 5-mm-diameter circumcised papules containing serous material, whereas *bullae* are larger than 5 mm.
- **Wheals** are irregularly elevated edematous skin areas that are often erythematous.
- **Telangiectasia** is a small superficial dilated blood vessel.
- Secondary lesions are considered evolved lesions or changes. This is due to not having the initial primary disorder not treated.
- **Excoriation** is a linear skin erosion caused by scratching.
- **Lichenification** increases skin thickening with induration secondary to chronic inflammation.
- **Edema** is swelling due to accumulation of water in the tissue.
- **Scale** is superficial dead epidermal cells that are cast off from the skin.

- **Crust** is a scab or dried exudate.
- **Fissure** is a deep skin split that extends into the dermis.
- **Erosion** is a loss of part of the epidermis. These lesions heal without scarring.
- **Atrophy** is decreased skin thickness due to skin thinning.
- **Scar** is an abnormal fibrous tissue that replaces normal tissue after an injury.
- **Hypopigmentation** is a decrease in skin pigment, whereas *depigmentation* is a total loss of skin pigment.

Lesion Location or Distribution

- The distribution of certain lesions is based on the propensity of certain types of lesions or conditions to present in a particular part of the body as well as at a certain age and in certain ethnic groups.
- It is necessary to consider the type of primary lesion, the nature of the secondary lesion, and the distribution of the lesion.

HISTORY OF COMPLAINT
Symptomatology

Ask about the following characteristics of each symptom using open-ended questions:

- Onset (sudden or gradual)
- Chronology
- Current situation (improving or deteriorating)
- Location
- Radiation
- Quality
- Timing (frequency, duration)
- Severity
- Precipitating and aggravating factors
- Relieving factors
- Associated symptoms
- Effects on daily activities
- Previous diagnosis of similar episodes
- Previous treatments
- Efficacy of previous treatments

Directed Questions to Ask

- How long has the rash/lesion been present?
- How did it look when it first appeared?
- Where did it first appear and where is it now?
- What treatments have been used and what was the response, this time and previously?
- Are any other family members affected or does any family member have a similar history?
- Previous history of similar rash for the patient.
- According to the patient's perspective, what caused the rash?
- Are there any new or different medications, personal care products, occupational or recreational exposures that may have caused the skin lesions/rash?
- Has been there been any increase in stress in his or her life?
- It is important to obtain a very thorough social history of occupation, hobbies, travel.
- Ask about sun exposure and use of sun protection strategies

- Does the patient have any allergies or potential allergies?
- Have there been any new growths/skin changes?
- Any history of acute blistering sunburns or chronic sun exposure?
- Any history of prior radiation, thermal injury, and cigarette smoking?

Assessment: Cardinal Signs and Symptoms

In addition to the general characteristics outlined previously, additional characteristics of specific symptoms should be elicited.

Skin
- Description of lesion in patient's own words
- Distribution of lesions
- Onset of lesions
- Location of lesions

Other Associated Symptoms
- Fever
- Malaise/fatigue
- Nausea or vomiting

Medical History: General

- Medical conditions and surgeries
- Allergies (seasonal as well as others)
- Medication currently used (prescription, birth control pill [BCP], and over-the-counter [OTC] drug)
- Herbal preparations and traditional therapies

Medical History: Specific to Complaint

- Chronic illness: diabetes, obesity
- Autoimmune disorders
- Skin cancer

PHYSICAL EXAMINATION

Vital Signs

- Temperature
- Pulse
- Respiration
- Oxygen saturation (SpO_2)
- Blood pressure (BP)

General Appearance

- Apparent state of health
- Appearance of comfort or distress
- Color
- Nutritional status
- State of hydration
- Hygiene
- Match between appearance and stated age

Skin

- Type of lesion (see the preceding)
- Shape of individual lesions
- Arrangement of multiple lesions
- Distribution of lesions
- Color
- Consistency

CASE STUDY

History

Directed Question	Response
How long has the rash/lesion been present?	*For about 2 weeks or so.*
How did it look when it first appeared?	*Fine slightly raised red dots.*
Where did it first appear and where is it now?	*It first appeared on my forearms and now has spread to my abdomen and legs.*
What treatments have you used and what was the response, this time and previously?	*I have used aloe vera gel and antibiotic ointment. Aloe vera seems to have helped with the itching.*
Are any other family members affected or have a similar history?	*No.*
Have you ever had a rash like this before now?	*I had eczema as a young child; no problem with it as an adult.*
What do you think could have caused the rash?	*I think I might have a sun allergy.*
Are there any new or different medications, personal care products, occupational or recreational exposures that may have caused the skin lesions/ rash?	*I don't take a regular medication, and I work at home as a biller for a physician's office. I was wondering about new spray-on sunscreen.*
Has there been any increase in stress in your life?	*No unusual stress.*
Do you have any hobbies or do you travel?	*No new hobbies and I do travel.*
Have you had any exposure to the sun and, if so, what form of protection have you used?	*I did go to a local pool with children a lot this summer. I always wore sunscreen and a sun hat.*
Do you have any allergies or potential allergies?	*Some hay fever in the spring; well controlled with antihistamines.*
Have there been any new growths/skin changes?	*No.*

Directed Question	Response
Any history of acute blistering sunburns, chronic sun exposure?	*No.*
Any history of prior radiation, thermal injury, and cigarette smoking?	*I smoked in high school and college.*

Physical Examination Findings

- VITAL SIGNS: temperature 98.8°F; respiratory rate (RR) 20; heart rate (HR) 88, regular; BP 120/82
- GENERAL APPEARANCE: well-developed, healthy-appearing female in no acute distress
- SKIN: inflammation and mild edema are located on forearms, upper arms, and chest wall, thighs, and knees; primary lesions are a macular papular rash with secondary linear excoriations on forearms and legs

DIFFERENTIAL DIAGNOSIS

Clinical Observations	Pain	Color	Configuration	Location
Dermatitis	Pruritic	Pink to red	Skin eruptions resembling rash	Typically moist areas such as creases of groin or neck or under breasts
Impetigo	Pruritic, burning, stinging	Yellow pus-filled vesicles	Leaking pus or fluid, and forms a honey-colored scab, followed by a red mark that heals without leaving a scar.	Nose or mouth
Herpes zoster	Painful	Yellow fluid-filled blisters	Skin rash with blisters	Limited area on one side of the body (left or right), often in a stripe
Eczema	Pruritic	Erythematous	Vesicular, weeping, and crusting patches	Face, inside of elbows, under breasts, groin area
Actinic keratosis	None	Dark or light, tan, pink, red, a combination of all these	Thick, scaly, or crusty areas	Sun-exposed areas of body—face, head, neck, arms
Psoriasis	Are usually pruritic	Erythematous	Scaly, patches, papules, and plaques	Elbows, knees, but can affect any area, including the scalp, palms of hands, and soles of feet, and genitals

DIAGNOSTIC EXAMINATION

Exam	Code	Cost	Results
Skin biopsy (punch)	11100 11101	$100 $150	• A punch biopsy is considered an excisional biopsy or removes an entire lesion. • This is a procedural code reimbursed at different rates based on the insurance provider. The initial punch is 11100 and each additional is a 11101 code. • A punch biopsy is the primary technique to obtain diagnostic, full-thickness skin specimens. The biopsy is performed using a circular blade. The instrument is rotated down through the dermis and into the subcutaneous fat. The punch biopsy yields a cylindrical core of tissue that must be gently handled to prevent crush debris, which can impact the evaluation of cell pathology. • Large punch biopsy sites can be closed with a single suture and produce a minimal scar. • Punch biopsies are not useful in the evaluation of rashes. They are useful in the differential diagnosis of inflammatory lesions. Punch biopsies are necessary in the evaluation of potentially malignant lesions. If there is a positive finding of malignancy, then additional surgical intervention is necessary and a referral to a dermatologist may be necessary.
Skin biopsy (shave)	11305 (lesion ≤0.5 cm) 11306 (lesion 0.6–1 cm) 11307 (lesion 1.1–2 cm) 11308 (lesion >2 cm)	$150–$1,000 depending on area	• A shave biopsy is an incisional biopsy because it removes only a small part of the lesion. The shave biopsy is used for lesions that are predominantly epidermal without extension into the dermis, such as warts, papillomas, skin tags, superficial basal, or squamous cell carcinomas. A superficial shave removes a thick disk of tissue, often by scalpel (usually no. 15 blade). • Excisional biopsies should be performed for any lesions perceived to be melanomas.

CLINICAL DECISION MAKING

Case Study Analysis

The advanced practice provider performs the assessment and physical examination on the patient and finds a macular papular rash with erythematous base with secondary lesions of excoriations on forearms and legs. The rash has been present for 2 weeks and with discovery of a more detailed history, exposure to spray-on sunscreen appears to be the culprit. Pustules leaking fluid around the nose and mouth are not present, ruling out impetigo. Painful, yellow fluid-filled blisters occurring in one area are absent, which rules out herpes zoster. Since the rash is over the arms and legs and not localized to the face, elbows, breasts, and groin area, eczema can be ruled out. The rash is not thick or crusty and localized to the face, neck, head, and arms, which rules out actinic keratosis. Absence of scaly patches, papules, and plaques on the elbows, knees, or other body areas rules out psoriasis.

Diagnosis: *Irritant contact dermatitis (chronic)*

Since the rash is a new onset the patient was counseled to avoid using spray-on tanning products and avoid applying any products with similar chemicals until the rash heals. Should the rash persist after 1 to 2 weeks the patient was encouraged to make an appointment with a dermatologist for further examination and testing to include a biopsy.

SLEEP DISTURBANCES

Case Presentation: A 32-year-old African American man complains of sleep disturbances.

INTRODUCTION TO COMPLAINT

- Sleep disturbance is considered insomnia when a patient complains of a difficulty falling asleep, staying asleep, or waking up earlier than desired *despite* ample opportunity and time for sleep *and* it interferes with daytime functioning.
- Insomnia is a very common complaint in the United States. A national survey found 35% of adults reported insomnia in the previous year and half of them described it as serious.
- A systemic review of 50 studies found that around 10% of adults develop chronic insomnia with daytime consequences.
- Women are 50% more likely to develop insomnia than men.
- Studies have found a correlation between insomnia and hypertension, myocardial infarctions, anxiety, depression, and diabetes. Many patients do not complain of insomnia at their appointments, so it is important to ask questions related to sleep.
- There are two types of insomnia: short term and chronic.
- Short term lasts less than 3 months and causes significant concern to the sufferer. It is often tied to specific events, such as job changes or grief and is expected to resolve when the stressor is resolved or adapted to.
- Chronic lasts longer than 3 months, at least three times a week, not related to another sleep disorder. Periods of sleep disturbance should last longer than 30 minutes at a time.

HISTORY OF COMPLAINT

Symptomology

Ask about the following characteristics of each symptom using open-ended questions:

- Onset
- Duration and progression of symptoms
- Timing
- External stressors
- Effect on daytime performance
- Associated symptoms, including mood
- Medication use
- Use of alcohol and/or drugs

Directed Questions to Ask

- When did you first notice these sleeping problems?
- Have these problems lasted since then or do they fluctuate?
- Does it happen more when you're trying to fall asleep or do you wake up often?
- Has it gotten worse over time?
- Have you had any big changes or stressors in your life recently?
- How does this affect you during the day?
- Have you noticed any changes to your health or mood since this started?
- Did you start any new medications around the time this started?
- Are you using any alcohol or drugs to help you sleep?
- Do you look at a phone or TV while in bed?
- Do you have any chronic pain?

Assessment: Cardinal Signs and Symptoms

General

- Fatigue
- Confusion
- Terse or anxious affect
- Sleepiness
- Weight changes

Head, Eyes, Ears, Nose, Throat (HEENT)

- Goiter
- Irritated or inflamed nasal membranes
- Enlarged tonsils or uvula
- Vision changes

Cardiac

- Hypertension
- Tachycardia
- Angina
- Palpitations

Respiratory

- Wheezing
- Sneezing
- Dyspnea

Gastrointestinal (GI)

- Heartburn
- Changes in stool or bowel habits

Genitourinary (GU)

- Nocturia

Musculoskeletal

- Low back pain
- Chronic pain
- Arthritis
- Weakness

Neurologic

- Tremors
- Restless legs

Skin

- Painful blisters or rash
- Texture
- Hair loss
- Pruritus

Medical History

- Medical conditions: seasonal allergies, gallstones
- Surgeries: appendectomy age 12, cholecystectomy age 29
- Allergies: seasonal, penicillin—anaphylaxis
- Medication use, including illicit drugs: Zyrtec 10 mg daily (takes when allergies bother him), Ambien 5 mg some nights (not prescribed), occasional marijuana
- Exercise and diet: no planned exercise, no specific diet

Family History

- Mother—hypertension, macular degeneration
- Father—thyroid disorder
- Brother—died at 33 from brain aneurysm

Social History

- Patient is married with two young children
- He is a middle school math teacher, drives semitrucks in the summer
- He denies tobacco use, drinks alcohol most nights (usually one beer, but up to five), occasional marijuana use
- He mentions increased anxiety and stress
- Denies suicide ideation, domestic violence

Sexual History

- In a monogamous relationship

PHYSICAL EXAMINATION

Vital Signs

- Temperature
- Pulse
- Blood pressure (BP)
- Respiration
- Oxygen saturation (SpO_2)
- Body mass index (BMI)

General Appearance

- Affect
- Coloring
- Orientation
- Muscle atrophy
- Nutritional status

HEENT

- Eye movement
- Lid drag
- Pupil response
- Nasal membrane irritation

- Thyroid size
- Exophthalmos
- Large neck size

Respiratory
- Lung sounds
- Chest expansion and symmetry
- Cough
- Crackles
- Wheeze

Cardiovascular
- Rate
- Rhythm
- Hypertension
- Peripheral edema
- Jugular venous distention (JVD)

GI
- Tenderness on palpation

Musculoskeletal
- Extremity weakness
- Inflammation
- Tremors
- Hyperreflexia

Skin
- Color
- Texture
- Hair

CASE STUDY

History

Directed Question	Response
When did you first notice these sleeping problems?	*About a year ago. I didn't think much of it, but now I'm exhausted all the time.*
Have these problems lasted since then or do they fluctuate?	*They've lasted the whole time.*
Does it happen more when you're trying to fall asleep or do you wake up often?	*I wake up a lot and can't get back to sleep.*
Has it gotten worse over time?	*Yeah. It used to only happen a couple times a month and now it's more days of the week than not.*
Have you had any big changes or stressors in your life recently?	*I have young kids and I teach middle school kids. That's pretty stressful. But I wouldn't say it's changed.*

Directed Question	Response
How does this affect you during the day?	*I'm shaky, exhausted, and I feel like I can't concentrate. I'm more short with the kids at work.*
Have you noticed any changes to your health or mood since this started?	*Yes. I've been more stressed out and anxious, so that may be what's causing this. I've lost some weight too, even though I feel like I eat more.*
Did you start any new medications around the time this started?	*No. I've tried some over-the-counter stuff to help me sleep, but I didn't start any new meds.*
Are you using any alcohol or drugs to help you sleep?	*Well, recently. My friend gave me some Ambien and that seems to help, and sometimes I'll get drunk just so I can sleep. But I don't do that often.*
How much coffee, sodas, or energy drinks do you drink in a day?	*I usually will have one or two of all of those every day. I feel like they help me focus and stay awake.*
Do you look at a phone or TV while in bed?	*No.*
Do you have any chronic pain?	*No.*

Physical Examination Findings

- VITAL SIGNS: temperature 99.0°F; RR 22 breaths per minute; pulse 110 beats per min; BP 134/68; SpO$_2$ 99% on RA; BMI 20
- GENERAL APPEARANCE: patient appears thin, anxious, stated age, well groomed; alert and oriented four times
- HEENT: pupils equal, round, and reactive to light and accommodation (PERRLA), ocular movement intact, lid lag present, vision 20/20; nasal membranes moist and pink; thyroid gland enlarged, firm, smooth; thymus gland and cervical lymph nodes nonpalpable; trachea midline
- RESPIRATORY: lungs clear to auscultation bilaterally; symmetric chest rise; tachypnea
- CARDIAC: tachycardia, regular rhythm; radial and dorsalis pedis pulses 2+ bilaterally; capillary refill <2 sec; no JVD noted; no peripheral edema noted; elevated BP with widened pulse pressure
- GASTROINTESTINAL: bowel sounds present in all four quadrants; abdomen soft, nontender; no organomegaly noted; patient endorses more frequent bowel movements, denies diarrhea
- MUSCULOSKELETAL: strength 4/5 in bilateral lower extremities
- NEUROLOGIC: tremor of upper extremities when outstretched; reflexes of Achilles and patellar tendons 3+ bilaterally
- SKIN: warm, dry, intact; lower extremities with hair loss

DIFFERENTIAL DIAGNOSIS

Clinical Observations	Thyroid Disorder	Excessive Caffeine Intake	Pheochromocytoma
Effect on sleep	Difficulty staying asleep	Difficulty falling asleep	Difficulty falling and staying asleep
Weight loss	Yes	No	Yes
Anxiety, irritability	Yes	Yes	Yes
BP changes	Widened pulse pressure	Possible rise in systolic pressure	Hypertension
Cardiac effects	Tachycardia, possibly irregular	Tachycardia, palpitations	Tachycardia, palpitations
Sweating	Yes	Yes	Yes
Vision changes	Yes/No	Hallucinations	Yes
Bowel changes	More frequent	Diarrhea	Constipation
Possible symptoms	Hair loss, weakness of hips or shoulders, dyspnea, tremor	Diuresis, dizziness, muscle twitching, dyspnea	Headaches, abdominal pain, dizziness, tachypnea

BP, blood pressure.

DIAGNOSTIC EXAMINATION

Exam	Code	Cost	Results
Sleep log	NK	$0	Looks at sleep–wake patterns and day-to-day variability. Include bedtime, time to fall asleep, number and duration of awakenings, total time awake at night after initially falling asleep, time in bed, total sleep time, sleep efficiency (total sleep time divided by time in bed), and naps (time, duration, frequency). Can also include medications, caffeine, and alcohol. Less reliable.
Epworth Sleepiness Scale	NK	Free (costs vary) for patient, licensing fee for practice	This is a questionnaire with eight items that patients use to self-report subjective sleepiness. It rates the answers for a possible total of 0–24. Normal is <10.
Polysomnography	99213	$1,500	Used when obstructive sleep apnea is suspected, when behavior or psychological treatment fails, or when awakenings occur with violent or injurious behavior.

(*continued*)

Exam	Code	Cost	Results
Actigraphy	95803	$250–$750 Part of many commercial activity trackers	Gives you the ability to monitor circadian rhythm patterns or sleep disturbances, especially in those with depression. Usually worn on the wrist and detects movement. Can be used 24 hours a day.
TSH	R94.6	$44	This detects the level of TSH in the blood, which is released by the pituitary gland. It responds to the T3 and T4 in your blood and will increase hormone production to stimulate the thyroid if T3 and T4 levels are low, or decrease production to hinder the thyroid gland if T3 and T4 levels are high.
Free T4	84479	$17	Detects the amount of thyroxine in the blood. A high level indicates too much thyroid-stimulating immunoglobulins is secreted and the thyroid is hyperactive. A low level is due to a deficiency of the pituitary gland or thyroid gland (if TSH is normal, points to pituitary).

TSH, thyroid-stimulating hormone.

CLINICAL DECISION MAKING

Case Study Analysis

Due to family history, patient complaint of insomnia, and physical findings, a suspicion of hyperthyroidism was evaluated. Patient had thyroid-stimulating hormone (TSH) level of 0.28 mIU/L (normal 0.35–5.0) and T4 level of 14.7 mcg/dL (normal 4.5–11.2). This points to an overactive thyroid gland. The caffeine, alcohol, and sleeping pill use all points to self-medicating to alleviate symptoms. The sleep log indicates that the patient did have trouble staying asleep and was getting about 5.5 hours of sleep on nights he was affected. No further sleep testing was warranted as a clinical diagnosis was determined to be the cause of the insomnia. Elevated T4 and decreased TSH levels eliminated the need to test for pheochromocytoma.

> ***Diagnosis:*** *Insomnia r/t hyperthyroidism*

Patient ought to be sent to an endocrinologist for further evaluation of symptoms and pre-scription of appropriate medication to regulate TSH and T4 levels. Also given metoprolol 25 mg BID to take until follow up and Ambien 5 mg qhs to help with sleep. If hyperthyroid symptoms reoccur, the patient may need a second dose. Patient educated that treatment can take up to 3 months to be effective and needs to be monitored for hypothyroid disorder and will need lifelong medication to regulate thyroid hormone levels. The patient was counseled to limit alcohol intake, avoid marijuana, and ensure an adequate dietary intake. Follow up at 1 month to reassess TSH, T4, BP, pulse, and weight. Once euthyroid state achieved, begin weaning metoprolol and Ambien. The patient was encouraged to seek treatment sooner if symptoms worsened or new ones developed before the follow-up appointment. Radioactive iodine treatment or surgery are last resort options in cases where the thyroid does not respond appropriately to medication.

SORE THROAT

Case Presentation: A 35-year-old Asian college student presents to the clinic with a complaint of a sore throat.

INTRODUCTION TO COMPLAINT

Pharyngitis is caused by the following problems.

Viral Infections

- Respiratory syncytial virus
- Influenza A and B
- Epstein–Barr virus (mononucleosis or "kissing disease")
- Adenovirus
- Herpes simplex virus

Bacterial Infections

- Group A beta strep (the most common)
- *Neisseria gonorrhoeae*
- *Mycoplasma pneumonia*
- *Chlamydophila pneumoniae*

Irritants and Injuries

- Low humidity, smoking, air pollution, yelling, or nasal drainage down the back of the throat (postnasal drip)
- Breathing through the mouth when the patient has allergies or a stuffy nose
- Gastroesophageal reflux disease (GERD)
- An injury to the back of the throat, such as a cut or puncture as a result falling with a pointed object in the mouth

HISTORY OF COMPLAINT

Symptomatology

Ask about the following characteristics of each symptom using open-ended questions:

- Onset (gradual or sudden)
- Current situation (improving or deteriorating)
- Location
- Radiation
- Quality

- Timing (frequency, duration)
- Severity
- Precipitating and aggravating factors
- Relieving factors
- Associated symptoms
- Effects on daily activities
- Previous diagnosis of similar episodes
- Previous treatments
- Efficacy of previous treatments

Directed Questions to Ask

- Do you have any fevers?
- Do you have any aches?
- Is it hard to swallow?
- Are you able to drink fluids?
- On a scale of 0 to 10, if 10 is the worst, what number is this pain?
- Do you have a headache?
- Do you have a rash?
- Do you have fatigue?
- Do you have nasal congestion?
- Do you have a cough?
- Do you have vomiting?
- Have you been exposed to anyone who has sore throat or strep throat?

Assessment: Cardinal Signs and Symptoms

Mouth and Throat

- Hoarseness or recent voice change
- Dental status
- Oral lesions
- Bleeding gums
- Sore throat
- Uvula midline
- Dysphagia

Neck

- Pain
- Swelling
- Enlarged glands

Other Associated Symptoms

- Fever
- Malaise
- Nausea or vomiting

Medical History: General

- Medical conditions and surgeries
- Allergies (seasonal, as well as others)
- Medication currently used (prescription, birth control pill [BCP], and over-the-counter [OTC] drug)
- Herbal preparations and traditional therapies

Medical History: Specific to Complaint

- Frequent throat infections
- Sinusitis
- Trauma to the throat area
- History of throat surgery
- Seasonal allergies

PHYSICAL EXAMINATION

Vital Signs

- Temperature
- Pulse
- Respiration
- Oxygen saturation (SpO_2)
- Blood pressure (BP)

General Appearance

- Apparent state of health
- Appearance of comfort or distress
- Color
- Nutritional status
- State of hydration
- Hygiene
- Match between appearance and stated age
- Difficulty with gait or balance

Mouth and Throat

- Lips: color, lesions, symmetry
- Oral cavity: breath odor, color, lesions of buccal mucosa
- Teeth and gums: redness, swelling, caries, bleeding
- Tongue: color, texture, lesions, tenderness of floor of mouth
- Throat and pharynx: color, exudates, uvula, tonsillar symmetry, and enlargement

Neck

- Symmetry
- Swelling
- Masses
- Active range of motion
- Thyroid enlargement

Palpation

- Tenderness, enlargement, mobility, contour, and consistency of nodes and masses
- Nodes: pre- and post-auricular, occipital, tonsillar, submandibular, submental, anterior and posterior cervical, supraclavicular
- Thyroid: size, consistency, contour, position, tenderness

Associated Systems for Assessment

- A complete assessment should include the respiratory system

CASE STUDY

History

Directed Question	Response
Was the onset sudden or gradual?	It was sudden.
Have you had any fever?	Yes, it was 101 this morning.
Do you have any aches?	Yes, I am very achy.
Is it hard to swallow?	Yes, it is so painful.
Are you able to drink fluids?	Yes, I am drinking some fluids, but it hurts.
If 10 is the worst pain you have ever had, what number is this pain?	9/10.
Do you have a headache?	Mild headache here [points to front of head].
Do you have a rash?	No.
Do you have fatigue?	Yes, I am so tired.
Do you have nasal congestion?	No, I'm not stuffy.
Do you have a cough?	No, I'm not coughing.
Do you have vomiting?	No, my stomach is okay.
Have you been exposed to anyone who has sore throat or strep throat?	No, not that I know of.

Physical Examination Findings

- VITAL SIGNS: temperature 101°F; respiratory rate (RR) 16; heart rate (HR) 110, regular; BP 100/60
- GENERAL APPEARANCE: well-developed, healthy-appearing female with slightly muffled voice in no acute distress
- EYES: no injection, anicteric, pupils even, round, reactive to light and accommodation (PERRLA), extraocular movements intact
- NOSE: nares are patent; no edema or exudate of turbinates
- MOUTH: no oral lesions; teeth and gums in good repair
- PHARYNX: tonsils are moderately enlarged, red with pockets of white exudate
- NECK: tonsillar nodes are 1.5 cm, round, mobile, tender bilaterally; no other cervical nodes are palpable; neck is supple; thyroid is not enlarged
- CHEST: lungs are clear in all fields; heart S1 and S2 has no murmur, gallop, or rub
- ABDOMEN: soft, nontender without mass or organomegaly
- SKIN: no rashes
- EXTREMITIES: no joint pain or swelling

DIFFERENTIAL DIAGNOSIS

Clinical Observations	Viral	Strep	Mono	Postnasal
Onset	Gradual	Abrupt	Either	Gradual

(continued)

Clinical Observations	Viral	Strep	Mono	Postnasal
Painful swallowing	Yes	Yes	Yes	Yes/No
Fever	Low	High	Either	Low or no
Chills	Rare	Yes	Either	No
Sweats	Rare	Yes	Either	No
Nasal congestion	Common	Rare	Rare	Common
Nasal discharge	Common	Rare	Rare	Common
Post nasal drip	Common	Rare	Rare	Common
Cough	Mild	Rare	Rare	Common
Fatigue	Common	Common	Common	Mild
Malaise	Common	Common	Common	Rare
Headache	Mild	Mild	Mild	Mild
Nodes in neck	Boggy	Enlarged tonsillar	Posterior	Boggy
Exposed to strep	No	Yes	No	No

DIAGNOSTIC EXAMINATION

Exam	Code	Cost	Results
Throat culture (culture usually done when rapid test is negative)	87880 87081	$80 $64	Rapid strep test Normal (negative results): No strep bacteria are present Abnormal (positive results): Strep bacteria are present • One problem with the test is that, though it has high specificity of approximately 95%–98%, the sensitivity is only 75%–85%. • This means that the odds of a false positive are lower than the odds of a false negative and one can be more confident about a positive result than a negative result. • If the rapid test is negative, a follow-up culture (which takes 24–48 hours) might be performed. • A negative culture could suggest a viral infection. • Works by detecting the presence of a carbohydrate antigen unique to group A *Streptococcus*. • If the test is performed before sufficient organisms are present in the throat, then the rapid strep test is less likely to detect the organism. • The clinician might still treat the throat infection based on his or her own judgment.

(*continued*)

Exam	Code	Cost	Results
			Throat culture Normal (negative): No bacteria or fungi grow in the culture. A negative throat culture may mean the infection is a virus, rather than bacteria or fungus, such as: • Enterovirus • Epstein–Barr virus • Herpes simplex virus • Respiratory syncytial virus Abnormal (positive): Bacteria grow in the culture. Some bacterial throat infections include: • Strep throat • Whooping cough (*Bordetella pertussis*) The most common fungal throat infection is thrush, caused by the fungus *Candida albicans*.
CBC	85025	$75	CBC The CBC typically has several parameters WBC count • High WBC count can be a sign of infection. • WBC count is also increased in certain types of leukemia. • Low WBC counts can be a sign of bone marrow diseases or an enlarged spleen. Hgb and Hct • Hgb is the amount of oxygen-carrying protein contained within the RBCs. • Hct is the percentage of the blood volume by RBCs. • Low Hgb or Hct suggests an anemia. • High Hgb can occur due to lung disease, living at high altitudes, or excessive bone marrow production of blood cells. MCV • Low values suggest iron deficiency; high values suggest deficiencies of either vitamin B_{12} or folate, ineffective production in the bone marrow, or recent blood loss with replacement by newer (and larger) cells from the bone marrow. Platelet count • High values can occur with bleeding, cigarette smoking, or excess production by the bone marrow. • Low values can occur from immune thrombocytopenia, acute blood loss, drug effects (such as heparin), infections with sepsis, entrapment of platelets in an enlarged spleen, or bone marrow failure from myelofibrosis or leukemia.

CBC, complete blood count; Hct, hematocrit; Hgb, hemoglobin; MCV, mean corpuscular volume; RBC, red blood cell; WBC, white blood cell.

CLINICAL DECISION MAKING

Case Study Analysis

The advanced practice provider performs the assessment and physical examination on the patient and finds the following pertinent positives: sudden onset of throat soreness, fever of 101.2°F, chills and malaise, painful swallowing, tonsillar adenopathy, and mastoid adenopathy. Pertinent negatives are absence of runny nose, sinus pain, or cough. Since the fever and throat pain had a sudden onset, a viral or postnasal cause can be ruled out. The presence of a fever also rules out a viral or postnasal cause. The absence of nasal congestion, nasal discharge, postnasal drip, and cough rules out a viral or postnasal cause. The presence of enlarged tonsillar lymph nodes indicates a strep infection of the throat. A rapid strep test completed during the examination was positive, which confirmed the diagnosis.

Diagnosis: *Strep throat*

The patient was provided with a prescription for antibiotics, and was counseled to increase oral fluids, and to use OTC analgesics for pain control and as an antipyretic. The patient was also encouraged to avoid crowds and stay indoors until the fever and throat pain subside. Oral lozenges were suggested to help with the throat pain. The patient was encouraged to complete the entire course of antibiotics and to return if symptoms did not subside or became worse after 2 weeks.

TREMORS

Case Presentation: A 40-year-old male presents with a complaint of tremors.

INTRODUCTION TO COMPLAINT

- Occurs when the body moves in an uncontrollable and unintended way
- Can be quick with jerking movements
- Can also be long-lasting tremors and seizures
- Also known as "dyskinesias"
- Chorea: continuous jerky movements in which each movement is sudden and may result in posturing for a few seconds
- Usually affects the head, face, or limbs
- Cerebrovascular diseases are common causes
- Inherited:
  - Huntington's disease
  - Benign hereditary chorea
  - Wilson's disease
- Acquired:
  - Stroke
  - Encephalitis
  - Lupus
  - Parkinson's disease
  - Multiple sclerosis
  - Meningitis
  - Lyme disease
  - Subacute bacterial endocarditis
  - Pregnancy
  - Electrolyte disturbance (hypernatremia, hyponatremia, hypomagnesemia, hypocalcemia, and hypercalcemia)
  - Polycythemia
  - Hepatic and renal failure
  - Vitamin B_1 and B_{12} deficiency
  - Trauma (cerebral palsy)
  - Toxins: carbon monoxide, cyanide, methanol
  - Alcohol
  - Medication induced

HISTORY OF COMPLAINT

Symptomatology

Ask about the following characteristics of each symptom using open-ended questions:

- Onset
- Chronology
- Location
- Timing and duration
- Quality
- Severity
- Precipitating factors
- Relieving factors
- Associated symptoms
- Effects on daily activities
- Previous diagnosis of similar episodes
- Previous treatments and efficacy of previous treatments
- Family history

DIRECTED QUESTIONS TO ASK

- When does this tend to occur?
- How quick is the onset?
- How long does it last?
- Does anything seem to make it occur?
- Can you describe the tremors?
- Does it affect one muscle or group of muscles?
- What makes it worse?
- Does anything make it better?
- How long have you had the tremors?
- Does it affect your daily activities?
- Does it cause you pain? If so, rate your pain on a scale of 0 to 10, with 0 being no pain and 10 being the most pain.
- Any family history of neurological or muscular diseases?
- Important past medical history (stroke, trauma, hormonal disorders)?
- Any change in medications (start or stop)?
- Any other symptoms associated with the tremors?
- Have you been sick recently (dehydration)?

Assessment: Cardinal Signs and Symptoms

General

- Fatigue
- Irritability
- Anxious

Head, Eyes, Ears, Nose, Throat (HEENT)

- Facial twitching
- Facial droop
- Ptosis
- Dysphagia
- Facial weakness
- Slow or abnormal eye movements
- Difficult with production of speech

Cardiac
- Chest pain

Respiratory
- Shortness of breath

Gastrointestinal
- Abdominal pain
- Diarrhea
- Constipation
- Vomiting

Genitourinary
- Dysuria
- Excessive urination
- Loss of bowel or bladder control

Musculoskeletal
- Impaired gait
- Rigidity
- Muscle contracture
- Impaired posture and balance
- Pain
- Tenderness
- Neuropathy

Neurologic
- Difficulty organizing, prioritizing, and focusing
- Lack of impulse control
- Lack of awareness
- Slowness in processing or "finding" words
- Difficulty learning new information

Medical History

- Surgeries: cholecystectomy, appendectomy
- Allergies: penicillin
- Medication: atorvastatin, ibuprofen for pain
- Health maintenance: received flu shot this year and is up to date on childhood vaccinations

Current Medical History
- Hyperlipidemia

Family History
- Father: diagnosed with Huntington's disease at age 50, currently in a nursing home
- Mother: coronary artery disease (CAD) and hypertension (HTN)

Social History
- Nonsmoker
- No drug/alcohol
- Married and currently working in the banking industry

PHYSICAL EXAMINATION

Vital Signs

- Temperature
- Pulse
- Respiration
- Oxygen saturation (SpO$_2$)
- Blood pressure (BP)

General Appearance

- State of health
- Any distress
- Difficulty sleeping
- Fatigue

HEENT

- Eye: ptosis, twitching
- Facial droop
- Movement of neck and head
- Speech

Cardiac

- Palpitations
- Chest pain

Respiratory

- Shortness of breath

Musculoskeletal

- Rigidity
- Balance and gait
- Posturing
- Grip strength

Psychology

- Mood
- Thinking pattern

CASE STUDY

History

Directed Question	Response
When does this tend to occur?	I experience throughout the day, morning, afternoon, and night.
How quick is the onset of the movements?	Sudden onset of jerking, became progressively worse.
How long do the movements last?	A few seconds at a time.
What aggravates it?	When I get nervous or more anxious sometimes.

Directed Question	*Response*
What alleviates it?	*Nothing.*
Does it affect one muscle or group of muscles?	*The movements affect my neck and tremors in my hands.*
How long have you had the tremors?	*The movements have progressively set in over the past year.*
Does it affect your daily activities?	*Yes, it is difficult to hold objects and focus when speaking to someone. Sometimes I forget what I was talking about.*
Does it cause you pain? If so, rate your pain on a scale of 0 to 10, with 0 being no pain and 10 being the most pain.	*Yes, my muscles in my hands get very painful at the end of the day, probably about an 8/10.*
Have you ever been diagnosed with a neurological or muscular disease? Any family history of neurological or muscular diseases?	*My father was diagnosed with Huntington's disease at the age of 50.*
Important past medical history (stroke or trauma)?	*No major past medical history that would cause the involuntary movements.*
Any changes in medication (start or stop)?	*No changes in medication.*
Any other symptoms associated with the tremors?	*I feel less able to focus, and my wife says I've become very impulsive.*

Physical Examination Findings

- VITAL SIGNS: temperature 98.5°F; respiratory rate (RR) 15; heart rate (HR) 85, regular; BP 128/80; SpO$_2$ 97% room air
- GENERAL APPEARANCE: anxious and fidgety
- EYES: pupils equal, round, and reactive to light and accommodation (PERRLA); extraocular movements intact
- NECK: no enlarged lymph nodes palpable; neck is supple; thyroid is not enlarged; involuntary movement of head and neck
- CHEST/CARDIOVASCULAR: lung sounds are clear in all fields; regular rate and rhythm (RRR); heart S1, S2 no murmur, gallop, or rub
- EXTREMITIES: uncontrollable twitching of hands, stable gait, unable to hold items in each hand; rigidity in bilateral shoulders
- NEUROLOGIC: fixated on pamphlets in room, unable to focus on answering questions completely

DIFFERENTIAL DIAGNOSIS

Clinical Observations	Parkinson's Disease	Huntington's Disease	Stroke
Onset	Gradual	Gradual	Sudden
Pain	Yes	Yes	Yes/No

(continued)

Clinical Observations	Parkinson's Disease	Huntington's Disease	Stroke
Inherited	No	Yes	No
Movement location	Typically in hands	Nonspecific (can occur in multiple extremities)	No
Change in mood/behavior	No	Yes	Possible
Other symptoms	Writing changes	Insomnia, mania	Unilateral symptoms

DIAGNOSTIC EXAMINATION

Exam	Code	Cost	Results
CBC without differential	68.89	$25–$100	**CBC** **WBC count** • White blood cell count • High WBC count can be a sign of infection (bacterial or viral) • WBC count is also increased in certain types of leukemia • Low white blood cell counts can be a sign of bone marrow diseases, possible HIV infection, or an enlarged spleen **Hgb and Hct** • Hgb is the amount of oxygen-carrying protein contained within the red blood cells • Hct is the percentage of the blood volume occupied by red blood cells • Low Hgb and Hct suggest an anemia • Anemia can be due to nutritional deficiencies, blood loss, destruction of blood cells internally, or failure to produce blood in the bone marrow **PLT** • This is the number of cells that collect in blood vessels and prevent bleeding • High values can occur with bleeding • Low values can occur with anticoagulant use or forms of leukemia
Complete metabolic panel	I10	$28–$46	A comprehensive metabolic panel is a group of blood tests. They provide an overall picture of the body's chemical balance and metabolism. **Normal levels** • Albumin: 3.4–5.4 g/dL • Alkaline phosphatase: 44–147 IU/L • ALT: 10–40 IU/L • AST: 10–34 IU/L • BUN: 6–20 mg/dL • Calcium: 8.5–10.2 mg/dL • Chloride: 96–106 mEq/L • CO_2: 23–29 mEq/L

(continued)

Exam	Code	Cost	Results
			• Creatinine: 0.6–1.3 mg/dL • Glucose: 70–100 mg/dL • Potassium: 3.5–5.0 mEq/L • Sodium: 135–145 mEq/L • Total bilirubin: 0.3–1.9 mg/dL • Total protein: 6.0–8.3 g/dL **Decreased potassium:** suggests dehydration **Elevated sodium:** suggests dehydration **Elevated BUN/creatinine:** suggests kidney damage/disease **Elevated ALT/AST:** suggests liver damage/disease
CT of head	R93	$1,200	CT images of internal organs, bones, soft tissue, and blood vessels typically provide greater detail than traditional x-rays, particularly of soft tissues and blood vessels. CT scanning provides more detailed information on head injuries, stroke, brain tumors, and other brain diseases than regular radiographs (x-rays). CT scanning of the head is typically used to detect: Bleeding, brain injury, and skull fractures in patients with head injuries • Bleeding caused by a ruptured or leaking aneurysm in a patient with a sudden severe headache • A blood clot or bleeding within the brain shortly after a patient exhibits symptoms of a stroke • A stroke, especially with a new technique called perfusion CT • Brain tumors • Enlarged brain cavities (ventricles) in patients with hydrocephalus • Diseases or malformations of the skull
MRI	94.02	$600–$1,550	MRI of the body uses a powerful magnetic field, radio waves, and a computer to produce detailed pictures of the inside of your body Unlike conventional x-ray examinations and CT scans, MRI does not utilize ionizing radiation. Instead, radio waves redirect alignment of hydrogen atoms that naturally exist within the body while you are in the scanner without causing any chemical changes in the tissues. As the hydrogen atoms return to their usual alignment, they emit energy that varies according to the type of body tissue from which they come. The magnetic resonance scanner captures this energy and creates a picture of the tissues scanned based on this information **Head.** MRI can look at the brain for tumors, an aneurysm, bleeding in the brain, nerve injury, and other problems, such as damage caused by a stroke. MRI can also find problems of the eyes and optic nerves, and the ears and auditory nerves.
HD genetic test (CAG repeat)	Z13.79	$2,000 or greater	Tests for the number of repetitive CAG groups in genes Number of CAG repeats: 26 or less (normal risk); patient will not develop HD 27–35 (intermediate risk); patient will not develop HD 36–39 (increased risk with reduced penetrance); patient is likely HD at some point in their lifetime, but it may be mild or later in life 40 or more (faulty gene with HD range with full penetrance); patient will almost likely to develop HD if they live a normal life span

ALT, alanine amino transferase; AST, aspartate amino transferase; BUN, blood urea nitrogen; CBC, complete blood count; Hct, hematocrit; HD, Huntington's disease; Hgb, hemoglobin; PLT, platelet count; WBC, white blood cell.

CLINICAL DECISION MAKING

Case Study Analysis

After history and examination were obtained, the patient continued to have tremors of his hands and involuntary movement of his neck. He also became manic and had to seek psychiatric care for impulsive behavior and suicidal ideations. Complete blood count (CBC) was normal; no anemia or infection was suggested by results. Complete metabolic panel (CMP) suggests normal kidney and liver function and no signs of dehydration or electrolyte imbalance. MRI of the brain showed atrophy of the caudate nucleus with concomitant enlargement of the frontal horns of the lateral ventricles. Huntington's disease genetic test revealed the presence of 42 CAG repeats in the HD gene. The patient's symptoms and results of diagnostic testing ruled out Parkinson's disease and stroke.

> **Diagnosis:** *Huntington's disease*

The diagnosis is Huntington's disease. He has familial traits for Huntington's disease and his involuntary movements have progressed over time. The patient also experienced psychological changes with increased manic behavior. The patient is likely to experience more progressive symptoms that will become completely debilitating and require him to receive 24-hour care. There is no cure for Huntington's disease. There are medications that can reduce the magnitude of tremors and help with the psychological changes, but there is not a medication or therapy to cure the disease.

The patient is being watched by the neurology clinic.

UNSTEADY GAIT

Case Presentation: A 68-year-old female reports to the office with a complaint of "not feeling steady" on her feet.

INTRODUCTION TO COMPLAINT

An unsteady gait can be the result of disease or conditions that result in an imbalance of/or damage to the musculoskeletal structures of the hips, legs, or feet. Additionally, disease or conditions that result in damage to the nervous system that controls movement necessary for walking can cause an unsteady gait.

Severity of the gait problem can vary from barely detectable to severely impacting the activities of daily living for the affected individual.

HISTORY OF COMPLAINT

Symptomatology

Ask about the following characteristics of each symptom using open-ended questions:

- Onset (sudden or gradual)
- Chronology
- Current situation (improving or deteriorating)
- Location
- Radiation
- Quality
- Timing (frequency, duration)
- Severity
- Precipitating and aggravating factors
- Relieving factors
- Associated symptoms
- Effects on daily activities
- Previous diagnosis of similar episodes
- Previous treatments
- Efficacy of previous treatments

Directed Questions to Ask

- When did you first notice the problem with your walking?
- Have you recently had an accident or sustained injury to your hips, legs, or feet?
- Do you have any pain?
- Are you experiencing any dizziness?

- Have you experienced any visual disturbances?
- Do you have diabetes?
- Have you had any recent changes in your medications?
- Have you had any recent serious viral illnesses?
- Is there a history of any neuromuscular disorders or diseases in your family?
- Are you having headaches?
- Do you drink alcohol? If yes, what and how often?
- Are you experiencing any tremors or shakes?
- Have you been undergoing cancer treatment with chemotherapy?

Assessment: Cardinal Signs and Symptoms

- Impaired walking mechanics

Medical History: General

- Medical conditions and surgeries
- Allergies (seasonal, as well as others)
- Medication currently used (prescription, birth control pill [BCP], and over the counter [OTC])
- Herbal preparations and traditional therapies

Medical History: Specific to Complaint

- Recent injury
- Recent infection
- Diabetes
- Visual disturbances
- Dizziness
- Headaches
- Personal and/or family history of neuromuscular diseases/disorders

PHYSICAL EXAMINATION
Vital Signs

- Temperature
- Pulse
- Respiration
- Oxygen saturation (SpO_2)
- Blood pressure (BP)

General Appearance

- Apparent state of health
- Appearance of comfort or distress
- Color and temperature of skin
- State of hydration

Musculoskeletal

- Inspect for size and symmetry of knees and ankles; lower extremities for signs of injury
- Palpate for height of iliac crest bilaterally with the patient standing
- Evaluate range of motion (ROM) hips, knees, ankles

Neurologic

- Test cranial nerves (CNs) II to XII
- Test sensory capability of lower extremities
- Testing of extremity strength
- Observe the patient walk

CASE STUDY

History

Directed Question	Response
When did you first notice the problem with your walking?	I have been feeling a little less "stable" on my feet for a few months now.
Have you recently had an accident or sustained injury to your hips, legs, or feet?	No.
Do you have any pain?	I have some nagging low back pain all the time.
Are you experiencing any dizziness?	No.
Have you experienced any visual disturbances?	No.
Do you have diabetes?	No.
Have you had any recent changes in your medications?	No.
Have you had any recent serious viral illnesses?	No.
Is there a history of any neuromuscular disorders or diseases in your family?	No.
Are you having headaches?	No.
Do you drink alcohol? If yes, what and how often?	No.
Are you experiencing any tremors or shakes?	No.
Have you been undergoing cancer treatment with chemotherapy?	No.

Physical Examination Findings

- VITAL SIGNS: temperature 97.4°F; respiratory rate (RR) 14; heart rate (HR) 62, regular; BP 108/67; SpO$_2$ 97%
- GENERAL APPEARANCE: well-developed, healthy-appearing female in no acute distress
- MUSCULOSKELETAL: no joint deformities or major limitations of ROM of hips, knees, or ankles noted; iliac crest higher on the right than the left
- NEUROLOGIC: CNs II to XII grossly intact, no diminished sensory capacity noted, strength testing lower extremities 5/5

DIFFERENTIAL DIAGNOSIS

Clinical Observations	Physical Injury Lower Extremity	Postviral	Neuropathy	Structural	Other Etiologies
Gait disturbance	Yes	Yes/No	Yes/No	Yes/No	Yes/No
Pain	Yes/No	Yes/No	Yes	Yes/No	Yes/No
Dizziness	No	Yes/No	No	Yes/No	Yes/No

DIAGNOSTIC EXAMINATION

Exam	Code	Cost	Results
Comprehensive metabolic panel	80053	$49	May identify hyperglycemia, which is a common cause of peripheral neuropathy; may identify electrolyte disturbances such as hyponatremia, which can impact neurologic function
CT scan	70450	Varies by market—$270–$4,800	CT of head to detect a causative factor for the unsteady gait

CLINICAL DECISION MAKING

Case Study Analysis

The patient's complete metabolic panel (CMP) was within normal limits. CT scan of the head was negative for pathology. The absence of a traumatic injury ruled out a physical injury as the cause for the symptoms. The absence of dizziness and radiating pain ruled out a postviral disorder and neuropathy. Uneven iliac crests support the diagnosis of pelvic rotation.

The patient is provided with instruction and printed materials on daily exercise to address her pelvic rotation. She is to follow up in 1 month. The patient may need a referral to orthopedic or neurologic clinic if symptoms persist after 1 month of exercises. The patient is also encouraged to wear low-heeled shoes and use OTC analgesics for pain management. Heat application was also recommended for lower back muscle tension/pain. Unsteady gait can be secondary to a wide range of etiologies; beyond initial screening and planning, patients with unresolved gait disturbances should be referred to a medical specialist for evaluation.

> **Diagnosis:** Gait disturbance, low back pain, pelvic rotation

VAGINAL DISCHARGE

Case Presentation: *A 33-year-old married female presents to the clinic with a vaginal discharge associated with a strong odor for the past 3 days.*

INTRODUCTION TO COMPLAINT

A vaginal discharge may be caused by a bacterial infection, a retained tampon, or vaginal dryness from atrophic vaginitis.

Infectious Process

Bacterial Vaginitis
- Alkaline vaginal pH due to menstrual blood, semen, or decrease in lactobacilli
- Poor perineal hygiene, especially in patients who are incontinent or have limited mobility
- Chemicals in the bubble bath or soap
- Introduction of foreign objects
- Low estrogen can be a predisposing factor for vaginitis
- Use of antibiotics
- Pregnancy
- Diabetes mellitus

Candida Vaginitis
- An overgrowth of bacteria of the normal flora
- Causes alteration in vaginal pH
- Discharge looks like cottage cheese and adheres to the vaginal wall
- Sometimes worsens after intercourse and before menses
- Common result of recent antibiotic use or history of diabetes
- Identified by a vaginal pH <4.5 with identifications of yeast or hyphae on a wet mount or potassium hydroxide (KOH) preparation

Trichomonal Vaginitis
- Caused by the protozoan *Trichomonas vaginalis*
- A sexually transmitted disease (STD) that presents with discharge that is diffuse, malodorous, and yellow–green with irritation

Atrophic Vaginitis
- Most common cause of vaginitis
- Discharge associated with atrophic vaginitis
- May be initially misdiagnosed as a yeast infection
- Discharge does not have a foul odor
- The microscopic examination is negative for findings indicative of yeast or common bacterial infections

Cervicitis

- Resembles vaginitis
- Abdominal pain, cervical motion tenderness, or cervical inflammation suggests pelvic inflammatory disease (PID)

Noninfectious Process

- Hypersensitivity or irritant reactions to hygiene sprays or perfumes, menstrual pads, laundry soaps, bleaches, fabric softeners, fabric dyes, synthetic fibers, bathwater additives, toilet tissue, or, occasionally, spermicides, vaginal lubricants or creams, latex condoms, vaginal contraceptive rings, or diaphragms
- A retained tampon is another common cause of vaginal odor and discharge

HISTORY OF COMPLAINT

Symptomatology

Ask about the following characteristics of each symptom using open-ended questions:

- Onset, gradual or abrupt
- Location of the discharge, vaginal or rectal
- Timing and frequency
- Aggravating or triggering factors
- Alleviating factors
- Pain associated with the discharge
- Effects on daily life

Directed Questions to Ask

- When did the change or abnormal vaginal discharge begin?
- Do you have the same amount and type of vaginal discharge throughout the month?
- What does the discharge look like (color and consistency)?
- Is there an odor?
- Do you have pain, itching, or burning?
- Does your sexual partner have a discharge as well?
- Do you have multiple sexual partners or sexual partners whom you do not know very well?
- What type of birth control do you use?
- Do you use condoms?
- Is there anything that relieves the discharge?
- Have you tried over-the-counter creams? Have they helped?
- Do you douche?
- Do you have any other symptoms like abdominal pain, vaginal itching, fever, vaginal bleeding, rash, genital warts or lesions, or changes in urination like difficulty, pain, or blood?
- Have you recently changed the detergents or soaps that you use?
- Do you frequently wear very tight clothing?

Assessment: Cardinal Signs and Symptoms

- Foul-smelling, white, cheesy discharge
- Painful intercourse

Medical History: General

- Current medical problems
- Past medical problems
- Past surgeries
- Current medications
- Medication allergies
- Family history
- Social history

Medical History: Specific to Complaint

- Menstrual history
- History of numerous sex partners
- Unprotected sex
- History of STDs in past 2 years

PHYSICAL EXAMINATION

Vital Signs

- Temperature
- Pulse
- Respiration
- SpO_2
- Blood pressure (BP)

Inspection and Palpation of the External Genitalia

- The external genitalia are examined, some mild erythema and irritation noted on the labia
- There is no swelling or blood noted
- The inguinal nodes are palpated and no tenderness noted
- Some discharge is noted on the vagina that is thick, milky, and gray in color, with a fishy odor

Speculum Assessment of the Internal Genitalia and Inspection of the Vaginal Wall

- The vaginal is wall noted to have some discharge
- No pain on insertion of the speculum, the cervix is normal in color
- Vaginal pH is measured and samples and secretions are taken for assessment. A high pH above 4.5 is associated with bacterial vaginosis. A pH below 4.5 is normal

Bimanual Examination

- No cervical motion tenderness and adnexal or uterine tenderness; the uterus is palpable

CASE STUDY

History

Directed Question	Response
Describe the discharge	*It was gray to greenish.*
When was the onset and duration?	*About 3 days ago.*

Directed Question	*Response*
Is there an odor?	*Yes.*
Are the symptoms associated with your period?	*No.*
Are you experiencing pain? If yes, when?	*No, no pain, perhaps a little irritation in the vagina with sex.*
Do you have itching, rash?	*No.*

Physical Examination Findings

- VITAL SIGNS: temperature 98.6°F; respiratory rate (RR) 18; heart rate (HR) 68; blood pressure (BP) 120/80
- GENERAL APPEARANCE: healthy young female; skin is warm, dry; no lesions, or acne; good hygiene; weight 123 lb; height 5′2″
- Has sexual intercourse with husband at least once a week, not using any lubricant
- Last Pap smear was a year ago and was normal
- Vaginal discharge is milky, gray in color with a "terrible," fishy odor; denies any blood, pain, or burning when urinating; no noticeable redness, irritation, lesion, or wound in the vaginal area
- Current medications include calcium pills

DIFFERENTIAL DIAGNOSIS

Clinical Observations	Bacterial Vaginitis	Candida	Trichomoniasis
Discharge	Yes	Yes	Yes
Color/characteristics	White, gray, or yellow	White, cheesy	Frothy yellow or greenish
Odor	Fishy	No	Foul
Pain	No	On intercourse, around vulva	On urination
Other symptoms	Itching, burning, redness, swelling of vulva/vagina	Itching, burning, vulvar swelling	Itching, burning

DIAGNOSTIC EXAMINATION

Exam	Code	Cost	Results
KOH	87210	$10.53	• Two-slide preparation: (a) 10% KOH, (b) NS • 10% KOH slide: will be positive for fishy odor 76% of the time in the presence of BV (whiff test) • Examine under microscope for branching and budding hyphae—characteristic of yeast (*Candida*) infection

(continued)

Exam	Code	Cost	Results
			• Clue cells (epithelial cells imbedded with bacteria) are characteristic of BV • NS slide: Examine under microscope for motile trichomonads that signal the presence of *Trichomonas*
pH testing	83986	$7.90	• Using litmus paper: normal vaginal secretions have pH <4.5 • A higher pH is consistent with BV, trichomoniasis, or atrophic vaginitis • pH of 4.0–4.7 consistent with *Candida* • pH of 6.5–7.0 may indicate atrophic vaginitis (if few WBCs and negative for pathogens)
Wet mount	87070	$23.26	• If pH <4.5, wet mount reveals up to three to five WBCs/high power field and the presence of epithelial cells and lactobacilli (may be physiological discharge) • WBCs high in the presence of foreign body

BV, bacterial vaginitis; KOH, potassium hydroxide; NS, normal saline; WBC, white blood cell.

CLINICAL DECISION MAKING

Case Study Analysis

The following pertinent positives were found: patient reports milky gray fishy-smelling discharge ongoing for 3 days. Menses are regular. pH of vaginal secretions is elevated and there is a positive whiff test with clue cells present on microscopy. Pertinent negatives are no pain with sexual intercourse, no itching, burning, or swelling of vagina. No new sexual partner. No budding yeast or mycelia present on microscopic examination. A candida infection is ruled out because the discharge is not white or cheesy appearing. A trichomoniasis infection is ruled out because the discharge is not frothy and the patient has no pain upon urination.

> ***Diagnosis:*** *Bacterial vaginosis*

The patient is prescribed an oral antibiotic for 7 days and counseled to complete the entire prescription. Reinforced information on female hygiene practices to include wearing loose-fitting cotton underwear, cleansing from front to back when toileting, and avoiding douching and bubble baths. The patient was also counseled to follow up if the symptoms do not subside or worsen. Additional testing for pregnancy or diabetes may be indicated if the condition persists.

VAGINAL ITCHINESS

Case Presentation: A 27-year-old female reports experiencing vaginal itchiness for the past 2 weeks.

INTRODUCTION TO COMPLAINT

Vaginal itching can be the result of numerous etiologies. The most common cause is a yeast infection.

Infections

- Yeast: A small number of yeast organisms share a symbiotic relationship with our bodies. When shifts in vaginal conditions occur (e.g., change in pH, mechanical irritation, hormonal shifts) the number of yeast organisms increases resulting in an infection
- Bacterial vaginosis: Bacteria, often referred to as "normal flora," share a symbiotic relationship with our bodies. When shifts in vaginal conditions occur (e.g., change in pH, mechanical irritation, hormonal shifts) imbalance in the normal flora in the vagina often results. Often this shift results in symptoms of "itching" and development of a "fishy odor"

Parasitic

- Trichomoniasis (trich): a sexually transmitted disease (STD) caused by the protozoan organism, *Trichomonas vaginalis*; often results in a watery, malodorous discharge
- Pinworms: *Enterobius vermicularis,* infection in children more common than adults; adult women can be infected and the worms migrate to the perineum, which can cause itching

Viral

- Herpes simplex virus: an STD

Noninfectious

- Often secondary to an allergic or "irritation" reaction to vaginal sprays, douches, spermicides, soaps, detergents, fabric softeners, or retained feminine hygiene products. Additionally, decreases or imbalances of hormones can result in atrophic vaginitis

HISTORY OF COMPLAINT

Symptomatology

Ask about the following characteristics of each symptom using open-ended questions:

- Onset (sudden or gradual)
- Chronology

- Current situation (improving or deteriorating)
- Location
- Radiation
- Quality
- Timing (frequency, duration)
- Severity
- Precipitating and aggravating factors
- Relieving factors
- Associated symptoms
- Effects on daily activities
- Previous diagnosis of similar episodes
- Previous treatments
- Efficacy of previous treatments

Directed Questions to Ask

- When did you first note the vaginal itching?
- Do you have a vaginal discharge?
- Do you have a vaginal odor?
- Do you have multiple sex partners?
- Do you have a history of genital herpes?
- Do you know if any of your sexual partners have genital herpes?
- Do you use condoms and/or spermicides when having intercourse?
- Do you use tampons?
- Are you using any new personal hygiene products, laundry detergents, soaps, perfumes?
- Do you wear very tight pants routinely?
- Do you douche?
- Have you noted any worms in your bowel movements?
- Have you used anything to help relieve the itching?

Assessment: Cardinal Signs and Symptoms

- Vaginal itching

Medical History: General

- Medical conditions and surgeries
- Allergies (seasonal as well as others)
- Medication currently used (prescription, birth control pill [BCP], and over the counter [OTC])
- Herbal preparations and traditional therapies

Medical History: Specific to Complaint

- Genital herpes or other STDs
- Multiple sex partners

PHYSICAL EXAMINATION
Vital Signs

- Temperature
- Pulse
- Respiration

- Oxygen saturation (SpO$_2$)
- Blood pressure (BP)

General Appearance

- Apparent state of health
- Appearance of comfort or distress
- Color
- State of hydration

External Genitalia

- Inspect for signs of irritation, lesions, erythema, swelling, discharge, atrophic changes
- Palpate for enlarged lymph nodes or tender glands

Internal Genitalia

- Inspect for signs of irritation, lesions, erythema, discharge, atrophic changes, or retained tampon
- Consider measuring the pH of the vaginal discharge; >4.5 associated with bacterial vaginosis

CASE STUDY

History

Directed Question	Response
When did you first note the vaginal itching?	*A couple weeks ago.*
Do you have a vaginal discharge?	*Not really.*
Do you have a vaginal odor?	*Not noticed an odor.*
Do you have multiple sex partners?	*No.*
Do you have a history of genital herpes?	*No.*
Do you know if any of your sexual partners have genital herpes?	*My current partner doesn't have genital herpes. Not aware that any of my sexual partners have had herpes.*
Do you use condoms and/or spermicides when having intercourse?	*No, I am on birth control pills.*
Are you using any new personal hygiene products, laundry detergents, soaps, perfumes?	*No.*
Do you wear very tight pants routinely?	*Yes, I practically live in my yoga pants.*
Do you douche?	*No.*
Have you noted any worms in your bowel movements?	*Uh, no!*
Have you used anything to help relieve the itching?	*Tried some over-the-counter "stuff" that really didn't help much.*

PHYSICAL EXAMINATION FINDINGS

- VITAL SIGNS: temperature 98.0°F; respiratory rate (RR) 15; heart rate (HR) 82, regular; BP 100/58; SpO$_2$ 98%
- GENERAL APPEARANCE: well-developed, healthy-appearing female in no acute distress
- EXTERNAL GENITALIA: erythema and mild swelling noted, no lesions noted, no atrophic changes noted, mild discomfort with palpation, no enlarged lymph nodes
- INTERNAL GENITALIA: no irritation, lesions, swelling, atrophic changes or discharge noted

DIFFERENTIAL DIAGNOSIS

Clinical Observations	Yeast	Bacterial Vaginosis	Parasitic	Viral	Noninfectious
Itching	Typically	Typically	Typically	Typically	Typically
Discharge	White, cheesy	White, gray, or yellow	Trich: frothy yellow or greenish; pinworms—none typical	No	No
Lesions	No	No	No	Yes	No
Burning	Possible	Possible	Possible	Possible	Possible

Trich, trichomoniasis.

DIAGNOSTIC EXAMINATION

Exam	Code	Cost	Results
pH testing	83986	Cost of pH paper, which is minimal	Normal is <4.5; higher pH is associated with bacterial vaginosis, trich, or atrophic vaginitis; based on pH value further testing may be indicated—including KOH or wet mount

Trich, trichomoniasis; KOH, potassium hydroxide.

CLINICAL DECISION MAKING

Case Study Analysis

Visible inflammation and mild swelling of the external genitalia. There is an absence of discharge, which rules out yeast, bacterial vaginosis, parasitic, and viral as a source of infection. Recommended that the patient not wear her yoga pants except for when she is doing a yoga routine. Also recommended that she wear underpants with a natural, cotton lining until the symptoms resolve. The patient was also counseled to avoid douching and taking bubble baths since these chemicals are irritating to vaginal tissues. A follow-up in 2 weeks is suggested if symptoms do not subside or persist.

Diagnosis: Noninfectious vaginitis

VAGINAL LESIONS

Case Presentation: A 19-year-old female reports that she has "sores" on and in her vagina. She tries to practice safe sex but has a steady boyfriend and figures she does not need to be so careful since she is on the birth control pill (BCP).

INTRODUCTION TO COMPLAINT

Sores in the perineal area can be painless or painful. Several sexually transmitted infections (STIs) are the most common cause of these sores.

Viral Infections

- Caused by a viral infection, such as herpes simplex virus (HSV-I, HSV-II) or human papillomavirus
- Transmitted through intimate contact with a person who is shedding the virus
- Herpes simplex viral infection can be triggered by stress
- Other viral infections, such as molluscum contagiosum

Bacterial Infections

- A bacterial infection, such as syphilis
- Transmitted through unprotected sexual intercourse with an infected person
- Other infections, such as chancroid or granuloma inguinale

Irritants and Injuries

- Sores in the perineal area also can be caused by some kind of trauma
- These are usually transmitted from person to person through unprotected sex
- A person can be infected and not know it; the sores may be triggered by some kind of event, such as hormonal stimuli, stress, or menstruation

HISTORY OF COMPLAINT

Symptomatology

Ask about the following characteristics of each symptom using open-ended questions:

- Chronology
- Current situation (improving or deteriorating)
- Location
- Radiation
- Quality
- Timing (frequency, duration)
- Severity

- Precipitating and aggravating factors
- Relieving factors
- Associated symptoms
- Effects on daily activities
- Previous diagnosis of similar episodes
- Previous treatments
- Efficacy of previous treatments

Directed Questions to Ask

- When did you first notice the sores?
- Was the onset sudden or gradual?
- Are the sores itchy?
- Have you had any swelling, burning, or redness?
- Are the sores painful?
- If 10 is the worse pain you have ever had and 0 is no pain, what number is the pain?
- Do you have any drainage from the sores?
- Do you have any rashes on your palms or soles of your feet?
- Have you had any fever?
- Have you noticed these sores anywhere else?
- Have you noticed a foul-smelling discharge?
- Do you use condoms during sexual intercourse?
- Have you ever been diagnosed with an STI? If so, what was it?
- Has your boyfriend ever been diagnosed with an STI? If so, what was it?
- Are both you and your boyfriend committed to a monogamous relationship?
- When was your last Pap smear? Have you ever had any abnormal results?

Assessment: Cardinal Signs and Symptoms

Genital/Urinary
- Pain or difficulty when urinating
- Urinary tract infection
- Blood in urine
- Length and time of menstrual cycle
- Vaginal bleeding: how long and how much?
- Foul or yellow/green vaginal discharge
- Vaginal lesions
- Vaginal infections

Medical History: General

- Medical conditions and surgeries
- Allergies
- Medications currently prescribed and over the counter (OTC)
- Herbal preparations and traditional therapies

Medical History: Specific to Complaint

- Vaginal infections
- Trauma to vaginal area
- Surgery in vaginal area
- Urinary tract infections
- STIs
- Last pap smear: What were the results?

- Have you ever been pregnant? If so, how many children? Any miscarriages?
- Have you ever had an abortion?

PHYSICAL EXAMINATION
Vital Signs
- Temperature
- Pulse
- Respiration
- Blood pressure (BP)
- Weight
- Height

General Appearance
- Apparent state of health
- Appearance of comfort or distress
- Color
- Nutritional status
- State of hydration
- Hygiene

Genital/Urinary Inspection
- Skin: note the color, texture
- Mons pubis, labia majora and minora, urethral meatus, clitoris, vaginal introitus, and perineum: note any inflammation, excoriation, ulceration, discharge, swelling, or nodules
- Vagina, vaginal walls: note the color, and any inflammation, ulceration, discharge, swelling, or nodules
- Cervix: note the color, position, characteristics of the surface, and any ulcerations, nodules, masses, bleeding, or discharge; palpate the cervix to check position, shape, consistency, regularity, mobility, and tenderness
- Uterus, ovaries: palpate the size, shape, consistency, and mobility; note any tenderness or masses
- Pelvic muscles: check for strength, tenderness during contraction, appropriate relaxation after contraction and endurance

Palpation
- Any nodules or lumps (inguinal nodes); note the size, consistency, position, and tenderness

CASE STUDY
History

Directed Question	Response
When did you first notice the sores?	*Three months ago.*
Was the onset sudden or gradual?	*Gradual.*
Are the sores itchy?	*No.*

Directed Question	*Response*
Have you had any swelling, burning, or redness?	*Swelling and burning during urination.*
Are the sores painful?	*Yes, very, during intercourse and urination.*
If 10 is the worse pain you have ever had and 0 is no pain, what number is the pain?	*5.5.*
Do you have any drainage from the sores?	*Yes, there is yellowish discharge from the sores that comes and goes.*
Do you have any rashes on your palms or soles of your feet?	*No.*
Have you had any fevers?	*Yes, I have a fever now and had a fever of 100°F yesterday.*
Have you noticed these sores anywhere else?	*Yes, I have bumps on the inner creases of my thighs and pelvic area.*
Have you noticed a foul-smelling discharge?	*No.*
Do you use condoms during sexual intercourse?	*No.*
Have you even been diagnosed with an STI?	*No.*
Has your boyfriend ever been diagnosed with an STI? If so, what was it?	*Not that I know of.*
Are both you and your boyfriend committed to a monogamous relationship?	*Yes, we have been committed for the past year.*
When was your last Pap smear?	*My first and only Pap smear was 3 years ago when I was 16 years old. I received birth control from a free clinic that does not require pelvic examinations for prescription refills.*
Have you ever had any abnormal results?	*No.*
What types of food do you usually eat?	*I eat a lot of junk food.*
How many glasses of water do you drink a day?	*I don't drink water, but drink a lot of Diet Coke.*

STI, sexually transmitted infection.

Physical Examination Findings

- VITAL SIGNS: temperature 100.2°F; respirations 18; pulse 72; BP 130/88; weight 156 lb, 25 lb overweight; height 5′3″
- GENERAL APPEARANCE: patient appears to have good hygiene; minimal makeup, pierced ears, no tattoos; well nourished (slightly overweight); no obvious distress noted
- CARDIAC: within normal limits, heart rate regular in rhythm

- RESPIRATORY: within normal limits, appropriate lung sounds auscultated, clear and equal bilaterally
- GASTROINTESTINAL: tender during palpation; the left lower quadrant was very tender during palpation; patient denies nausea or vomiting
- INTEGUMENTARY: hot and dry; skin turgor has fast recoil, no tenting noted
- MUSCULOSKELETAL: poor muscle tone; full range of motion of all extremities; no muscle deformities; no history of broken bones prior to fractured femur
- VAGINAL: labia major and minor: numerous ulcerations, too many to count; some ulcerations enter the vaginal introitus; no ulcerations in the vagina mucosa; cervix is clear, some greenish discharge; bimanual exam reveals tenderness in left lower quadrant; able to palpate the left ovary; unable to palpate the right ovary; no tenderness; uterus is normal in size, slight tenderness with cervical mobility; no odor; whiff test is negative; no history of pregnancy or abortion
- INGUINAL LYMPH NODES: tenderness bilaterally, numerous, 1 cm in size; four palpated on right side and three palpated on left side

DIFFERENTIAL DIAGNOSIS

Clinical Observations	Syphilis	Genital Warts	Herpes	Pelvic Inflammatory Disease	Molluscum Contagiosum
Painful	No	No	Yes	Yes	No
Lesions	Yes	Yes	Yes	No	Yes
Itchiness	No	Yes	Yes	No	Yes
Vaginal discharge	No	Yes	Yes	Yes	No
Sexually transmitted	Yes	Yes	Yes	Yes	Yes
Rashes	Yes	No	No	No	No

DIAGNOSTIC EXAMINATION`

Exam	Code	Cost	Results
Serology for syphilis	RPR VDRL EIA 2007443	$49–$79	Detects antibodies for the bacteria that cause syphilis Results in 1–4 days
Viral culture; Tzanck smear	88160	$80–$100	Rapid diagnostic test used to identify multinucleated giant cells from suspected herpes lesions Results available in 1–5 days

(continued)

Exam	Code	Cost	Results
PAP smear ThinPrep	2000137	$5–$33	A microscopic examination of the cells scraped from the cervical opening Results in 1–14 days
Beta hCG, urine qualitative	81025	$45	Tests for pregnancy results available in 24 hours

hCG, human chorionic gonadotropin.

CLINICAL DECISION MAKING

Case Study Analysis

Patient has a fever of 100°F, ulcerated sores with a yellowish discharge causing pain of 5 out of 10, lower left abdominal pain, cervix with greenish discharge, tenderness with cervical mobility, burning on urination, and tenderness of inguinal nodes (~1 cm in size)—four on right side and three on left side. Painful lesions rule out syphilis, genital warts, and molluscum contagiosum as a source of the infection. The presence of lesions rules out PID. The presence of vaginal discharge rules out syphilis and molluscum contagiosum. Absence of a rash rules out syphilis.

> *Diagnosis:* *Genital herpes*

Provided with a prescription for antiviral medication. Counseled to avoid sexual intercourse while lesions present. Additional counseling included taking showers, avoiding tub baths, avoiding douching, personal hygiene approaches when toileting, and wearing loose-fitting clothing with cotton underwear. A follow-up appointment is recommended in 2 weeks if the lesions persist or worsen.

VOMITING

Case Presentation: A 16-year-old female comes to the clinic with her mother because of frequent vomiting for the past 4 months.

INTRODUCTION TO COMPLAINT

Vomiting is a symptom and is associated with the following disorders.

- **Peptic ulcer disease:** This is a constant burning pain that may be accompanied by nausea and/or vomiting.
- **Viral gastroenteritis:** This can occur at any age and usually involves a diffuse, cramping pain along with nausea, vomiting, diarrhea, and low-grade fever. It usually resolves on its own.
- **Bowel obstruction:** Sudden onset of crampy pain usually in umbilical area of epigastrium. Vomiting occurs early with small intestinal obstruction and late with large bowel obstruction.
- **Ileus:** Abdominal distention, vomiting, obstipation, and cramping due to a decreased peristalsis.
- **Acute pancreatitis:** Usually presents with a history of cholelithiasis or alcohol abuse. Pain is steady and boring and is unrelieved by change in position, located in the left upper quadrant and radiates to back; nausea, vomiting, and diaphoresis.
- **Acute cholelithiasis or cholecystitis:** Appears in adults more than children, females more than males, colicky pain progressing to constant pain; located in right upper quadrant that may radiate to right scapular area; pain of cholelithiasis is constant, progressively rising to plateau and falling gradually; nausea, vomiting, and history of dark urine and/or light stools.
- **Renal calculi:** Sudden-onset, excruciating colicky pain that may progress to constant pain. Pain in lower abdomen and flank and radiates to groin; nausea, vomiting, abdominal distention, chills and fever, and increased frequency of urination.
- **Pyelonephritis:** Fever, chills, back pain, nausea and vomiting, toxic appearance. Sometimes frequency and dysuria are associated with pyelonephritis.
- **Salmonella food poisoning:** Acute onset 12 to 24 hours after exposure; lasts 2 to 5 days; moderate to large amounts of nonbloody diarrhea, abdominal cramping, and vomiting.
- **Entamoeba histolytica:** Acute onset 8 to 18 hours after ingestion of contaminated food or water, large amounts of bloody diarrhea, abdominal cramping, and vomiting.
- **Diabetic enteropathy:** Nocturnal diarrhea, postprandial vomiting, fatty stools from malabsorption caused by poorly controlled diabetes.
- **Diabetic ketoacidosis:** Excessive thirst, frequent urination, nausea and vomiting, abdominal pain, weakness or fatigue, shortness of breath, fruity scented breath, and confusion.

- **Pregnancy:** Delayed or irregular menses with sexual activity and no contraception.
- **Brain tumor:** Headaches; nausea and vomiting; changes in speech, vision, or hearing; problems balancing or walking; changes in mood or personality; problems with memory; muscle jerking or twitching; numbness, or tingling in the arms or legs.
- **Appendicitis:** Peaks at age 10 to 20 years. Sudden onset of colicky pain that progresses to a constant pain. The pain may begin in epigastrium or periumbilicus and later localizes to the right lower quadrant (RLQ). Pain worsens with movement or coughing. Vomiting after the onset of pain sometimes occurs. The patient will demonstrate involuntary guarding. Classically, pain occurs in the RLQ. Tests for peritoneal irritation will be positive. Rebound tenderness will be present. Variation in presentation is common, especially in infants, children, and older adults.

HISTORY OF COMPLAINT
Symptomatology

Ask about the following characteristics of each symptom using open-ended questions:

- Gradual or abrupt onset
- Duration, timing, and frequency
- Presence of abdominal pain and location
- Characteristics of emesis
- Triggers
- Medication
- Activities of daily living

Directed Questions to Ask

- Are you sexually active?
- When was your last period?
- Have you had any pain with intercourse?
- Have you had a vaginal discharge or abnormal bleeding?
- Do you vomit at certain times of the day, such as the morning?
- Do you wake up at night to vomit?
- Do you vomit more when you eat certain foods, like fatty or fried foods?
- Do you have any burning in the stomach or chest?
- Is there pain anywhere in your abdominal area?
- Do you have any pain in the back?
- Do you have pain with urination?
- Is there any stress in your life right now?

Assessment: Cardinal Signs and Symptoms

Genitourinary
- Description of any pain
- Last menstrual period
- Regularity of periods

Gastrointestinal
- Bowel function
- Appetite
- Weight loss

Medical History: General

- Surgical history
- Family history
- Social history, including smoking, alcohol, use of drugs, occupation, hobbies, and marital status
- Allergies to medications
- Medication currently used

Medical History: Specific to Complaint

- New medications such as aspirin, ibuprofen, or Naprosyn
- Family history of gastrointestinal diseases
- Exposure to anyone with similar symptoms

PHYSICAL EXAMINATION

Vital Signs

- Temperature
- Blood pressure (BP), supine, sitting, and standing

General Appearance

Eyes
- Observe for icteric sclera

Mouth
- Observe for dry mucous membranes

Neck
- Inspect for abnormal lymph nodes

Chest
- Listen to heart for the rate and rhythm, and the presence of abnormal sounds

Lungs
- Listen for crackles that may indicate a lower lobe pneumonia

Abdomen
- Inspect for previous scars, abdominal distention, or hernias
- Listen to the bowel tones in all quadrants and note if active, hyperactive, or hypoactive
- Palpate the last painful area first with light and then deep palpation
- Assess for enlargement of the liver, spleen, or kidneys as well as any unusual masses

Rectal Examination
- Check for frank or occult blood in the stool

Extremities
- Note whether edema is present

CASE STUDY

History

Directed Question	Response
When did you start vomiting?	A few months ago.
Was it sudden?	Yes, I woke up one morning with it.
Is there a color?	It is clear, or it is what I just ate.
Is there any blood in it?	No, never.
Do you have any fever?	No, I feel okay otherwise.
Do you have any pain in your belly area?	No, nothing hurts.
Does anything make it worse?	Yes, the smell of bacon or fried meats.
Does anything make it better?	Yes, resting or sipping cola.
Do you have any diarrhea or constipation?	No, I go okay.
Is it worse with fried foods?	I don't like fried foods.
Is it worse with milk?	No, milk is fine.
Do you keep any food or fluids down?	Yes, small amounts, I nibble.
Do you have a burning feeling anywhere?	No.
Do you have menstrual periods?	Yes, since I was 14.
Are they regular?	No, they have never been regular.
Have you ever had sex with anyone?	No, that would be against our religion.
Do you have any vaginal discharge?	No.
Do you have any unusual bleeding?	No.
Do you have any back pain?	No.
Do you have any pain with urination?	No.
Do you drink alcohol?	No.
Do you smoke?	No.
Do you use any drugs?	No.
Do you take any medications?	No.
Have you had any surgery on your belly?	No.
Mom, is there any family history of vomiting?	No, she's the only one like this.

Physical Examination Findings

- VITAL SIGNS: temperature 97°F; respiratory rate (RR) 16; heart rate (HR) 88; BP 110/70
- GENERAL APPEARANCE: anxious shy female; mom is asked to leave the room during the examination

- EYES: anicteric
- MOUTH: mucous membrane is moist
- NECK: no lymphadenopathy
- CHEST: heart has normal S1 and S2, no murmur
- LUNGS: clear and resonant without labored breathing
- ABDOMEN: soft, flat with normal bowel tones; nontender, no organomegaly or masses
- PELVIC: external, shows no abnormal lesions; bulbourethral and Skene's glands negative
- VAGINAL: smooth walls with normal rugae; no vaginal discharge
- CERVIX: nulliparous, no cervical motion tenderness
- OVARIES: nonpalpable
- UTERUS: enlarged, smooth, nontender, size 12 weeks
- EXTREMITIES: no edema

DIFFERENTIAL DIAGNOSIS

Clinical Observations	Infection	Food Poisoning	Obstruction	Metabolic Disorder	Appendicitis	Pregnancy	Cholecystitis/Pancreatitis
Onset: gradual/rapid	Rapid	Rapid	Gradual	Gradual	Gradual	Gradual	Rapid
Nausea/vomiting	Nausea and vomiting	Nausea and vomiting	Nausea and possible vomiting depending on location of obstruction	Nausea and vomiting	Nausea and vomiting	Nausea, vomiting intermittent, typically in the morning	Nausea, vomiting intermittent
Malaise	Yes	Yes	Yes	Yes	Yes	None	None
Fever	Possible	Possible	Possible	None	Typically low grade	None	Possible
Diarrhea	Possible	Possible	Possible	None	None	None	None
Bowel sounds, positive or negative	Hyperactive	Hyperactive	Areas of hyperactivity and hypoactivity	Hyperactive	Hyperactive	Normal	Normal
Abdominal pain, positive or negative	All quadrants	All quadrants	Possible around obstruction	Upper abdominal pain	Midline initially, then moves to RLQ	None	Upper right quadrant or epigastric
Liver enlarged	Possible	Possible	Possible	Possible	None	None	Possible
Abnormal laboratory parameters	Elevated WBC count	Elevated WBC count	Elevated WBC count	Elevated WBC count	Elevated WBC count	None	Elevated WBC count, elevated lipase

RLQ, right lower quadrant; WBC, white blood cell.

DIAGNOSTIC EXAMINATION

Exam	Code	Cost	Results
CBC	85025	$10.69	CBC • WBC count: WBCs protect the body against infection. When there is an infection present, the WBC count rises very quickly. The WBC count includes a differential white count • WBC differential: ▪ Neutrophils: The most abundant of the white blood cells. They respond more rapidly to areas of tissue injury and are active during an acute infection ▪ Eosinophils: Are active during allergic or parasitic illnesses ▪ Basophils: Will increase during the healing process ▪ Monocytes: The second defense mechanism against bacterial and inflammatory illnesses; monocytes are slower to respond than neutrophils but are bigger and can ingest larger molecules ▪ Lymphocytes: Become increased after chronic bacterial and viral infections • RBCs: These cells carry O_2 from the lungs to the body • Hematocrit: This is the measure of the amount of space the RBCs take up in the blood • Hemoglobin: This is the molecule that fills up the RBCs • MCV: Shows the size of the RBCs • MCH: Shows the amount of hemoglobin contained in the average RBC • MCHC: Measures the concentration of the hemoglobin in an average RBC • Platelets: The platelets play an important role in blood clotting
Lipase	83690	$9.47	• Elevated level: Indicates possible acute pancreatitis, chronic pancreatitis, cancer of the pancreas, obstruction of the pancreatic duct, perforated ulcer, and acute renal failure
CMP	80053	$14.53	• Glucose level: Is used to determine a possible diagnosis of a prediabetic state or diabetes mellitus • Creatinine clearance: Decreased levels could be an indicator of renal impairment • Alkaline phosphatase, alanine aminotransferase, aspartate aminotransferase: These are all diagnostic tests that indicate how the liver is functioning
Urine pregnancy	84703	$10.33	• Determines whether patient is pregnant
Urinalysis	81003	$3.09	• Color ▪ Red or red–brown: Indication of possible blood in urine, foods such as beets, or medication ▪ Orange: Restricted fluid intake, concentrated urine, medications, and foods such as carrots ▪ Blue or green: *Pseudomonas* toxemia, medications, or yeast concentrate ▪ Black or dark brown: Lysol poisoning, melanin, bilirubin, medications

(*continued*)

Exam	Code	Cost	Results
			• Appearance: Hazy or cloudy appearance can indicate bacteria, WBCs, phosphates. Milky appearance indicates fat or pyuria • Odor: Ammonia—urea breakdown by bacteria; foul—due to bacteria; sweet or fruity—diabetic ketoacidosis • Foam: Liver cirrhosis, bilirubin, or bile • pH: <4.5 = acidosis or diet high in meat; >8 = bacteriuria, UTI • Specific gravity: <1.005 = diabetes insipidus, excess fluid intake, overhydration, renal disease, severe potassium deficit; >1.026 = decreased fluid intake, fever, diabetes mellitus, vomiting, diarrhea, dehydration • Protein: >8 = proteinuria, exercise, severe stress, fever, acute infectious disease, renal disease, lupus, cardiac disease, septicemia • Glucose: >15 = diabetes mellitus, CNS disorders, stroke, Cushing's syndrome, glucose infusions, severe stress, infections • Ketones: +1 to +3 = ketoacidosis, starvation, diet high in proteins • RBCs: >2 = trauma to kidneys, renal diseases, excess aspirin, infection, menstrual contamination • WBCs: >4 UTI, fever, strenuous exercise, lupus, nephritis, renal disease • Casts: Fever, renal diseases, heart failure
Ultrasound abdomen/ pelvis	76700	$158	• Determines presence of masses
CT scan abdomen/ pelvis	74178	$818	• Useful for diagnosing tumors, obstructions, cysts, hematomas, abscess, bleeding perforation, calculi, fibroids, and other pathologic conditions that appear in the abdomen and pelvis

CBC, complete blood count; CMP, complete metabolic panel; CNS, central nervous system; MCV, mean corpuscular volume; MCH, mean corpuscular hemoglobin; MCHC, mean corpuscular hemoglobin concentration; RBC, red blood cell; UTI, urinary tract infection; WBC, white blood cell.

CLINICAL DECISION MAKING

Case Study Analysis

The clinical finding of significance is uterine size of 12 weeks. Because of this the advanced practice provider discusses the possibility of pregnancy after the examination and the patient beings to cry and admits to having a boyfriend with whom she has had intercourse. The patient agrees to have a urine pregnancy test and this is positive. There is no abdominal pain to suggest an ectopic pregnancy or an infection. Other etiologies of vomiting are eliminated in the history and examination. There is no evidence to support an infection, food poisoning, obstruction, metabolic disorder, appendicitis, cholecystitis, or pancreatitis. The patient agrees to discuss the pregnancy with her mother with the advanced practice provider present. They are referred to a local obstetrics and gynecology clinic for further evaluation.

Diagnosis: Pregnant

WEIGHT GAIN

Case Presentation: A 66-year-old African American male presents to the acute care practice complaining of weight gain "approximately 15 lb over the past month." During the examination Mr. Braswell seems to have labored breathing and shortness of breath. He endorses bilateral lower extremity swelling. Mr. Braswell has a history of type 2 diabetes and coronary artery disease (CAD). Patient denies recent traveling. Patient denies change in eating habits.

INTRODUCTION TO COMPLAINT

- Could be a symptom: edema in heart failure
- Could indicate a problem: hypothyroidism, Cushing's syndrome, or obesity
- Lack of exercise
- Side effects of some drugs

HISTORY OF COMPLAINT

Symptomatology

Ask about the following characteristics of each symptom using open-ended questions:

- Onset of noticed weight gain
- Current life events
- Effects on daily activities
- Diet changes
- Associated symptoms

Directed Questions to Ask

- Was the onset of the weight gain steady or did you notice your weight fluctuating up and down?
- When did you notice this started?
- Has your food intake changed?
- Do you use more salt than you used to?
- How often do you weigh yourself?
- Has your weight been steady before the onset of the weight gain?
- Have you noticed a change in the way your clothes fit?
- Have you noticed yourself more fatigued than normal?
- How is your breathing today? Are you short of breath?
- Have you had any coughing? Are you producing any sputum?
- Have you had any nasal congestion?
- Have you been eating out more than normal? Fast food places?
- Have you traveled anywhere recently? Long distances?

- Have you ever been told you have high blood pressure (BP)?
- Have you ever been tested for sleep problems like snoring? Did you see a medical provider for the snoring?
- Have you noticed a change in your bowel habits? Any constipation?
- Have you had any nausea or vomiting?
- How far would you say you are able to walk in one period of time?
- Have you had to use extra pillows at night if you are in the bed sleeping?
- Have you had any pain in your legs? Specifically your calves? While walking?
- Have you noticed any numbness or tingling in the legs or feet?
- Have you felt your heart beating faster than usual?
- Have you ever been told you have heart problems?
- Have you had any chest pain?
- Have you had trouble completing your daily activities?
- Have you ever been told you have a thyroid issue?
- Have you ever had stents placed or open heart surgery?

Assessment: Cardinal Signs and Symptoms

General
- Weight gain
- fatigue
- clothes fitting tighter

Skin
- Assess skin for any changes/abnormalities

Head, Eyes, Ears, Nose, Throat (HEENT)
- Assess neck for jugular venous distention (JVD) or bruits

Cardiovascular
- Assess heart for abnormalities

Respiratory
- Assess lungs for abnormalities

Gastrointestinal
- Assess abdomen for signs of constipation

Medical History

- Current medications: metformin 1,000 mg oral BID; atorvastatin 40 mg oral daily
- Allergies: sulfa: hives
- Medical: CAD, type 2 diabetes
- Surgical: hernia repair in his 20s
- Psychological: none
- Health maintenance: flu vaccine the past year. Pneumonia vaccine the past year as well. Colonoscopy done at the age of 60, it was normal. He does not exercise daily

Family History
- Mother died from stroke at age 60
- Father alive, has hypertension (HTN) and prostate cancer
- Brother alive, has HTN
- Sister died from motor vehicle accident (MVA) in her 30s
- Patient lives with his wife, they have one child in the military in Germany

Social History
- Tobacco: never smoked
- Ethanol (ETOH): consumes the occasional beer, approximately four a month
- Sexual: sexually active with his wife of 35 years
- Illicit drugs: denies
- Diet: eats red meat, likes to eat out at the Golden Corral at least once a week, and Bojangles' ham biscuit every morning
- Occupational: retired from the military after 30 years

PHYSICAL EXAMINATION

Vital Signs
- Temperature
- Pulse
- Respiration
- SpO_2
- Blood pressure (BP)

General Appearance
- Apparent state of health
- Appearance of comfort or distress
- Color
- Nutritional status
- State of hydration
- Hygiene
- Match between appearance and stated age
- Difficulty with gait or balance

Mouth and Throat
- Lips: color, lesions, symmetry
- Oral cavity: breath odor, color, lesions of buccal mucosa
- Teeth and gums: redness, swelling, caries, bleeding
- Tongue: color, texture, lesions, tenderness of floor of mouth
- Throat and pharynx: color, exudates, uvula, tonsillar symmetry and enlargement

Neck
- Symmetry
- Swelling
- Masses
- Active range of motion
- Thyroid enlargement

Palpation
- Tenderness, enlargement, mobility, contour and consistency of nodes and masses
- Nodes: pre- and post-auricular, occipital, tonsillar, submandibular, submental, anterior and posterior cervical, supraclavicular
- Thyroid: size, consistency, contour, position, tenderness

Associated Systems for Assessment
- A complete assessment should include the cardiac and respiratory system

CASE STUDY
History

Directed Question	Response
Was the onset of the weight gain steady or did you notice your weight fluctuating up and down?	*This was sudden. I have never noticed my weight fluctuating before.*
When did you notice this started?	*It happened last month.*
Has your food intake changed?	*I haven't noticed my food intake changing.*
Do you use more salt than you used to?	*No more than I used to use, I don't salt everything, but I do add some to my food.*
How often do you weigh yourself?	*I only weigh at the doctor's office each year.*
Has your weight been steady before the onset of the weight gain?	*I am usually the same weight every year, maybe gaining a few pounds yearly.*
Have you noticed a change in the way your clothes fit?	*My pants are tighter, that's why I thought I gained weight.*
Have you noticed yourself more fatigued than normal?	*Yes.*
How is your breathing today? Are you short of breath?	*I think my breathing is okay. I am a little short of breath, but I thought it was because I walked into the office from the parking lot.*
Have you had any coughing? Are you producing any sputum?	*I have a dry cough at night.*
Have you had any nasal congestion?	*No.*
Have you been eating out more than normal? Like fast food places?	*Our kids are grown and gone, so it is easier to eat out than cook for ourselves.*
Have you traveled anywhere recently? Long distances?	*No.*
Have you ever been told you have high blood pressure?	*Seems like I might have heard that awhile back.*
Have you ever been tested for sleep problems like snoring? Did you see a medical provider for the snoring?	*No.*
Have you noticed a change in your bowel habits? Any constipation?	*No.*
Have you had any nausea or vomiting?	*No.*
How far would you say you are able to walk in one period of time?	*Maybe to the mailbox and I get out of breath.*
Have you had to use extra pillows at night if you are in the bed sleeping?	*Two pillows at night.*

Directed Question	Response
Have you had any pain in your legs? Specifically your calves? While walking?	No pain, but I think they look bigger.
Have you noticed any numbness or tingling in the legs or feet?	No.
Have you felt your heart beating faster than usual?	No.
Have you ever been told you have heart problems?	I have a history of CAD, that's all.
Have you had any chest pain?	No.
Have you had trouble completing your daily activities?	I get short of breath in the shower, but I bought a shower chair so I can sit down while I wash.
Have you ever been told you have a thyroid issue?	No.
Have you ever had stents placed or open heart surgery?	No.

CAD, coronary artery disease.

Physical Examination Findings

- VITAL SIGNS: temperature 98.7°F; respiratory rate (RR) 30; heart rate (HR) 110; BP 140/90; SpO_2 92% on room air; height 5'8"; weight 220 lb
- GENERAL APPEARANCE: obese African American male who appears his stated age; he is alert and oriented; he is a good historian; he has labored breathing and dyspnea on exertion
- SKIN: warm, dry, and normal color with 2 + pitting edema noted to the bilateral lower legs; fingers and nails are negative for clubbing or cyanosis
- NECK: positive for JVD and carotid bruit noted; thyroid midline
- HEENT: head normocephalic and atraumatic, pupils equal, round, and reactive to light and accommodation (PERRLA), nares patent, oral mucosa intact; thyroid midline
- RESPIRATORY: lungs positive for crackles in bilateral lower bases; percussion produces dullness at the bases
- CARDIOVASCULAR: tachycardiac; no rubs or gallops; normal S1, S2, murmur noted
- GASTROINTESTINAL: abdomen obese, soft, and nondistended; normal bowel sounds; organs not palpable

DIFFERENTIAL DIAGNOSIS

Clinical Observations	Heart failure	DVT	Thyroid	Obesity
Onset	Sudden	Sudden	Gradual	Gradual
Elevated BNP	Yes	No	No	No

(continued)

Clinical Observations	Heart failure	DVT	Thyroid	Obesity
CXR (pulmonary congestion)	Yes	No	Yes	No
Pain	No	Yes	No	No
Fatigue	Yes	Yes	Yes	No
Dyspnea	Yes	Yes	No	No
Lower extremity edema	Yes	Yes	Yes	No

BNP, brain natriuretic peptide; CXR, chest x-ray; DVT, deep vein thrombosis.

DIAGNOSTIC EXAMINATION

Exam	Code	Cost	Results
CBC	R68.89	$12	Show severe anemia
Lipid panel	Z13.220	$29	Monitor cholesterol levels specifically LDL, HDL, and triglycerides
Cardiac enzymes, include troponin	R74.8, R79.89	$61	Check for damage in the heart
Ultrasound of lower extremities	M79.8	$308	Rule out DVT
Echocardiogram	R93.1	$1,000–$2,000	EF, heart function
BNP	R79.89	$79	Rule in heart failure
CMP	Z13.0	$12	Check for electrolyte abnormalities (Na or K)
Chest x-ray	R91.8	$200–$400	Rule in pulmonary venous congestion
TSH	Z13.29	$45	Rule out thyroid problems
EKG	R94.31	$50	Assess for arrhythmia, diagnose underlying issues
Urinalysis	Z13.89	$25	Rule out proteinuria
ABG	R79.81	$85	Acid–base evaluation

ABG, arterial blood gas; BNP, brain natriuretic peptide; CBC, complete blood count; CMP, complete metabolic panel; DVT, deep vein thrombosis; EF, ejection fraction; TSH, thyroid-stimulating hormone.

CLINICAL DECISION MAKING

Case Study Analysis

Sudden onset of weight gain up to 15 lb, labored breathing, shortness of breath, bilateral lower extremity edema, fatigue, dry cough, exercise intolerance, JVD, carotid bruit, crackles in lung bases, tachycardia, and a heart murmur. Blood samples sent for complete blood count (CBC), lipid panel, cardiac enzymes, brain natriuretic peptide (BNP), complete metabolic panel (CMP), and thyroid-stimulating hormone (TSH). Mild anemia noted on CBC. Lipid panel showed slightly elevated triglycerides, which could indicate the need to adjust statin medication dose. Cardiac enzymes and troponin were negative for cardiac muscle damage. BNP was elevated. Electrolyte levels within normal limits from the CMP, and TSH level was within normal limits. Based on the results of laboratory tests the patient is scheduled for an echocardiogram, EKG, and chest x-ray to be completed within the next 2 days.

Based on these findings, deep vein thrombosis and hypothyroidism as a cause for the weight gain can be ruled out. Since the weight gain was sudden, it is unlikely to be caused by increased food intake. Obesity can be ruled out.

> **Diagnosis:** *Heart failure*

Depending on the results of the echocardiogram, EKG, and chest x-ray the patient should be started on a diuretic and possible angiotensin-converting enzyme (ACE) inhibitor. Reviewed the importance of measuring weight daily and reporting a weight gain of 3 to 5 lb. Counseled on the need to reduce sodium in the diet and provided a list of high-sodium foods, which the patient has stated he eats on a regular basis (ham), to avoid eating. Appointment made with the cardiology clinic in 3 days at which time the results of the echocardiogram and chest x-ray will be available.

WEIGHT LOSS

Case Presentation: A 45-year-old Black woman is at the clinic for unexplained weight loss.

INTRODUCTION TO COMPLAINT

- Weight loss: Unexplained weight loss, or losing weight without trying, particularly if it is significant or persistent, may be a sign of an underlying medical disorder.
- The point at which unexplained weight loss becomes a medical concern is not exact.
- But many doctors agree that a medical evaluation is called for if you lose more than 5% of your weight in 6 months to a year, especially if you are an older adult. For example, a 5% weight loss in someone who is 160 lb (72 kg) is 8 lb (3.6 kg). In someone who is 200 lb (90 kg), it is 10 lb (4.5 kg).
- Your weight is affected by your calorie intake, activity level, overall health, age, nutrient absorption, and economic and social factors.

HISTORY OF COMPLAINT

Symptomatology

Ask about the following characteristics of each symptom using open-ended questions:

- Onset
- Chronology
- Current situation
- Timing
- Severity
- Precipitating and aggravating factors
- Associated symptoms
- Effects on daily activities
- Previous diagnosis of similar episodes
- Previous exams

Directed Questions to Ask

- When did the weight loss start?
- How much weight have you lost and how fast?
- Do you feel depressed, feeling of worthlessness?
- Are you having unprotected sex and how many partners do you have?
- Have you had any fevers?
- Have you had any shortness of breath (SOB)?
- Have you had any nausea and vomiting (N/V)?
- Have you noticed any chest pain?

- Have you noticed any swelling of your feet?
- Do you have any abdominal pain?
- Have you noticed any fatigue?
- Noticed any night sweats?
- Have you noticed a change in appetite?
- Have you had a change in how you smell or taste?
- What medications have changed?
- Any stressful events?
- Have you noticed dark or bloody stools?
- Have you been having diarrhea?

Assessment: Cardinal Signs and Symptoms

General
- Fatigue

Head, Eyes, Ears, Nose, Throat (HEENT)
- Inflammation
- Adenopathy
- Drainage
- Neck pain

Cardiac
- Chest pain

Respiratory
- Cough
- Sputum production
- SOB

Gastrointestinal (GI)
- Diarrhea
- Constipation
- Melena

Genitourinary
- Dysuria
- Hematuria
- Foul-smelling urine
- Urinary frequency/urgency

Musculoskeletal
- Pain
- Swelling
- Redness
- Hot/warm

Other Associated Symptoms
- Malaise
- Shaking
- Chills

Medical History

- Hypertension (HTN)
- Surgical: gallbladder removed 2 years ago

- Allergies: penicillin
- Medication: lisinopril 20 mg daily
- Psychosocial: one glass of wine a weekend; denies drug use

Family History
- Mother HTN
- Dad HTN

PHYSICAL EXAMINATION

Vital Signs
- Temperature
- Pulse
- Respiration
- SpO$_2$
- Blood pressure (BP)

General Appearance
- Oriented four times
- Looks well kept
- BMP 17

Eyes
- Pupils are a 3 bilaterally and are reactive

HEENT
- Normocephalic
- Oral mucosa is moist

Neck
- Supple
- Nontender
- No carotid bruit
- No jugular venous distention

Respiratory
- Clear lung fields
- No SOB

Cardiovascular
- Normal rate
- Regular rhythm
- No murmur, rubs, or gallops
- 0 pitting edema all extremities

GI
- Soft
- Tender
- Nondistended
- Normal bowel sounds

Genitourinary
- No costovertebral angle tenderness

Musculoskeletal
- Normal range of motion
- Normal strength

Integumentary
- Warm
- Dry

Cognition and Speech
- Speech clear

Psychiatric
- Cooperative
- Appropriate mood and affect

CASE STUDY
History

Directed Question	Response
When did the weight loss start?	I noticed it 3 months ago.
How much weight have you lost and how fast?	I've lost 30 lb in the past 3 months.
Do you feel depressed, feeling of worthlessness?	No, I'm doing great. My kids are about to go off to college and I can't wait to have my house without kids in it.
Are you having unprotected sex and how many partners do you have?	No and I only have sex with my husband.
Do you drink and how much?	A glass of wine a weekend.
Do you use drugs, if so what, and do you share needles?	No drugs.
Have you had any fever?	No.
Have you had any SOB?	No.
Have you had any N/V?	About three times a week, but it's been getting more frequent.
Have you noticed any chest pain?	No.
Have you noticed any swelling of your feet?	No.
Do you have any abdominal pain?	Usually when I have the N/V, and it's been getting more frequent too.
Have you noticed any fatigue?	Yes, and I've been trying to watch what I eat and do exercise, but nothing seems to help.

Directed Question	*Response*
Noticed any night sweats?	*Yes I have, I think I might be starting menopause.*
Have you noticed a change in appetite?	*No, I've been trying to eat more, but when I get nauseous I can't eat.*
Have you had a change in how you smell or taste?	*No.*
What medications have changed?	*No.*
Any stressful events?	*No, everything right now is exciting.*
Have you noticed dark or bloody stools?	*Not that I've noticed.*
Have you been having diarrhea?	*Yes, and I've tried several medications for it and they don't seem to work.*

N/V, nausea and vomiting; SOB, shortness of breath.

DIFFERENTIAL DIAGNOSIS

Clinical Observations	DM	HIV	COPD	Thyroid
Onset	Abrupt to gradual	Abrupt to gradual	Gradual	Gradual
Fever	No	Yes/No	No	No
SOB	No	Yes/No	Yes	No
Cough	No	Yes/No	Yes	No
Fatigue	Possible	Possible	Yes	Yes
Weight loss	Possible	Abrupt	Gradual	Gradual
Leveled WBC	No	Yes/No	No	No
Elevated A1C	Yes	No	No	No
TSH level	Normal	Normal	Normal	Abnormal
Western blot	No	Yes	No	No

COPD, chronic obstructive pulmonary disease; DM, diabetes mellitus; SOB, shortness of breath; TSH, thyroid-stimulating hormone; WBC, white blood cell.

DIAGNOSTIC EXAMINATION

Exam	Code	Cost	Results
A1C	R73.09	$35	The A1C test is a blood test that provides information about a person's average levels of blood glucose, also called blood sugar, over the past 3 months.
Western blot	A69.20	$128	This is an immunoassay test method that detects specific proteins in blood or tissue. It combines an electrophoresis step with a step that transfers (blots) the separated proteins onto a membrane. Western blot is often used as a follow-up test to confirm the presence of an antibody and to help diagnose a condition. Examples of its use include confirmatory HIV and Lyme disease testing.
TSH levels	Z13.29	$39	There are two types of thyroid hormones easily measurable in the blood, thyroxine (T4) and triiodothyronine (T3). For technical reasons, it is easier and less expensive to measure the T4 level, so T3 is usually not measured on screening tests. Additionally, most diseases impact both T4 and T3 similarly, so T4 is typically measured first. Please be clear on which test you are looking at. We continue to see a tremendous amount of confusion among doctors, nurses, laboratory technicians, and patients on which test is which. In particular, the "total T3," "free T3," and "T3 uptake tests" are very confusing, and are not the same test. **Thyroxine (TT4):** This shows the total amount of T4. TT4 consists of two portions: T4, which is bound to carrier proteins and is inactive; "free" or unbound T4, which is available to cells and therefore active. High levels may be due to hyperthyroidism; however, technical artifact occurs when the bound/inactive T4 is increased. This can occur when estrogen levels are higher from pregnancy, birth control pills, or estrogen replacement therapy. An FT4 (see the following) can avoid this interference.
			FT4: This test directly measures the FT4 in the blood rather than estimating it like the FTI. Because it is a more reliable test than the TT4, many labs such as ours do the FT4 routinely rather than the TT4. High levels suggest hyperthyroidism, and low levels are found in hypothyroidism and chronic illness. **TT3:** This is usually not ordered as a screening test, but rather when thyroid disease is being evaluated. T3 is the more potent and shorter lived version of thyroid hormone. Some people with high thyroid levels secrete more T3 than T4. In these (overactive) hyperthyroid cases the T4 can be normal, the T3 high, and the TSH low. The TT3 reports the total amount of T3 in the bloodstream, including T3 bound to carrier proteins plus freely circulating T3. **FT3:** This test measures only the portion of thyroid hormone T3 that is "free," that is, not bound to carrier proteins. **T3RU or thyroid uptake:** This is a test that confuses doctors, nurses, and patients. First, this is not a thyroid test, but a test on the proteins that carry thyroid around in your bloodstream. Not only that, a high test number may indicate a low level of the protein! The method of reporting varies from lab to lab. The proper use of the test is to compute the FTI.

(continued)

Exam	Code	Cost	Results
			FTI or T7: A mathematical computation allows to estimate the FTI from the T4 and T3 uptake tests. The results tell us how much thyroid hormone is free in the bloodstream to work on the body. In contrast to the TT4 alone, it is less affected by estrogen levels. While this test is less commonly ordered, it is still of use in special situations such as pregnancy.
			TSH: This protein hormone is secreted by the pituitary gland and regulates the thyroid gland. A high level suggests your thyroid is underactive, and a low level suggests your thyroid is overactive. This test can vary by time of day, so a single abnormal measurement does not always mean there is a problem. Also, levels tend to be higher in older people, so it is not uncommon to see mild elevations in people in their 70s or 80s, which do not necessarily indicate a medical problem.
CBC	R69.89	$33	**WBC count** is the number of white cells. High WBC count can be a sign of infection. WBC count is also increased in certain types of leukemia. Low white blood cell counts can be a sign of bone marrow diseases or an enlarged spleen. Low WBC count is also found in HIV infection in some cases. (Editor's note: The vast majority of low WBC counts in our population is *not* HIV-related.)
			Hgb and Hct: Hgb is the amount of oxygen-carrying protein contained within the RBCs. Hct is the percentage of the blood volume occupied by RBCs. In most labs the Hgb is actually measured, while the Hct is computed using the RBC measurement and the MCV measurement. Thus purists prefer to use the Hgb measurement as more reliable. Low Hgb or Hct suggests an anemia. Anemia can be due to nutritional deficiencies, blood loss, destruction of blood cells internally, or failure to produce blood in the bone marrow. High Hgb can occur due to lung disease, living at high altitude, or excessive bone marrow production of blood cells.
			MCV: This helps diagnose a cause of an anemia. Low values suggest iron deficiency, high values suggest either deficiencies of B_{12} or folate, ineffective production in the bone marrow, or recent blood loss with replacement by newer (and larger) cells from the bone marrow.
			PLT: This is the number of cells that plug up holes in your blood vessels and prevent bleeding. High values can occur with bleeding, cigarette smoking, or excess production by the bone marrow. Low values can occur from premature destruction states such ITP, acute blood loss, drug effects (such as heparin), infections with sepsis, entrapment of platelets in an enlarged spleen, or bone marrow failure from diseases such as myelofibrosis or leukemia. Low platelets also can occur from clumping of the platelets in a lavender-colored tube. You may need to repeat the test with a green-top tube in that case.
BMP	R79.89	$121	The BMP is used to check the status of a person's kidneys and their electrolyte and acid/base balance, as well as their blood glucose level—all of which are related to a person's metabolism. It can also be used to monitor hospitalized patients and people with certain known conditions, such as hypertension and hypokalemia.

CBC, complete blood count; BMP, basic metabolic panel; FT3, free T3; FT4, free T4; FTI, free thyroxine index; Hct, hematocrit; Hgb, hemoglobin; ITP, immune thrombocytopenia; MCV, mean corpuscular volume; PLT, platelet count; RBC, red blood cell; TSH, thyroid-stimulating hormone; T3RU, T3 resin uptake; TT3, total T3; TT4, total T4; WBC, white blood cell.

CLINICAL DECISION MAKING

Case Study Analysis

With the patient's symptoms of N/V, diarrhea, and extreme weight loss, and the physical examination of an underweight lady who is having GI issues and abdominal pains, it seems that there is a possibility of having contracted HIV. Diagnostic testing was negative for a thyroid disorder and diabetes. There are no symptoms to support a diagnosis of COPD. The Western blot was positive. Adding the patient's presenting symptoms and extreme sudden weight loss, the patient is HIV positive.

> ***Diagnosis:*** *HIV*

Additional laboratory testing was prescribed along with a chest x-ray and EKG to have as a baseline. The patient was counseled on the infection, modes of transmission, and method of treatment. Provided with names and contact information of clinic health care professionals who specialize in the treatment of patients with HIV. Encouraged patient to make an appointment as soon as possible, so antiretroviral therapy can begin. Encouraged patient to have spouse tested as soon as possible and reviewed approaches for safe intercourse. Provided the patient with the local HIV support group telephone number and HIV websites that provide information on the illness and treatment. The patient was encouraged to maintain all scheduled health care appointments going forward and to return to the clinic at any time with questions or issues with other health problems.

WHEEZING

Case Presentation: *A working 34-year-old Caucasian male presents to your acute care practice with the chief complaint of wheezing.*

INTRODUCTION TO COMPLAINT

The chief complaint of wheezing is a pulmonary and airway complaint. The key sign is a musical sound caused by the reverberations of the airway. The reverberations are caused by airway obstruction. This can be secondary to many items such as edema, increased secretion, and smooth muscle contraction. Physical examination is imperative to differentiate wheezing from stridor. While wheezing can occur anywhere in the airway and is mostly upon expiration, stridor is much louder and concentrated in the tracheal and laryngeal regions. The causes of stridor in adults are much different than those that cause wheezing, which include vocal cord paralysis, foreign body aspiration, and upper airway infection.

HISTORY OF COMPLAINT

Symptomatology

Ask about the following characteristics of each symptom using open-ended questions:

- Onset of complaint
- Sudden or gradual onset
- Chronology
- Improved, stable, or deteriorating situation
- Timing
- Precipitating or aggravating factors
- Relieving factors
- Effects on daily activities
- Medications or treatments

Directed Questions to Ask

- When did your wheezing start?
- Are you short of breath when this occurs?
- Was it sudden or gradual?
- What events have accompanied it?
- How often does it occur?
- When does it occur?
- Where does it occur?
- What other symptoms do you feel during the shortness of breath?

- Do you hear yourself wheezing?
- Have you ever been diagnosed with a congestive heart failure (CHF) or a pulmonary disorder?
- Have you coughed up anything?
- Have you coughed up any blood?
- Have you been running a temperature?
- How many pillows do you sleep with at night?
- Do you wake up short of breath?
- Have you been around anyone sick recently?

Assessment: Cardinal Signs and Symptoms

General
- Fatigue
- Fever

Head, Eyes, Ears, Nose, Throat (HEENT)
- Tonsillar enlargement
- Macroglossia
- Foreign body in airway
- Inflamed airway

Neuro/Mental
- Agitated
- Anxious

Cardiac
- Tachycardia
- Chest pain
- Palpitations
- Edema

Pulmonary
- Dyspnea
- Tachypnea
- Wheezing
- Crackles
- Rhonchi
- Absent breath sounds
- Accessory muscle use
- Sputum production
- Cough
- Chest tightness

Gastrointestinal (GI)
- Ascites
- Gastroesophageal reflux disease (GERD)

Hematological
- Active hemorrhage
- Bruising

Integumentary
- Cyanosis
- Clubbing

Medical History

- Allergies: penicillin
- Medical: hypertension (HTN)
- Surgical: knee replacement at 55 years
- Psychological: no previous history
- Current medications: ibuprofen 400 mg as needed, Benadryl 50 mg by mouth nightly PRN, hydrochloric thiazide 25 mg orally

Family History
- Unknown; patient states parents died of old age

Social History
- Tobacco: patient denies smoking
- Alcohol: patient states he drinks a beer or two on Sundays while watching football
- Sexual: patient sexually active with his wife
- Illicit drugs: patient denies
- Diet: patient states he does not follow a specific diet
- Emotional support: patient lives with his wife
- Occupational: construction foreman
- Exercise: patient states he does not participate in any
- Socioeconomics: employed; lives in a home with wife

PHYSICAL EXAMINATION

Vital Signs

- Temperature
- Pulse
- Respiration
- Oxygen saturation (SpO_2)
- Blood pressure (BP)

General Appearance

- Apparent state of health: well-developed male
- Appearance of comfort or distress: well relaxed
- Color: no signs of jaundice or hypoxia
- Nutritional status: patient appears to be undernourished
- State of hydration: no signs of dehydration or fluid overload
- Hygiene: patient well kept
- Match between appearance and stated age: patient appears to be his stated age
- Difficulty with gait or balance: no difficulty with gait

HEENT
- No thyroid enlargement. Neck supple, no tonsillar enlargement, Mallampati airway score 2, soft pallet low lying

Respiratory
- Chest expansion even, no cyanosis or pallor, lung sounds clear throughout, no crackles, rhonchi, or rales. Slight expiratory wheeze heard throughout. Cough productive with sputum, trachea midline

Cardiovascular

- Regular rate and rhythm, +2 radial pulses bilaterally. Point of maximum impulse (PMI) dime sized, fifth intercostal space, midclavicular line. No murmurs, rubs, or gallops. S1 and S2 clearly auscultated. No edema

Gastrointestinal

- Abdomen soft, flat, not distended. No fluid wave present. Bowel sounds active

Integumentary

- Partially balding, no cyanosis

Hematological

- No ecchymosis present

Neurologic

- Alert, oriented, tearful, emotionally distressed, and cooperative; thought process coherent; romberg: maintains balance with eyes closed; no pronator drift; gait with normal base; good muscle build and tone; strength 5/5 throughout; rapid alternating movements (RAMs): finger to nose; hand flip flop and serial finger opposition intact; cranial nerves (CNs) II through XII intact; deep tendon reflex (DTR): brachioradialis, biceps, triceps, patellar, Achilles all 2+ bilaterally; negative Babinski reflex

CASE STUDY

History

Directed Question	Response
When did your wheezing start?	*About 3 weeks ago.*
Are you short of breath when this occurs?	*Yes.*
Was it sudden or gradual?	*Sudden.*
What events have accompanied it?	*We've been using a new paint at work.*
How often does it occur?	*Two or three times a week.*
When does it occur?	*When we're spraying new paint at work.*
Where does it occur?	*At work.*
What other symptoms do you feel during the shortness of breath?	*I feel chest tightness.*
Do you hear yourself wheezing?	*Slightly.*
What relieves these signs and symptoms?	*Sitting down outside and getting some fresh air.*
How long do the signs and symptoms last?	*Varies, 15 minutes sometimes, 30 minutes.*
Have you ever been diagnosed with a CHF or a pulmonary disorder?	*No.*
Have you coughed up anything?	*Lots of phlegm.*

Directed Question	Response
Have you coughed up any blood?	*No.*
Have you been running a temperature?	*No.*
How many pillows do you sleep with at night?	*Just two.*
Do you wake up short of breath?	*No.*
Have you been around anyone sick recently?	*No.*

CHF, congestive heart failure.

DIFFERENTIAL DIAGNOSIS

Clinical Observations	Asthma	Acute Bronchitis	Chronic Bronchitis	Emphysema	Pneumonia
Dyspnea	Yes	Yes	Yes	Yes	Yes
Sputum	Yes	Yes	Yes	Yes	Yes
Expiratory wheezing	Yes	Yes	Yes	Yes	Yes/No
Chest tightness	Yes	Yes	Yes	No	No
Episodic signs and symptoms	Yes	No	Yes	Yes	No
Sudden episode	Yes	No	No	No	No

DIAGNOSTIC EXAMINATION

Exam	Code	Cost	Justification	Results
Spirometry	94010	$100	Spirometry evaluates for the severity of disease and allows for staging of asthma.	FEV_1 and total FVC should both be measured. A FEV_1/FVC ratio of ≤80% is indicative of asthma. Must be measured before and after SABA administration.

(*continued*)

Exam	Code	Cost	Justification	Results
Bronchial provocation	95070	$45–$800 depending on the diagnosis	Bronchial provocation and subsequent hypoxia is the hallmark diagnostic test for asthma. Reversibility of 15% or greater FEV_1/FVC ratio indicates asthma and rules out COPD	Bronchial hyperresponsiveness and then a reversibility as evidenced by an increase in FEV_1/FVC Ratio by at least 15% or greater indicates asthma and rules out COPD.
SABA reversibility	I67.841	Part of provocation cost		
Serum potassium	E87.5	$21	The administration of SABAs can cause hypokalemia. A BMP should be drawn to reduce the risk for further complications.	Normal levels: 3.5–5.0 mEq/L
BNP	83880	$50–$200 depending on the diagnosis	SOB can be caused by fluid overload. A BNP level can be used to evaluate the possibility of fluid overload and heart failure	≤100 pg/ml is within normal limits. Greater than 100 indicates fluid overload or heart failure
CXR	R91.8	$490–$1,100	A CXR can be used to diagnose a multitude of conditions such as pneumonia, asthma, pulmonary edema, PE, and effusions.	A CXR allows for visual diagnostics of the thoracic cavity. Helpful in the diagnosis of pneumonia, effusions, malignancies, heart failure, edema, among other disorders. Asthma and COPD will show hyperinflation and flattening of the diaphragm.
Sputum culture	R09.3	$25–$43	A positive sputum culture could indicate an infectious process.	Purulent sputum containing microorganisms is indicative of infectious process.
Allergen skin testing	Z01.82	$60–$300	If the SOB is caused by extrinsic asthma it is important to identify the trigger through allergen skin testing so that the patient may avoid those triggers.	Patient's skin is exposed to allergen. Within minutes skin will develop a weal around the exposed area. Antihistamines should be avoided 24–48 hours before testing.
ABGs	R79.81	$218	Tested to evaluate for the severity of an acute attack, as well as the patient's ability to ventilate and oxygenate.	The blood gas should be normal during this office setting because the patient is not having acute respiratory distress.

ABG, arterial blood gas; BMP, basic metabolic panel; BNP, brain natriuretic peptide; COPD, chronic obstructive pulmonary disease; CXR, chest x-ray; FEV_1, forced expiratory volume over 1 second; FVC, forced volume capacity; PE, pulmonary embolism; SABA, short-acting beta-agonist; SOB, shortness of breath.

CLINICAL DECISION MAKING

Case Study Analysis

The complaint of wheezing has a wide breadth of possible diagnoses and etiologies. For example, the complaint could be cardiac in origin, caused by increased secretions secondary to pulmonary edema in heart failure. The origin could be related to liver cirrhosis, in which the patient could develop ascites, elevating the diaphragm causing pulmonary edema. The respiratory diagnoses associated with wheezing are extensive. Airway obstruction should be immediately ruled out. Items such as pneumonia, pleural effusions, malignancies, hemothorax, and pneumothorax can be diagnosed quickly with a chest x-ray. In addition, these diagnoses can be ruled out by the episodic and self-limiting nature of this patient's complaints. Acute and chronic bronchitis and emphysema should be considered. However, their exacerbations usually correspond with sustained hypoxia.

The sudden onset associated with a change in a chemical/paint used at work strongly suggests the diagnosis of asthma. A chest x-ray ruled out bronchitis, emphysema, and pneumonia. The patient was scheduled for pulmonary function tests and provided with and instructed on a peak flow meter to use at home.

Prescribed with a rescue inhaler and instructed on its use. Scheduled for an appointment with the pulmonology clinic in 3 days. Encouraged to measure peak flow meter readings at home and at work for the next 2 days to provide the information during the pulmonology appointment. Anticipate further diagnostic testing and treatment to be provided through the pulmonologist.

Diagnosis: Asthma exacerbated by environmental factors

WRIST PAIN

Case Presentation: A 43-year-old woman presents to the clinic with a complaint of wrist pain for 2 days.

INTRODUCTION TO COMPLAINT

Wrist pain may be caused by trauma; overuse through activities, such as knitting or typing; inflammatory disorders, such as arthritis; or neurological problems, such as nerve entrapment.

Acute Pain

- Duration of pain observed is less than 2 weeks.
- Trauma
- Inflammation from gout, osteoarthritis, or rheumatoid arthritis

Subacute and Chronic Pain

- Duration of pain observed is 2 weeks to 3 months (subacute) or more than 3 months (chronic).
- Prior acute trauma
- Chronic repetitive trauma or overuse
- Degenerative disease, such as osteoarthritis
- Connective tissue disorders, such as rheumatoid arthritis

HISTORY OF COMPLAINT

Symptomatology

Ask about the following characteristics of each symptom using open-ended questions:

- Onset: sudden or gradual
- Trauma: if yes, have the patient describe specifics of fall or other injury
- Location
- Timing: Is the pain greater at a specific time of the day?
- Severity on a scale of 0 to 10, with 0 being no pain and 10 being the most pain
- Quality: Is the pain burning, aching, stabbing, hot, cold?
- Continual or intermittent pain
- Weakness during specific movements
- Instability: Does the wrist "give out?"
- Sensation: Numbness, tingling

- Stiffness
- Functional disability
- Skin color or temperature changes
- Recent trauma
- Course: worsening, improving, or stable
- Exacerbating factors
- Alleviating factors
- Self-treatment
- Occupational and recreational activities
- Recent unusual activities like overtime, repainting the house
- Dominant hand: if patient endorses ambidexterity, ask which hand is used to write
- Previous occurrences of similar complaint

Directed Questions to Ask

- Can you describe the injury from the beginning?
- Was there immediate pain?
- Was there immediate swelling?
- How has your pain changed since the injury?
- Can you point to the area of pain?
- Do you have weakness of your hand grip?
- Does the wrist or hand just give way?
- Do you have any numbness or tingling of the hand or wrist?
- If this is present, can you show me where it is?
- Does the wrist or hand feel cold?
- Have you had to change your normal activities?
- Do you do any type of work or hobby with your hands?
- Does your family have any history of arthritis or joint disease?

Assessment: Cardinal Signs and Symptoms

- Etiology
- Injury with swelling
- Sprain/fracture
- No trauma, heat, or swelling
- Gout
- Arthritis
- Numbness and tingling
- Nerve injury, carpal tunnel
- Weakness

Medical History: General

- Medications, including supplements and over-the-counter (OTC) medications
- Rheumatologic, inflammatory, or neuromuscular conditions
- Past trauma
- Any family history of rheumatologic, inflammatory, or neuromuscular conditions

Medical History: Specific to Complaint

- Any previous history of joint pain
- Any family history of gout, arthritis, or inflammatory joint diseases such as rheumatoid arthritis

PHYSICAL EXAMINATION

Vital Signs

- Blood pressure
- Heart rate
- Respiration
- Weight
- Level of pain

General Appearance

- Comfort
- Nutritional status
- Hygiene level
- Hydration

Hand and Wrist Exam

Inspection

Observe the patient's upper extremities bilaterally from fingertip to elbow and note:

- Skin color and turgor
- Presence or absence of normal hair growth
- Swelling or nodules
- Skin tightness or looseness
- Deformity
- Symmetry: dominant side is usually larger and stronger
- Ulnar or radial deviation
- Position
- Contractures
- Ease, smoothness, and dexterity of movement

Palpation

- Observe the patient's face for signs of discomfort during palpation rather than observing the area palpated
- Palpate hand, wrist, and forearm
- Palpate corresponding areas on contralateral extremity to note any differences
- Note temperature of skin
- Note any "bogginess" of tissue, especially tendons or ligaments
- Note any discrete firm masses: Are they movable or fixed?
- Crepitus
- Joint laxity
- Swelling: discrete or diffuse

Wrist Specific

Scaphoid: Use thumb on "anatomic snuffbox" and index finger on thenar eminence. Tenderness may indicate scaphoid injury.

Passive Range of Motion

Move the patient through range of motion, and watch patient's face for any sign of discomfort.

- Spasticity: difficulty in moving joint
- Crepitus
- Snapping or popping. A brief snap or pop that is only momentarily uncomfortable is not a concern.

Movement

Observe the patient during active range of motion.

- FINGER: flexion, extension
- WRIST: flexion, extension, ulnar deviation, radial deviation, pronation with flexed elbow, supination with flexed elbow
- ELBOW: flexion, extension, pronation, supination

Observe functional ability as the patient performs.

- FINE PINCH: picking up a paper clip
- FLAT PINCH: holding a key to unlock a door
- TRIPOD GRIP: using a pen
- WIDE GRIP: grasping the circumference of a mug
- POWER GRIP: holding a hammer

Tinel's test: Light tapping over volar wrist; sensation of tingling, electrical pain, or "pins and needles" may indicate nerve compression as in carpal tunnel syndrome.

Phalen's test: Have patient flex wrists and hold for 60 seconds. Sensations of tingling or numbness may indicate nerve compression. Negative results do not rule out nerve compression.

Ulnar Side

- Tendinopathy, subluxation, fibrocartilaginous injuries, especially from repetitive actions (from racquet sports, excessive computer keyboard/mouse use)
- Triangular fibrocartilage complex injury; suspect this if your dominant finding is ulnar-side wrist pain, or find instability of wrist. Most commonly occurs from trauma. May be caused by overuse injury in occupations like carpentry

Radial Side

- Scaphoid fracture; frequent after moderate trauma; tenderness at anatomic snuffbox. May cause avascular necrosis later. X-rays are usually initially negative
- de Quervain's tenosynovitis. Pain with grasp or pinch. Usually caused by overuse
- Osteoarthritis is rarely seen in the wrist unless there is a history of previous injury. If there is osteoarthritis of the wrist, you will see prominent carpometacarpal and metacarpophalangeal joint pain
- Rheumatoid arthritis frequently affects the wrist, is symmetrical and bilateral, and presents with ulnar deviation of fingers and metacarpals
- Inflammatory conditions, such as infections or gout, are rare in the wrist. If suspected, examine and aspirate

Volar Side

- Carpal or ulnar neuropathy: symptoms are worse at night; pain at hypothenar eminence (if ulnar). Positive Tinel's or Phalen's signs; wasting of thenar or hypothenar eminence
- Hamate bone fracture can mimic pain from strain/sprain. Pain is usually observed over the hypothenar eminence

Dorsal Side

- Ganglion cyst: discrete, spheroid mass, somewhat movable, not hard nor fixed; often returns after aspiration; may require referral to hand surgeon
- Degenerative osteophyte formation, usually occurs at base of second and third metacarpals; "carpal boss": fixed, bony mass

- Kienbock's disease of lunate: slow onset; chronic; mild swelling; progressive dorsal wrist pain
- Forearm tendinopathy or "intersection syndrome" is caused by friction where portions of the abductor pollicis longus and extensor pollicis brevis pass over the extensor carpi radialis longus and extensor carpi radialis brevis. Pain over distal, dorsal forearm, especially with wrist extension. Etiology is most often from overuse. Crepitation or tendonous "creaking" (use stethoscope) may be heard over area

CASE STUDY
History

Directed Question	*Response*
How did the pain begin?	*Suddenly.*
How did the injury happen?	*I was walking my lively young dog on a leash when the dog suddenly leapt to chase a squirrel. During the dog's maneuvers I tripped over the leash, fell, and attempted to break my fall with outstretched right hand, and I landed on hard-packed dirt.*
Where is the pain?	*Right side of wrist/base of palm.*
Is the pain greater at a specific time of the day?	*No.*
On a scale of 0 to 10, 10 being the most severe, how much pain do you have?	*4 to 6.*
Is the pain burning, aching, stabbing, hot, cold?	*Aching.*
Continual or intermittent pain?	*Continual.*
Weakness during specific movements?	*No loss of strength, but painful.*
Does the wrist "give out?"	*No.*
Do you have any numbness or tingling?	*No.*
Do you have any stiffness?	*No.*
Does the pain interfere with usual activities?	*I avoid any activity that increases the pain, especially gripping objects.*
Have you had any skin color or temperature changes?	*No.*
Has the pain worsened, improved, or is it stable?	*Stable.*
What makes it worse?	*Using my wrist.*
What makes it feel better; what have you tried?	*Acetaminophen or ibuprofen at OTC doses is moderately helpful.*

Directed Question	*Response*
What are your occupational and recreational activities?	*I am an interior designer and use my computer and mouse extensively, which has been painful since the injury. And I like gardening, which I have not been able to do since the injury.*
Any recent unusual activities like overtime, repainting the house?	*No.*
Which is your dominant hand?	*Right.*
Any previous occurrences of similar complaint?	*No.*

OTC, over the counter.

Physical Examination Findings

Observe a diffuse ecchymosis over proximal thenar eminence on the right hand. The patient moves her right hand and wrist gingerly. The right wrist appears mildly swollen during extension. She complains of increased pain when gripping with right hand, and with firm palpation of thenar eminence. She is mildly tender in the anatomical snuffbox. Otherwise there are no remarkable findings on the right side, and her left side is normal.

DIFFERENTIAL DIAGNOSIS

Clinical Observations	Trauma	Osteoarthritis	Rheumatoid Arthritis	Gout	Ganglion Cyst	Nerve Compression	Repetitive Trauma/ Overuse
Onset	Sudden	Rarely	Possibly	Possibly	No	Rarely	No
Bilateral	Variable	Rarely	Yes	No	No	Unlikely	Possibly dominant side most affected
Deformity	Variable	Hypertrophy of thumb, distal interphalangeal, metacarpophalangeal, carpometacarpal joints	Hypertrophy of proximal interphalangeal joints; ulnar deviation	Swelling	Swelling	No	Rarely; muscle wasting if chronic
Warmth	Variable	Unlikely	Yes	Yes	No	No	No
Stiffness	Variable	Yes	Yes	No	No	No	No

DIAGNOSTIC EXAMINATION

Exam	Code	Cost	Results
X-ray, plain film	733120	$200	<ul><li>Inexpensive</li><li>Fairly low radiation exposure</li><li>Correct positioning is essential for accurate diagnosis</li><li>Initial evaluation: posteroanterior, lateral, and oblique; if concern for scaphoid fracture, add scaphoid view</li></ul>Trauma, weakness, locking; may reveal calcification or fracture
MRI	74200	$850	<ul><li>Expensive</li><li>No exposure to radiation</li><li>Best for soft tissue assessment (ganglia, tendinitis, effusions)</li></ul>
CT	74202	$750–$950	<ul><li>Expensive</li><li>Exposes patient to increased radiation, although lower radiation techniques are increasingly used</li><li>Useful for assessment of bone healing</li></ul>

CLINICAL DECISION MAKING

Case Study Analysis

The patient has a 2-day history of acute trauma, and the examination shows predominantly radial-sided symptoms. Although tenderness at the anatomic snuffbox is mild, the scaphoid bone is a common area for fracture after a fall with outstretched hand. A plain film, including posterior–anterior, lateral, oblique, and scaphoid views was completed; however, the imaging is negative. The patient is scheduled for a CT of the hand/wrist to be completed in 3 days. The sudden onset of the pain and traumatic event rules out osteoarthritis, rheumatoid arthritis, gout, ganglionic cyst, nerve compression, and repetitive trauma as causes for the patient's symptoms.

Until the CT scan is completed the wrist is wrapped with an ACE bandage. The patient is instructed to remove the bandage several times a day and to not wear it during sleep. Elevating the extremity at rest will help reduce edema along with the application of ice for 20 minutes three to four times a day. The patient is instructed to continue to use OTC analgesics for pain control. An appointment with the orthopedic clinic is made to occur in 7 days at which time the results of the CT scan and other x-rays will be evaluated to determine further treatment.

> **Diagnosis:** Wrist pain, possibly contusion. Tenderness of the scaphoid area with negative x-ray does not rule out a fracture. Consider referral to a hand specialist. Another alternative is to repeat the x-ray in 2 weeks to see whether an occult fracture is identified.

INDEX